The Cult of Pharmacology

Duke University Press Durham + London 2006

Richard DeGrandpre

The Cult of Pharmacology

How America Became the World's Most Troubled Drug Culture

Designed by Jennifer Hill / Typeset in Galliard by Keystone Typesetting, Inc.

Library of Congress Cataloging-in-Publication Data appear
on the last printed page of this book.

Contents

E ngland began importing coffee from the Muslim East in the seventeenth century. At first many Britains viewed the brewed substance with suspicion, and some groups made efforts to demonize it. The "coffee house" was a threat to English ale houses, and thus the economy, and of course was counter to Christian values. Worse still, its stimulant actions caused impotence and "made men as unfruitful as the deserts whence that unhappy berry is said to be brought."[1] England eventually made peace with the popular and profitable bean, however, reclassifying it as a harmless beverage.[2] Today coffee is not just the working person's daily wake-up fix and the café philosopher's stimulant of choice—it is also a global billion-dollar business.

This about sums up the modern history of drugs: irrational and unpredictable, full of fear and loathing, with a strong theme of commerce running right through the center. Far from deviating from this norm, America in the twentieth century dealt with drugs in a fashion as irrational and as seemingly unpredictable as any nation in history. The only obvious constant in America's relationships with psychoactive substances, whether from the street, the store, or the pharmacy, was that, like coffee, nearly all these substances at some point carried a strong emotional charge in society. This was as true for heroin and alcohol as it was for popular "medicines" like Benzedrine, Miltown, and Prozac.

Drugs in twentieth-century America thus became a vast and layered realm of significance, a territory of meaning contested with great zeal. For the meaning of a drug determined not only its legitimacy but also who could use it and how, and who could not—at least not legally. By midcentury, drugs in America began to be divided up accordingly, as the market for mind-altering substances fractured into two and then three parts: the "illegal drugs" of the black market, the "ethical medicines" of the pharmaceutical market, and the drugs of the gray market, which by the end of the century included alcohol, tobacco, and caffeine. Whether a drug fell into one category or another at any particular time was viewed not as an irrational and unpredictable enterprise driven by the historically contingent forces of culture and commerce but as a straightforward scientific issue. Even respected drug scholars and researchers held throughout the century that by entering the bloodstream and thereby directly impacting the brain, drugs acquire special powers.

Modern science did not do away with myth, in other words, by tearing down the ancient view of drugs as powerful spirits. Instead, a cult of pharmacology emerged as pharmacological essences replaced magical ones. The former were said to act in much the same manner as the latter, in that a drug's powers were still viewed as capable of bypassing all the social conditioning of the mind, directly transforming the drug user's thoughts and actions. As "soul" was reinterpreted as "mind," and "spirit" was reinterpreted as "biochemistry," magical explanations of drug action fell out of use. Indeed, psychobabble and biobabble had taken their place.

But do not misunderstand me. In suggesting that a cult of pharmacology came to reign supreme over America, I am not also suggesting a conspiracy theory. In this book I describe various networks of understandings within which drug-related phenomena, both praised and condemned, were interpreted, and how these understandings caused the social and historical determinants of "drug effects" to be overlooked. The pharmaceutical industry, the tobacco industry, modern biological psychiatry, the biomedical sciences, the drug enforcement agencies, and the American judicial system — all these institutions were quick to embrace and promote a cult of pharmacology not as a conspiracy but as a belief system that served their own interests, albeit in varying ways. In fact, to suggest an active conspiracy would be to miss a central theme of this history, for the power of the cult of pharmacology to classify drugs as angels and demons stemmed largely from the fact that it was widely embraced. America became the world's most troubled drug culture not because the government conspired to allow access to drugs to some while denying access to others, but because more than any other nation, it was a full member of the cult — it truly believed.

Still, the ideology of the all-powerful drug, the cult of pharmacology, at times came into question, as in Peter Laurie's *Drugs*, Alfred Lindesmith's *Addiction and Opiates*, Stanton Peele's *The Meaning of Addiction*, Oakley Ray's *Drugs, Society, and Human Behavior*, Eric Schlosser's *Atlantic Monthly* essays on "reefer madness," Thomas Szasz's *Ceremonial Chemistry*, Andrew Weil's *The Natural Mind*, and Norman Zinberg's *Drugs, Set, and Setting*.[3]

These and other interrogations of drug issues implicated a variety of non-pharmacological factors in the shaping of drug outcomes and of America as a drug culture. Although they had little effect in tearing down the cult of pharmacology, they were nevertheless significant for promoting understanding of how drugs work.

Weil's *Natural Mind* (1972), for instance, lays out a first principle about drugs and society: the desire for altered states of consciousness is a natural drive among human beings (indeed, of all the cultures in the world, only the Eskimos lack a tradition of drug use).[4] Much of what has taken place in the name of drugs, throughout history and in twentieth-century America, boils down to this fact and one other, namely, that given the basic human tendency toward altered states, society is always confronted with the problem of how to deal with mind-altering substances and activities.

Weil later co-wrote *From Chocolate to Morphine*, an equally lucid work that, among other things, attempts to clarify the differences between *drug use* as a description of behavior and *drug abuse* as a moral judgment of that behavior. "Any drug can be used successfully, no matter how bad its reputation, and any drug can be abused, no matter how accepted it is. There are no good or bad drugs; there are only good and bad relationships with drugs."[5] Here Weil presents another basic principle for drugs and society: in its response to drugs, society has a tendency to load them with extraneous meaning — with myth. Gradually, but sometimes very quickly, this meaning joins the drug ritual itself, animating drug outcomes.

In looking at drugs in twentieth-century America, one must pick up where the nineteenth century left off, that is, in the middle of an ongoing drug drama, a drama that not only spilled over into the twentieth century with great impact but also clearly emerged from the two principles identified by Weil: drug use is ubiquitous, and the social meanings drugs acquire often transform their effects, their uses, and their users. But something specific to drugs in twentieth-century America was also evident by the end of the century. Below the surface of the influential pseudoscience of drugs that developed was a strong and growing undercurrent of understanding, both scientific and conceptual, that, had it been acknowledged in Western society, could have undermined the modern mythologizing of drugs as angels and demons.

Instead, America became the world's most troubled drug culture, never making peace with drugs. In much the same manner that the U.S. government protected settlers from the "transgressions" of American Indians more than a century ago, it came to defend one side of drugs (pharmaceutical drug use and "misuse") while trying to exterminate the other (illicit drug use and "abuse"). What is more, it did this in large part by promoting the mythology that "drugs" and their users, like the American Indians, are demons in need of total destruction.

That a cult of pharmacology continues to prevail reveals a final, basic principle about mind-altering drugs: any society that allows the meaning of drugs to unhinge from their everyday, human reality puts itself at risk for great misadventure and even unprecedented human tragedy.

Part One End of a Century

Ah, cocaine. Such an amusing drug, don't you think?
—Princess Margaret of Great Britain

I
magine that a collective of South American nations had control over coffee and oil imports into the United States. Imagine also that the peoples of these countries were increasingly given to drinking American spirits, leading to an epidemic of alcoholism in rural Andean society. Imagine finally that representatives of this collective came to America with the following ultimatum: either the U.S. government cease all production of distilled spirits, for both domestic and foreign markets, or member states of the collective would be forced to indefinitely prohibit all coffee and oil exports to the United States.

As strange as this story might sound, it is one that requires no imagination when the table is turned. Beginning in the 1970s, the United States pressured various South American nations — Bolivia, Colombia, and Peru — to prohibit a common traditional practice, the chewing of coca, and to eradicate an indigenous psychoactive substance, the coca plant. The United States did this by linking billions of dollars in economic aid with the mandatory adoption of American-style drug attitudes and drug policies. As a result, more than thirty U.S. government agencies had situated themselves in the Andean region by 1990, including the Drug Enforcement Administration (DEA), U.S. Customs, the U.S. Information Agency, the Bureau for International Narcotic Matters, the Federal Bureau of Investigation (FBI), the Central Intelligence Agency (CIA), and the Agency for International Development. Never mind that Bolivia, Colombia, and Peru were sovereign nations; more important, never mind that the oral consumption of coca had a great deal in common with the oral consumption of one of late-twentieth-century America's most popular pharmaceutical drugs: Ritalin.

A report published in 1995 in the prestigious *Archives of General Psychiatry* explains: "Cocaine, which is one of the most reinforcing and addictive of the abused drugs, has pharmacological actions that are very similar to those of methylphenidate [Ritalin], which is the most commonly prescribed psychotropic medication for children in the United States."[1] In the 1990s doctors annually wrote millions of Ritalin prescriptions for children of various ages, including growing numbers of toddlers and infants. During that decade, more American children were given Ritalin and other stimulants to modify their behavior than in the rest of the world combined. North America accounted for about 95 percent of worldwide Ritalin consumption in 1997, with Canada alone having a per-capita consumption comparable to that of the United States. In 1998 Canada consumed 1,000 times more Ritalin than did the more populated country of France.

The story of Ritalin in America, and how it befriended parents across the nation, began in the 1950s, when European scientists first synthesized the artificial angel. The story gained momentum in the 1970s, when the manufacturer of Ritalin hailed it as a panacea for such things as the so-called chronic fatigue syndrome.[2] The story peaked at the end of the twentieth century, with Ritalin not only having been widely adopted as a panacea for child-behavior problems but also having taken on a second life as a popular drug of misuse.

Consider Gerald Smith, once a principal at Aspen Elementary School in the Mormon town of Orem, Utah. While serving there as "a very good school principal," according to a local school-district spokesperson, Mr. Smith was also doing something very strange for a person of his position: he was sneaking into the school safe and replacing students' Ritalin pills with calcium and antihistamine pills.[3] Since Ritalin had by that time become a controversial drug, some might have assumed that Mr. Smith was swapping the pills as a moral act, that he felt, as many Christians do, that psychiatric drugs had usurped the role of family values in the American home. But this was not Mr. Smith's motivation: rather, he had secretly exchanged several hundred Ritalin pills because he wanted them for himself. The fifty-year-old man was stealing Ritalin for his own casual use.[4]

This was the late 1990s, and Gerald Smith was not alone. In 1997 the

Milwaukee police charged an elementary-school teacher with possession of Ritalin, which he had stolen from a school office.[5] In 1999 police arrested a computer technician at a junior-high school in Traverse City, Michigan, after school officials caught him on videotape in the act of stealing Ritalin.[6] The same year, Indiana authorities ordered a school nurse into treatment and fined her $1,300 after she admitted to stealing Ritalin and other prescription drugs.[7] In Nashville in 1995 James Smith became the second teacher at Grassland Middle School to be arrested for stealing Ritalin.[8] In 1987 authorities charged a physician in Orange County, California, with writing fraudulent prescriptions for Ritalin, which he used to obtain the drug for his own purposes.[9]

These anecdotes are consistent with a host of DEA findings during the 1990s, a time when drug agents began careful monitoring of Ritalin misuse.[10] From 1990 to 1995, they recorded 1,937 incidents of Ritalin theft. Most of these were night-time burglaries at pharmacies, but they also included a variety of armed robberies and employee thefts. Meanwhile, between 1987 and 1994, the Ohio Board of Pharmacy reported more than 100,000 Ritalin tablets stolen from Ohio pharmacies, with eighteen of the cases involving pharmacists. On one occasion, a store videotaped a pharmacist crushing Ritalin pills and snorting the powder. A similar study in Indiana described a physician who knowingly sold Ritalin prescriptions to members of a multistate drug-trafficking ring.[11]

From 1996 to 1998, about 700,000 Ritalin pills were reported missing from pharmacists and licensed handlers of the drug. In comparison, only 100,000 Ritalin pills were legally dispensed in all of France in 1998.[12] Numerous states have identified scams in which a parent drags his or her child to multiple physicians in order to obtain several Ritalin prescriptions, some or all of which are used or sold by the adult. In a report summarizing these findings Gretchen Feussner of the DEA concluded that "the magnitude and significance of diversion and trafficking of MPH [methylphenidate, or Ritalin] are comparable to those associated with pharmaceutical drugs of similar abuse potential and availability (e.g., morphine)."[13]

Adults supervising the culturally sanctioned use of Ritalin were not the only ones to appropriate it for their own use or to sell. The DEA reported that children and adolescents also diverted Ritalin for recreational use.[14] The following is a typical story.

Lauren was 13 when she began pilfering her brother's Ritalin pills, crushing a few at a time and snorting them. It wasn't really like taking drugs, she says, because lots of other teen-agers she knew either had prescriptions for the pills or knew someone who would share his or her supply. "I would take one pill in the morning, then snort one or two pills when I came home from school," says Lauren, now 17. . . . "Every once in a while, I'd take a whole bunch at once."[15]

As with reports of illicit Ritalin use by adults, and as suggested by the confession of Lauren, various statistics demonstrated that the stimulant had achieved a niche among children and teens similar to that among adults. One national survey found that the number of high-school seniors who misused Ritalin had nearly tripled from 1994 to 1996. In a 1996 phone survey in Georgia, more than 1 percent of the participating adolescents reported using Ritalin to get high.[16] When asked specifically about their misuse of Ritalin (versus stimulants or "drugs" generally), as they were in an Indiana survey in 1997, 7 percent of students reported having misused the drug in the previous year, and 2.5 percent reported using it on a monthly or more frequent basis. In a study published in the *Journal of Developmental Behavioral Pediatrics* in 1998, 16 percent of participating children reported having been approached at school to sell, trade, or give away their stimulant drugs.[17] Meanwhile, Ritalin-related emergency-room visits among children between the ages of ten and fourteen totaled about twenty-five in 1991; in 1995 this number topped 400; in 1996 the number of such visits among children from the ages of ten to seventeen was 630; in 1998 the number surpassed the same statistic for cocaine, jumping to 1,725.

Recreational Ritalin use also began showing up on college campuses in the 1990s, including top universities like Harvard. One young woman there acknowledged, "In all honesty, I haven't written a paper without Ritalin since my junior year in high school." Another reported, "I knew a girl in the freshman class who actually stole a script pad from the health center and faked her own prescription. She's an unbelievably smart girl, got a 1600 on her SAT, but is convinced she needs to snort Ritalin in order to do all her work. She's become an absolute speed freak—up all night and strung out all day. Ironically, she's failing two of her classes."[18]

Such stories gave sociological expression to what researchers had already established, namely, that all else being equal, Ritalin is the closest pharmacological substitute for cocaine.[19] Nora Volkow and her colleagues at Brookhaven National Laboratory in Upton, New York, reported in 1995 that Ritalin and cocaine have very similar pharmacological actions; furthermore, they showed two years later in the journal *Nature* that Ritalin could be substituted for cocaine in addiction research. Ritalin is "like cocaine," they wrote, in that it "increases synaptic dopamine by inhibiting dopamine reuptake, it has equivalent reinforcing effects to those of cocaine, and its intravenous administration induces a 'high' similar to that of cocaine."[20]

Volkow was not the first to pull back the curtain to reveal the truth about Ritalin. A 1975 study conducted by two pioneers in the study of drugs and behavior, Chris Johanson and C. R. Schuster, allowed rhesus monkeys to choose between Ritalin and cocaine. Because these studies were intended to test the drugs' liability for misuse, drug administration was typically intravenous. The study revealed that when one response led to administration of the drug and a different response led to administration of a placebo, animals responded for the drug. Furthermore, higher doses of one drug were preferred over lower doses of the other, and, most importantly, when they were delivered in comparable doses, no preference was found.[21] Other studies have replicated these findings in other species, showing that animals will respond in a similar or identical fashion to Ritalin and cocaine.[22] In fact, by the end of the twentieth century, more than a dozen studies had documented the comparability of these two drugs.[23]

The finding that animals in the laboratory do not prefer cocaine to Ritalin mirrors what animal "drug-discrimination studies" first showed in the 1970s. Animals in these studies were involuntarily administered both drugs and required to gives responses that identified which drug was which, with correct responses being rewarded with food; in other words, the animals relied on the drug's psychoactive effects to instruct them on which button to press to receive food. When trained in this way, animals are usually better "blind" discriminators of drug effects than humans. Drug-discrimination studies demonstrated, however, that animals cannot reliably differentiate the psychoactive effects of Ritalin, cocaine, and the amphetamines, although they can tell the difference between these stimulants and caffeine, as well as other drugs.[24]

Beginning in the 1990s, Volkow and her colleagues worked to clarify these findings. Measuring the effects of Ritalin in the human brain, they found that Ritalin was more akin to cocaine than to amphetamines—a dramatic set of findings in light of the fact that media reports had almost always characterized Ritalin's misuse as a cheap thrill and Ritalin itself as no more addictive than, say, caffeine and certainly no more powerful than amphetamines. A reporter covering the elementary-school principal who stole his students' Ritalin, for example, noted, "Ritalin is a mild stimulant usually given to children with attention deficit hyperactivity disorder, said Charles Ralston, a University of Utah pediatrician."[25] Another story noted, "According to medical texts, the drug is a more potent stimulant than caffeine and less potent than amphetamines."[26] Even the *New York Times* likened Ritalin to a "mild stimulant," "roughly [equivalent to] a jolt of strong coffee."[27] Ritalin's manufacturer claimed Ritalin to be a pharmacological middleweight, acting merely as "a mild central nervous system stimulant."

To understand why Ritalin is more akin to cocaine one needs to consider the actions of these two drugs in the brain in terms of pharmacokinetics and pharmacodynamics. Pharmacokinetics involves the study of processes that govern the fate of a drug once it is taken into the body, including its distribution, absorption, metabolism, and elimination. Once a drug enters the bloodstream, it is distributed more or less throughout the body and is absorbed into the body's tissues, where it is metabolized, or broken down so it can be expelled from the body. Pharmacokinetics differ for different drugs because of their varying chemical compositions. For instance, some drugs are readily absorbed into the brain, whereas others are excluded altogether. Among those that do have access, some will have longer-lasting effects than others, such as amphetamine versus cocaine. The bodily processes that govern these events also vary from person to person. Pharmacokinetics are thus determined by both the drug and individual physiology. The recommended dose of an over-the-counter analgesic will be by-and-large correct for most users, for example, but will be too low for some and too high for others.

Whether a drug has the capacity to enter the brain is a question of pharmacokinetics, but once it does, it enters the realm of pharmacodynamics. By definition, psychoactive drugs affect nerve cells in the brain to alter the ongoing processes of the central nervous system. As long as pharmacokinetic activities continue to distribute and redistribute a drug's molecules throughout the body (that is, until they are fully metabolized and eliminated), a portion of those molecules will permeate and act directly on the nervous system, including the brain, prompting pharmacodynamic processes regardless of whether or not enough drug remains in the body to produce its intended effects (relaxation, intoxication, anaesthesia, or analgesia).

The relationship between the chemistry of a drug and its pharmacodynamics is not a simple one. Whether naturally occurring or synthetic, any pharmacologically active substance has its own unique chemical structure. The antidepressant drugs Zoloft, Paxil, and Prozac are all selective serotonin reuptake inhibitors (SSRIs), but each has a more-or-less unique chemical structure — which is prerequisite for patenting a drug and getting it on the market. It is perhaps natural to assume that drugs with similar pharmacological actions will have similar chemical structures, and vice versa, but this is often not the case. Sometimes drugs of the same class do have similar structures, as is true of tricyclic antidepressants, benzodiazepines, and the amphetamines. But broader drug classes, such as antidepressants, stimulants, or hallucinogens, can include drugs with quite different structures; mescaline, lysergic acid (LSD), and psilocybin, for example, produce similar hallucinogenic effects in humans, all else being equal, but they are highly dissimilar in structure. Furthermore, drugs with similar structures will sometimes vary considerably in their effects. Amphetamine and tranylcypromine illustrate this, where a slight structural difference causes the latter to act not as a stimulant but as an antidepressant. Classifications based on chemical structure would therefore bear little relationship to classifications based on uses or effects.

Pharmacodynamics helps clarify why not all stimulants act on the brain in the same way. Caffeine, for example, acts on brain cells by affecting the metabolism within nerve cells (neurons). Ritalin, the amphetamines, and cocaine, by contrast, affect the release of neurochemicals between neurons; these central-nervous-system stimulants can also be grouped loosely together in that they directly promote the activity of two neurotransmitter systems, norepinephrine and dopamine, albeit not exactly in the same way or to the same degree.

Until late in the twentieth century, cocaine was believed to have greater activity in the dopamine system of the brain, while Ritalin was assumed to be, like the amphetamines, efficacious in the norepinephrine system.[28] Research has since demonstrated that Ritalin's pharmacology is actually more akin to cocaine's.[29] When Volkow and her colleagues first addressed this issue, they commented that "although socioeconomic factors . . . could account for the higher rate of cocaine abuse than methylphenidate abuse, it is possible that pharmacological differences between the drugs are responsible."[30] In other words, might pharmacokinetic differences in how rapidly Ritalin enters the brain account for the radically different understandings and uses that distinguish Ritalin from cocaine in American society?

Using the positron emission tomography (PET) scan, a brain-imaging technology, Volkow and colleagues found, to their surprise, that Ritalin's pharmacology is best compared not to amphetamine but to cocaine. Ritalin and cocaine were strikingly similar in their uptake into the brain, their distribution within it, and their actions on it. The rush experienced by snorting, smoking, or injecting cocaine was already known to result from the inhibition of dopamine reuptake. Volkow and colleagues found that, contrary to the claims made by experts and textbooks in the field of psycho-pharmacology at that time, Ritalin produced its psychoactive effects in the same way. Just as drugs like Prozac and Paxil selectively block the "reuptake" of the neurotransmitter serotonin, both cocaine and Ritalin block the reup-take of dopamine. Thus, from a perspective that deems pharmacology all-important in classifying drugs as good or evil, as "medicines" or as "drugs," Ritalin cannot be grouped as an amphetamine-type drug, which acts on dopamine by causing its release from neurons. All else being equal, Ritalin is nothing less than synthetic cocaine.

As Volkow and others have pointed out, however, such studies compare Ritalin and cocaine when delivered rapidly into the brain via intravenous injection. Children usually take their Ritalin orally, which dramatically changes the pharmacokinetics of the drug by slowing down its absorption into the bloodstream and thus into the brain. This fact led Volkow and colleagues to ask another risky question: how similar are the physiological effects of oral Ritalin compared to those of snorted or injected cocaine? The results of the study were published in 1999 in the *American Journal of Psychiatry*.[31]

At the outset of this study Volkow and colleagues still clung to the popular understanding of Ritalin and cocaine; that is, they "hypothesized that oral methylphenidate [Ritalin], at doses prescribed therapeutically, would not induce a 'high' because it would not achieve sufficient levels of dopamine transporter blockade."[32] And again they were surprised. Therapeutic-level doses of Ritalin did in fact inhibit the reuptake of dopamine, and to a degree that was comparable to intravenous cocaine. "This study measures for the first time the levels of dopamine transporter blockade achieved after therapeutic doses of oral methylphenidate. . . . It shows that oral methylphenidate is very effective in blocking dopamine transporters."[33] At two of the doses studied, both of which fell within the range of Ritalin's therapeutic use (given in tablet form to children), oral Ritalin affected dopamine transporters to the degree that would be necessary to produce a drug high if snorting or injecting cocaine.

The actions of oral Ritalin were found to be almost identical to those of intravenous cocaine, both qualitatively and quantitatively, except for one important feature: the time required to produce the same magnitude of effect with prescribed doses of oral Ritalin was considerably greater than would be required if cocaine was snorted or injected. Of course, the same would be true for cocaine if it were taken in pill form. As one media report summarized, "Dr. Nora Volkow and her colleagues have found that the oral medication, with similar pharmacology to cocaine, does not trigger a 'high' because it takes about an hour to make its way into the brain in sufficient levels to help children focus."[34] As real and important as this difference is, it is a difference only in how Ritalin and cocaine are used — a historical and contingent fact — not a difference in the pharmacology of the two drugs.

If Ritalin could legally be given to millions of American children despite the fact that its effects were indistinguishable from cocaine when taken in comparable doses and via the same route of drug administration, then popular and scientific beliefs concerning these two drugs in the twentieth century were nonsensical. In fact, either cocaine is not the inherent demon drug it was made out to be, or Ritalin is incorrigibly evil and corrupting. If the former sounds more plausible, it is perhaps because only a small percentage of the millions of children who take Ritalin orally find themselves wanting to crush up their tablets and snort them.

Still, Ritalin did spill out of its accepted medical boundaries, garnering considerable casual use by the end of the twentieth century. Meanwhile, the similarities that existed between North America's Ritalin trade and South America's coca trade passed without notice: both were viewed traditionally as beneficial for their "native" users; both were diverted into other, nontraditional practices by "outsiders"; and both were manipulated by their unintended users to intensify their pharmacological effects. The political contradiction suggested by these similarities also went unnoticed: if America could have its Ritalin, why couldn't South Americans have their indigenous coca, or even their cocaine?

On 29 February 1996, the retired army general Barry McCaffrey was sworn in as President Bill Clinton's new director of the Office of National Drug Control Policy, a position he occupied longer than any of his predecessors, stepping down in January 2001 after five years of service.[35] McCaffrey, a twenty-nine-year army veteran at the time of his appointment, had received two Distinguished Service Crosses, a Bronze Star, and three Purple Hearts during his military career. He had served as a combat soldier in Vietnam, as well as the commander of the Twenty-fourth Mechanized Infantry Division during Operation Desert Storm.[36] Having also served as the commander-in-chief of the U.S. Southern Command (SOUTHCOM) from February 1994 to February 1996, McCaffrey was an obvious choice to be the nation's fourth drug czar; as SOUTHCOM's commander, he had been responsible for overseeing counter–drug operations in Central and South American countries, which had familiarized him with the drug trade in those regions.

As drug czar, McCaffrey appointed Col. James Hiett to head the U.S. Army's expanding anti-drug control operations in Colombia. Like McCaffrey, Hiett had served a tour of duty in SOUTHCOM. In the summer of 1998, while stationed at Ft. Bragg, North Carolina, following his SOUTHCOM assignment, the colonel was awarded the coveted antidrug position. The appointment sent him to the U.S. embassy in Bogotá, making him the top military official in charge of "counternarcotics" operations in Colombia. Commanding a unit of 200 army troops, the colonel's top responsibility was to train and assist the Colombian army in mobilizing operations against the indigenous cocaine trade, as well as the growing heroin trade. Between 80 and 90 percent of the cocaine, as well as some 60 percent of the heroin, consumed in the United States at the time was produced and / or distributed in Colombia.

But Colonel Hiett remained at his post in Bogotá for just one year before being returned stateside to sit idle at a desk at Ft. Monroe, Virginia. The reason was neither his performance as a military officer — Hiett's twenty-four-year record was spotless — nor his behavior off duty. The reason was his wife. As Mike Wallace later remarked in an episode of *60 Minutes*, "In

Colombia, the wife of America's top military drug-fighter was herself a drug smuggler."

A few years before his assignment to Colombia, when he and his wife were still at Ft. Bragg, Hiett and the U.S. Army first became aware of Laurie Anne Hiett's drug problem. The problem involved the same white powdery substance that had for more than twenty years financed, via the demand of the American illegal drug market, a brutal civil war in Colombia, and the same substance that had brought Colonel Hiett to Colombia: cocaine.

James Hiett met Laurie, who was twelve years younger, when serving in the Canal Zone in Panama. At that time, Laurie worked as a secretary at SOUTHCOM and lived with her mother, a Panamanian, and her father, an American engineer. During the time when Jim and Laurie courted, and then married a year or so later, in 1989, Laurie says she had recreated with cocaine but not to excess. Living the cloistered life of an army wife, however, brought her drug habits to the fore, she later admitted, and blurred out most everything else. Not unlike the domestic housewives of the 1960s and 1970s, who took the edge off their staid lives with daily doses of barbiturates (Seconal) or benzodiazepines (Valium), Laurie Hiett developed her own domestic drug habit, albeit one more perilous for her husband, the army, and America's drug war.

Laurie Hiett first received treatment for her cocaine problem in the mid-1990s at the army hospital in Ft. Bragg, followed by a brief stay in a private drug rehab center. Her husband was fully aware of all this, as was army and drug czar McCaffrey when he appointed Colonel Hiett to the Bogotá position. The colonel also knew that his wife had strayed back into her drug lifestyle well before their departure to Colombia. Drug treatment had kept her clean for only a few months. She taught Spanish in a local high school, and fellow teachers later reported having known of her drug habits; according to one of her drug-using friends, these habits sometimes included lunches that began with marijuana and rum-and-Cokes, and ended with amphetamines or cocaine.[37] When Laurie told a friend about her husband's promotion and that she would be moving to Bogotá, the friend's first thought was, "Oh wow, that's where cocaine comes from. This ain't gonna be good."

By the age of thirty-six, Laurie was a compulsive drug user. Only four months before the colonel's promotion to Colombia, she snorted a line of cocaine in front of him. His response was to walk out of the room in silence. The colonel was in denial of his wife's habit, relying on the familiar military policy of don't ask, don't tell. The army was in denial, as well. Not long after the Hietts were transplanted to Bogotá, McCaffrey reported to the Senate Committee on Foreign Relations that the members of a new Colombian antidrug battalion "have been carefully selected, fully vetted, and are being trained and equipped with U.S. support."[38] He failed to mention that this was not entirely true for Colonel Hiett, the chief U.S. military officer advising the battalion.

Not long after the colonel's arrival in Colombia the actions of his wife appeared to confirm the stereotype that drug availability leads inevitably to drug problems. In fact, Laurie's lifestyle in Colombia was anything but the norm. A rather unsuitable candidate for the straight-and-narrow world inhabited by the spouses of diplomats, Laurie was described by others as a young, giggly, out-of-control party girl. Like the teachers at the Fayetteville school where she had taught, embassy officials, diplomats, spouses of diplomats, and business associates had little trouble remembering her comportment, and few were surprised by the international scandal that followed.

In Bogotá, with her leopard-skin blouses, miniskirts, and casual references to cocaine, Laurie quickly found herself excluded from the diplomatic soirees attended by her husband and purged from the daily social functions of the wives' club. Shunned from the diplomatic social scene, she turned to her Colombian driver, Jorge Ayala, who obligingly took her away from the high-security embassy compound, across its encircling moat, and into the Bogotá night.

Laurie Hiett's forays into Bogotá's nightclub scene included visits to the infamous La Zona Rosa, a district filled with casinos, clubs, and cocaine. It was there that she first asked her driver whether he could score some cocaine for her. When he returned with a one-pound brick of high-grade cocaine, Laurie was amazed. Expecting to pay her usual $100 for a single gram, she ended up paying only $1,000 for 500 grams—a mere $2 per gram. Reflecting on the cocaine binge that followed, which began only minutes later when she snorted a few lines in the embassy bathroom, she remembers thinking, "'Oh my God, I'm so wired.' . . . It was this beautiful thing, you know?"[39]

After that night in La Zona Rosa, and with cocaine back in her life in a big way, the colonel's wife also began venturing into other high-risk environments. She is even reported to have visited an underground nightclub district where a U.S. DEA agent had been shot a year earlier. While her husband was off waging America's drug war in the Andean mountains, which was most of the time, Laurie indulged in weekend drug binges at her favorite Andean resort, a drug haven that could only be accessed via a mountain road known for the frequency of its guerrilla kidnappings. The colonel's wife had unwittingly stumbled into a world that placed essentially no financial limits on cocaine consumption, a situation that, in the case of the Hietts, ended badly for everyone.

Laurie Hiett's coke habit was an embarrassment, but, like the other nefarious activities said to occur regularly in the U.S. embassy in Bogotá, it might have been kept short of public scandal. However, when Laurie the habitual drug user became Laurie the drug trafficker, the stage was set for a personal tragedy — the Hietts had two young boys — as well as for what could easily have been a public-relations disaster for America's international drug war. As it turned out, most Americans did not hear the news until months after it was initially reported in the *Village Voice* and well after the multibillion dollar militarization of America's drug war in Colombia, known as "Plan Colombia," had been "debated" and approved on Capitol Hill.[40]

The three-month investigation into Laurie Hiett's drug trafficking began on 24 May 1999, when a drug dog showed interest in a package sent to Miami from the U.S. embassy via diplomatic post. Noticing the dog's interest in the package, a U.S.-customs agent decided to open it, against standard procedure for handling embassy parcels. What was first believed to be a shipment of pure cocaine — it was declared on the package to be coffee, candy, and a T-shirt — actually turned out to be almost three pounds of high-grade heroin. In conspiring with her driver and his friend in New York, Laurie had put her faith in the unspoken rule that customs agents do not inspect diplomatic mail; but she and her colleagues did not know that customs drug dogs sometimes do.

As reported by Gabriella Gamini in the *London Times*, the discovery of Laurie's drug shipment came just days after Colonel Hiett had been nominated for a post that would involve him even more deeply in the Andean drug war.[41] The assignment, had it not been revoked, would have placed him in charge of U.S. troops stationed at two new anti-drug bases located in Colombia's southern jungles. One was established in the area of Tres Esquinas, an air base for counter-drug operations in the center of the coca-growing region; the other was set up in the area of Tolemaida. The colonel could not keep cocaine out of his own home, but apparently the army still thought he could keep it out of America.

After the May discovery of what was later found to be Laurie Hiett's seventh shipment of drugs to New York, an undercover agent delivered the intercepted package to its Queens address, followed by an arrest of one of Laurie's partners and soon thereafter of her friend and driver in Bogotá. The army's Criminal Investigation Division (CID) then showed up to question the colonel's wife (the colonel had been given advanced warning of a prop-erty search). This led two months later to her voluntary arrest in Brooklyn, where the case was eventually heard in U.S. federal court.

As court records later showed, Laurie Hiett made two trips to New York during her brief tenure as a drug trafficker, bringing to Colombia a sum of about $40,000 in cash, which she admitted giving to her husband. And in a move perhaps more surprising than anything Laurie herself did, the colonel accepted the drug money, no questions asked, which he then laundered — or "dissipated," as he put it — by paying off Laurie's exorbitant shopping bills and by placing small amounts of cash in various bank accounts. At one point while the investigation was still ongoing, he met her in Florida with $11,000 of the cash still in hand.

A year after the initial discovery by customs agents, Laurie Hiett pleaded guilty in U.S. federal court to distributing cocaine. She received a five-year sentence, meaning she would be out in three. The sentence, delivered by Judge Edward Korman, was two years shy of the term required by federal sentencing guidelines, and while certainly punishing, it was much shorter than those typically given for a first-offense felony charge of this sort: an unsympathetic trafficker can receive ten to fifteen years imprisonment for the same. Judge Korman, for instance, handed down a longer sentence to the middleman in Laurie's drug-dealing scheme, her driver's friend in New York.

The colonel, too, may have hoped for light punishment — forced retire-ment from the army, rather than felony charges of laundering drug money — and, indeed, the CID initially cleared him of any wrongdoing. But pres-sure eventually mounted, and in the same courtroom in which his wife had been sentenced to five years, the colonel received a sentence of five months.

The Hiett affair was a bizarre scandal that threatened the U.S. drug war, but it was not surprising. Laurie Hiett was a party girl who liked shopping and taking drugs that she viewed as benign, someone who exploited an unlikely situation that was hardly of her own making. Her husband found himself in an absurd position, but he managed to compartmentalize it in much the same way as did the rest of America: when those involved in using and selling drugs are close to us, or have ties to the powers that be, they are treated in an understanding way; when they have no such status or access to power and privilege, they are made "examples of," punished in the most draconian fashion. That the wife of America's top military drug fighter in Colombia could be a drug trafficker did not prove to America that its drug war was a hopeless debacle or suggest that perhaps Colombia's drug problems hailed from America's drug demand.[42] Rather, being viewed through the prism of drugs as inherently good or evil, these events fueled the opposite argument: that cocaine was so corrupting that it had to be fought with even greater fury.

"One of the things that have always made drugs so powerful," wrote Malcolm Gladwell in the *New Yorker*, "is their cultural adaptability, their way of acquiring meanings beyond their pharmacology."[43] There does seem to be something about substances that produce mind-altering effects via an invisible set of molecules that both inspires myth making and leads to elaborate social regulations and rituals. One result is that most psychoactive drugs eventually acquire their own social histories, their own mythologies, which often turn into self-fulfilling prophecies. As with oral coca and oral Ritalin, the existence of different histories and myths for comparable pharmacological substances makes compartmentalization not only possible but also necessary. "Allegories and myths are ways that societies keep track of their contradictions," wrote the cultural theorist Laura Kipnis, continuing, "new ones are constructed as required."[44]

Because drugs occupy a socially animated realm, it is difficult, if not impossible, to know how much of what is observed as a drug effect is due to the drug as a pharmacological agent and how much is due to the drug as an object to which a whole set of beliefs, rituals, and expectations have been attached. This is a recurring theme in drug histories. When steeped in drug mythology, whether on the streets of America or in the ceremonies of an Amazonian tribe, people are consumed as much by "drugs" as drugs are consumed by people.

So concluded Craig Van Dyke and Robert Byck, researchers from Yale University who conducted a series of experimental investigations into the pharmacological and psychological effects of cocaine. Summarizing their findings in a 1982 essay in *Scientific American*, they noted, "It is all too easy to suppose the physiological and social consequences of the use of cocaine are commensurate with its popularity and economic importance. [In truth,] 'recreational' users who take the drug under controlled conditions often cannot distinguish it from other drugs or even from a placebo."[45]

Studies conducted at the University of Chicago and at Johns Hopkins University reported equally surprising results after asking experienced cocaine users to report on the effects of different drugs taken in a controlled context in which the users were blind to what they were taking. Researchers employed the concealment in these studies as a method for teasing pharmacology from myth, as it allowed them to remove or at least undermine people's beliefs and expectations with regard to the different drugs. In the Yale study by Van Dyke and Byck, drug users sometimes mistook a placebo for cocaine. The placebo in the study, a local anesthetic called lidocaine, was used because it produces the same numbing effect in the nose but does not have any of cocaine's psychoactive effects.[46]

In the 1976 University of Chicago study, users often could not discriminate between the initial high produced by intravenous cocaine and the high that was produced by intravenous amphetamine.[47] Similarly, in the Johns Hopkins study, published in 1995, recreational cocaine users mistook relatively high doses of intravenous caffeine for cocaine.[48] The Johns Hopkins researchers noted that, as the dose increased, study participants rated caffeine's effects more and more positively, an effect that peaked two minutes after the injection; increases in the dosage of caffeine also increased the frequency with which the participants believed the drug might be cocaine or amphetamine.[49] As Van Dyke and Byck concluded with regard to their own findings, "Such results are the first steps toward distinguishing the almost overwhelming mythology that surrounds cocaine from reliable information about its effects."[50]

While some of the study participants were no doubt more discriminating about drug and nondrug effects than others, just as some users find the sensory effects of snorted or smoked cocaine to be much more pleasurable than others, the findings of these studies were nevertheless surprising: cocaine's reputation seemed to have more to do with its self-perpetuating status as a uniquely powerful drug than it did with its basic pharmacological effects. Although beliefs, expectations, and context may not be considered drugs per se, there are times when it appears that the drug context, with all its layers of meaning, is at least as efficacious in producing druglike effects. This is demonstrated not only in laboratory investigations but also in the rituals of drug taking itself.

Cocaine was not always an international cult commodity sought by the rich and famous or by those who wanted to feel as though they were rich and famous. For more than four thousand years, and perhaps as long as seven thousand years, Indians living in the Andean mountain regions of present-day South America used cocaine in the form of coca, taking it for a variety of religious, medicinal, physical, and social purposes. "The Incas regarded it as a gift from the gods intended to improve human life," Andrew Weil wrote. "They have personified the spirit of the plant as Mama Coca, a divine and beneficent aspect of nature."[51]

South American Indians bring the drug into the body by chewing a preparation made in part from the leaves of the coca plant, which is indigenous to the tropical Andean regions. While this substance produces noticeable psychoactive effects, these effects have always been structured by the various social norms and environs in which coca has been chewed. The traditional use of coca—whether for sacred rituals, to curb hunger, or to energize the body or mind—did not give rise to health problems, drug policies, or drug wars. Nor did it produce escalating drug use or any kind of dependence that could be labeled addiction. Researchers found that some Indians achieved daily blood levels of cocaine as high as those obtained today with powder cocaine, yet these levels were not associated with physical or psychological dependence. Men within Indian communities would sometimes go without coca for months while labouring in the jungle forest; during this time they showed no obsession with or impairment due to the absence of coca.[52]

This is not to say, however, that the traditions that have governed the use and experience of coca by Amazonian tribes have been invulnerable to outside influence. Weil visited the Cubeos Indians in southeastern Colombia several times, beginning in the 1970s. On his first visit to the remote tribe he found widespread coca chewing, a practice that he interpreted as healthy and sacred. The tribe was very welcoming, and Weil came to realize how coca chewing contributed to the healthy functioning of the society. In the years that followed, however, Weil observed the devastating impact of the urban drug trade on the tribe: as traffickers came to the Indians with money in hand, asking them to produce cocaine for export, the stability and structure of the tribe rapidly deteriorated. "On my last visit to the Rio Cuduyari," Weil wrote, "the whole settlement was in disarray, with the moloca untended and food scarce. On one occasion, when the Indians tried to hold a fiesta to celebrate my return, cane whiskey appeared instead of chicha and coca, and the fiesta was over in less than an hour, with many of the men lying drunk on the ground. One of these was the oldest man in the village, whose health and vigor I had so admired; when I last saw him, he was semiconscious, with blood streaming down his face as a result of a fall." The demon drug for the Cubeos Indians of the Rio Cuduyari was not coca or cocaine — it was alcohol.

The chief pharmacological ingredient in Mama Coca was first isolated in the mid-nineteenth century, in Germany. Before then, cocaine in the form of coca had not been particularly popular in Europe, even though Spanish colonialists had first imported coca leaves from South America in the sixteenth century. At that time, Europeans seemed to find the idea of "chewing" anything, let alone coca, to be primitive and distasteful. This problem was solved three hundred years later when the alkaloid known as cocaine hydrochloride was extracted from coca in pure form.

While the isolation of cocaine from nature was immediately recognized as a scientific and medical achievement, the symbolic significance of the advance went virtually unnoticed. Whereas New World Indians had kept the plant intact, which mirrored the unity and strength of their social communities, North Americans and Europeans isolated the drug from the plant, which mirrored the disunity and isolating nature of their societies. It is difficult to assess the degree to which a direct cultural link might exist between the isolation and reduction of a drug from the natural world and the isolation and reduction of the individual from the social world; however, at least in hindsight, one thing seems clear: the likelihood of developing a compulsive attitude toward a psychoactive drug increases the more the drug is concentrated in substance and then taken — as in the case of Laurie Hiett, or the street addict, or the domestic housewife — as a substitute for, rather than as a complement to, a meaningful social existence.

In *Tastes of Paradise* Wolfgang Schivelbusch presented this argument as a model for understanding alcohol use in eighteenth-century England.[53] As the industrial revolution undermined traditional ways of living and working, the traditions around drinking beer and wine also began to break down, with a sudden and dramatic increase in the consumption of distilled spirits. "Liquor thus represents a process of *acceleration* of intoxication intrinsically related to other processes of acceleration in the modern age. . . . The maximized effect, the acceleration, and the reduced price made liquor a true child of the Industrial Revolution."[54] As drinking and intoxication lost their traditional role of establishing social bonds or connections, Schivelbusch noted, drinking began to function for many as an antagonist of, rather than as a complement to, a harmonious social existence.

Coca experiences a similar fate in industrial societies. Soon after cocaine was isolated from coca, it was added to various popular concoctions. One of these was the patent medicine Vin Tonique Mariani (Mariani Wine Tonic), a prescription cure-all that contained French wine and an extract of coca leaves. Angelo Mariani was a well-known promoter of his European product, often obtaining and publishing testimonials from respected users, including Pope Leo VIII and Thomas Edison. Cocaine also found its way into American products. Parke Davis and Company, for instance, sold a tincture of cocaine, which although widely used was not nearly as successful as the product known today as Coca-Cola. Just as powder cocaine took hold of the American drug scene after a crackdown on street amphetamine and marijuana use in the late twentieth century, the tonic Coca-Cola was born during the rise of the Temperance movement and the prohibition of alcohol in Atlanta in 1888. To preserve his market, the Atlanta-based inventor John Pemberton removed the red wine from his popular French Wine Cola, added cocaine, and changed its name to Coca-Cola.

Along with the widespread availability of popular tonics in Europe and America came a growing respectability for the oral consumption of cocaine. This was especially true after the publication of Freud's 1884 paper on the subject, "Über Coca" (On coca). The conclusions of the paper, including the suggestion that cocaine might be an effective treatment for morphine addiction, then called morphinism, were immediately seized on and promoted by the German pharmaceutical manufacturer E. Merck and Company. Merck, which remains prominent in the pharmaceutical industry today, had begun to produce and sell cocaine in 1862 but increased production dramatically after the release of Freud's report.[55] The popularity of cocaine as a medical panacea peaked by the end of the nineteenth century. By the 1930s the first era of fashionable cocaine use had passed.

The myth of cocaine as a wonder drug remained in suspended animation for almost half a century, only to awaken, fresh and renewed, in the early 1970s, a time when the belief in cocaine as a medical panacea was long forgotten and a new myth of illicit potency and excitement was born. (This was also the period when George W. Bush was recreating with it.) And just as the demand for cocaine as the drug of the socially elite made it a major American import, the idea of cocaine as a chic commodity also become a major cultural export of the United States—a cultural meme that would spread to and infect other societies around the globe.

The international effect of America's commodification of cocaine was not singular or absolute, however. Even at the end of the twentieth century, the uses of coca and cocaine remained varied, as did social and political attitudes regarding its use. This was the conclusion of the largest international study of cocaine ever conducted. The 1992–94 study was first announced by Dr. Niroshi Nakajima, then the director-general of the World Health Organization (WHO), at the April 1990 World Summit on Drugs in London.[56] Financial support for the study came from the Italian Ministry of the Interior, and it was jointly organized and executed by WHO and the United Nations Interregional Crime and Justice Research Institute (UNICRI). Referred to as the WHO/UNICRI Cocaine Project, it was an immense study, and one in which the U.S. government was not involved.

The objectives of the cocaine initiative were fairly simple: to obtain data on the use of coca-related drugs in both coca-producing and nonproducing countries; and to examine the effectiveness of different strategies seeking to curb cocaine use and cocaine-related harms. Several features of the study made it historically significant, including its scale and scope. Researchers directly investigated drug use and other cocaine-related practices in twenty-two sites across nineteen countries, spanning all continents save Antarctica. The study was also unique in that it focused on the need for reducing drug demand rather than on law-enforcement practices that sought to curb drug supplies, which ensured original and detailed information about cocaine culture from around the globe.

Among the study's notable findings was that even late in the twentieth century there remained a great diversity in the kinds of relationships people had with cocaine, including how it affected them, both as individuals and as societies. "One of the main conclusions of the study is that there is no 'average cocaine user,'" a WHO press release noted after the study's completion. "There is an enormous variety in the types of people who use cocaine, the amount of drug used, the frequency of use, the duration and intensity of use, the reasons for using cocaine and any associated problems that users experience."[57] Brazilian researchers, for example, reported that cocaine use was heavy among street children in São Paulo, whereas Cairo researchers reported that use was confined mainly to affluent adults. Mexican researchers found use in Mexico City to be concentrated in twenty- to twenty-four-year-old males. And in Korea cocaine was traced to Korean nationals who traveled not to South America but to the United States — one example of how, as drugs are imported to the United States, American drug myths and drug practices are exported in return.

Researchers also reported differences in the manner in which cocaine was used. In Mexico City use among young adult males was restricted primarily to the homeless, and cocaine was injected rather than snorted or smoked. In contrast, throughout Bolivia and Peru traditional coca chewing was found not only to still exist but also to be quite common. In Nigeria researchers reported that cocaine was smoked in the form of crack cocaine, a crystalline "rock" substance that forms when cocaine hydrochloride is mixed under heat with other chemicals. Similar to cocaine use in Korea, crack use in Nigeria was restricted not to the poor and desperate but to wealthy Nigerians described as living in the "fast lane." Colombian prostitutes smoked coca-paste (a crude intermediary product in the making of cocaine hydrochloride). In Harare, Zimbabwe, and São Paulo, Brazil, day-laborers like taxi drivers and garbage collectors used cocaine to prolong work capacity and stay alert, an extension of the traditional use of coca. In the urban scene of Sydney, researchers reported, cocaine snorting was especially popular among the regulars at gay nightclubs.

The WHO/UNICRI Cocaine Project found, in other words, that cocaine use varied within and across almost every possible demographic category. If one knew the right places to look in the world, one could find cocaine use in nearly every segment of human society: from children to the elderly, from straights to gays (and bisexuals), from single to married, from men to women, from homeless to professional, and from rural to urban. Frequently, researchers found cocaine to be concentrated in a particular segment of one population but then restricted to an entirely different segment in another, perhaps even neighboring population. Overall, a variety of cultural factors seemed to influence cocaine-related practices. And because these factors varied significantly across cultures and subcultures, the meaning, the use, and the significance of the drug known as "cocaine" also varied significantly.

There can be little doubt that cocaine is a highly efficacious substance. What the laboratory studies and the WHO/UNICRI project brought into question, however, was whether the molecular powers of the drug are so specific and powerful in their effects that they are immune to the historical and cultural factors that mediate all other kinds of human experiences. What the WHO/UNICRI report also brought into question was whether use in a society necessarily has a deleterious effect, inevitably leading to the escalation of drug problems. The societal pattern of cocaine use in the study was reported to be stabilizing or decreasing in most countries. As the WHO later summarized, while cocaine use had not "exploded," use was indeed "diffusing" throughout the world. The largest group of users worldwide were found to be casual users of powder cocaine, and the vast majority of these users were found to suffer few, if any, ill effects. In particular, cardiac arrest was found to be "very rare," and casual cocaine use that escalated into excessive or addictive use was the exception, not the rule. Quite like the perceptions of American parents handing out Ritalin to their children, between 50 and 75 percent of users across the cocaine study found the drug to be "harmless" and "beneficial" to them.[58]

Documenting the cult standing of powder cocaine exported from the United States, users in the WHO/UNICRI study tended to associate the drug with enhanced status and believed that the drug made them more sociable, relaxed, and stimulated — a description that would be heard a decade later in America for the antidepressant drug Prozac. Researchers found as well that the smoking of cocaine in the form of coca paste or crack was largely associated with the poorest and most marginalized segment of society, Nigeria being the exception. This appeared to be simple economics. If powder cocaine was glamorized as a high-society drug and priced accordingly, "discounted" versions of the drug, in the form of crack rocks or crude coca paste, would have appeared on the market to capitalize on drug use in socially and economically impoverished areas. Indeed, the WHO/UNICRI study consistently found that the using and selling of coca paste and crack was most common among those who wanted but could not afford powder cocaine.

In the United States the rise of the secondary market for cocaine began in the 1980s — a trend that threatened the purity of cocaine's reputation. While powder cocaine continued to be associated with status and vitality, this stood in growing contrast to the image, however exaggerated, of the poor, habitual, inner-city cocaine or crack addict. Drug researchers eager to be in the public light, or at least in the public monies, followed up on this development with a popular characterization of crack as somehow hyper-addictive. This theory sat atop of a heap of contradictions that were never considered, let alone resolved: to wit, crack differs from cocaine only in the rate of drug absorption; many inner-city crack users were found to use the drug only recreationally; and many first-time crack users describe the experience as overwhelming and unpleasant.[59]

The contrasting images of the desperate crack addict versus the casual cocaine user in America did reinforce one of the WHO/UNICRI findings, namely, that at the end of the twentieth century the image of cocaine varied dramatically across the global social landscape. What this finding did not affirm was the theory that drug effects flow directly and decidedly from the chemistry or pharmacological actions of the drug. Such a perspective fails to explain the coexistence of multiple and conflicting meanings and drug effects for the same basic chemical substance, sometimes even within the same population. For Ritalin and cocaine, as well as for cocaine and crack, this contradiction was glossed over by constructing a myth around each drug's pharmacology that coupled its putative powers with the accepted, popular wisdom about it. The WHO/UNICRI study clearly demonstrated, however, that coca and cocaine existed in the world not as pure substances, free of all pride and prejudice, but rather as socially defined commodities, with all the added significance of any commodified substance, from Coca-Cola to Prada bags.

This sociological view of "cocaine" contradicted the popular understanding of drugs in twentieth-century America, wherein drugs were to be classified as pharmacological angels and demons, not as generic substances that lacked moral significance independent of social practices. Thus, the results of the WHO/UNICRI Cocaine Project did not bode well for its own future. Although a 1995 press release announced that the complete findings of the study were to be made available in a series of papers, and although full reports were in fact scheduled for publication in public journals, this never took place.[60] The U.S. government, it turned out, was less than pleased with the study's main conclusions.

Neil Boyer, a U.S. representative for the State Department at the time, raised his government's concerns at a meeting in Geneva shortly after the WHO's initial report of the findings. Minutes from the meeting note matter-of-factly, "The United States government has been surprised to note that the [WHO/UNICRI study] seemed to make a case for the positive uses of cocaine."[61] That is, the U.S. government did not find the conclusions of the study, however valid, to be consistent with U.S. policy concerning cocaine. Although the cocaine study was the result of intensive investigations in twenty-two sites and nineteen countries around the world, the U.S. government did not want the study's research to jeopardize or complicate the globalization of American drug policy, which by the end of the century was represented by DEA offices in seventy-nine cities and fifty-six countries across the globe. Patricia Erickson, an international expert on cocaine from the University of Toronto who served as a project advisor for the study, drew her own conclusion: "Of course, many of the findings [of the study] have gone totally against the image of cocaine as this evil drug that enslaves people. This is the 1920s mythology. Sure, cocaine can get people in trouble and there are reasons to be concerned about it, but we found that people who otherwise are working and doing other things could use it recreationally. The study was not aimed at making cocaine look bad but getting a sense of the whole spectrum of how it was used in other countries."[62]

Meanwhile, Mr. Boyer was direct in delivering his government's message: "If WHO activities . . . failed to reinforce proven drug control approaches, funds for the relevant programs should be curtailed." Subsequent to such pressure, the WHO quashed all open discussion of the cocaine study, "convened a committee to review the findings," and never uttered another public word on the subject.[63] When I made inquiries a few years after Boyer delivered the American ultimatum, the WHO recommended via email that interested parties contact the U.S. State Department and provided a phone number—this despite the fact that the U.S. government had had no financial or administrative ties to the WHO/UNICRI Cocaine Project.

The WHO/UNICRI study showed cocaine to be not one thing—neither an angel nor a demon, neither good nor evil—but rather different things to different peoples, just as it was for Laurie versus James Hiett. Unfortunately, with compartmentalization in full force in America, little *apparent* progress was made in the twentieth century toward clarifying the dialectic of meaning involving drugs—the mutual exchange of influence between drugs, their users, and the contexts in which drugs acquire meaning and are used. In truth, considerable success *was* achieved in understanding psychoactive drugs, especially from the 1950s onward, but these clinical, empirical, and conceptual developments had little chance to shape common wisdom about drugs. Instead, perceptions of drugs became trapped within a bewildering and often-brutal differential system of prohibition—a labyrinth constructed around a black-and-white mythology of psychoactive substances.

The idea that a drug has an essence that the user inevitably consumes along with the drug itself is part of a system of "pharmacologicalism." Technically speaking, pharmacologicalism, like racism, is an ideological system rooted in a set of assumptions that, although false and exaggerated, govern a whole range of perceptions, understandings, and actions. A key supposition of pharmacologicalism is that pharmacological potentialities contained within the drug's chemical structure determine drug outcomes in the body, the brain, and behavior. Accordingly, nonpharmacological factors play little role, whether in the realm of the mind or of the world of society and culture. In this highly reductionist system drugs have moral attributes that stem not from social and psychological forces but rather from the sphere of molecules.[64] As a result, pharmacologicalism dictates that the moral status of a drug exists as a purely scientific question that can be documented and classified once and for all, not as a societal one that must be considered and reconsidered across time and place. Society, culture, and history can be ignored.

Drugs and the plants from which they derive have long been viewed as having special properties. In the twentieth century, this drug mythology did not disappear. Rather, it was transplanted from the realms of religion and mysticism to the kingdom of science. Preserving the myth of drugs as unique causes of experience required no insurmountable feat; it needed only to be modernized, with the magical essence being replaced by a molecular essence. Pharmacologicalism thus provided a scientific foundation for the moral orderings of drugs, which then allowed for a disparate, compartmentalized treatment of them as angels (Ritalin) or demons (cocaine). Pharmacologicalism only makes sense, though, when one refuses what the WHO/UNICRI cocaine study revealed: drug use and drug outcomes are ultimately artifacts of culture, not of the inherent pharmacological properties of drugs. Without a system of constructing the social meaning of drugs, Ritalin and cocaine could not be defined as two radically different drugs while sharing nearly identical pharmacological actions in the body when taken in comparable doses and circumstances.

Modern pharmacologicalism and the differential prohibition of drugs that it sanctions have not operated flawlessly. Some drugs of disrepute have turned out to possess properties too useful to be demonized, as was the case for opiate analgesics like morphine. Although synthetic opiates (opioids), such as Demerol, have been synthesized since the 1950s, morphine and codeine remained within the sanctioned pharmacopoeia throughout the twentieth century. At the same time, a number of pharmacological angels fell from grace in the twentieth century, a fact of history that according to the orthodoxy of pharmacologicalism should never occur. The list includes alcohol (during Prohibition), cocaine, heroin, marijuana, the amphetamines, barbiturates (Seconal), the benzodiazepines (Valium), and even the SSRI antidepressants (Paxil).

Of course, the United States did not invent the black-and-white ideology of drugs, just as it did not invent pharmacologicalism. Coca was proclaimed an angel by the Incan State in what is now Peru in the fifteenth century, as well as by South American tribes, including the Aymara and the Quechua. Indeed, many "primitive" cultures around the world have elevated psychoactive plant substances to a divine status.[65] Much the same applies to the demonization of drugs, one of the earliest modern instances of this originating not from the United States but from an American-educated brain researcher from Peru, Carlos Gutiérrez-Noriega. Conducting human and animal studies on cocaine in the 1940s, Gutiérrez-Noriega established an entire pseudoscience of cocaine dedicated to tearing down the positive image of coca that prevailed throughout Andean history and society.[66] In making his essentially political assessment of coca—that the Andean Indian population consisted primarily of coca addicts—Gutiérrez-Noriega relied almost exclusively on observations of Indian prisoners, since he had no firsthand knowledge of Indian culture and people. It was later revealed that he often had to ignore his own findings in order to uphold the position supported by the Peruvian government, that coca was an inherently harmful substance.[67]

What made the American angels-and-demons ideology unique, then, was not the idea of a drug having an inherent essence, but the successful effort to modernize the system by taking it out of the realm of magic and spirit and situating it within the sciences of pharmacology, thus giving political entities leverage over public understandings of drugs. For while the modern science of drugs was largely a pseudoscience, it presented drugs to the public as a technical and intimidating subject matter, open to question only by those who had the proper credentials. This was a significant achievement, especially given the fact that the modern cult of pharmacology emerged alongside a diverse array of empirical findings that flatly contradicted it. Most of these findings were ignored simply because they made no sense in light of the public attitude: some drugs were obviously good while others were clearly evil.

Between the years 1969 and 1984, a group of studies appeared to confirm cocaine's status as a demon drug.[68] These laboratory studies employed animals to test the abuse potential of cocaine and other misused drugs. Animals self-administer many or most of the psychoactive substances taken voluntarily by people, and these studies showed that monkeys and rats not only responded voluntarily to produce intravenous injections of cocaine but often administered the drugs to the point of death or near death.[69] On the surface, these studies seemed to support the U.S. government's attitude toward cocaine, like the Peruvian stance before it, as an inherently destructive drug.[70] And, not surprisingly, these studies were quickly seized on indisputable scientific evidence of the dangers of cocaine.

> Cocaine's power of reinforcement produces its most notorious effects: the desire to keep taking it as long as the drug is available. In one series of experiments . . . scientists let caged monkeys self administer . . . cocaine until they died. . . . The drug made them monomaniacal. (*Rolling Stone*, 1989)[71]

> Cocaine addicts tend to go on binges, and monkeys hooked up intravenously will inject themselves repeatedly, rejecting food, sex and sleep until they die. (*New York Times*, 1992)[72]

> Cocaine, says Michael Kuhar of the government's Addiction Research Center in Baltimore, "is the most powerful reinforcer known." That's animal researcher talk for the fact that a variety of species from mice to monkeys will learn to self-administer cocaine faster than any other drug and will do it until they die. (*Science*, 1989)[73]

While the early animal studies investigating cocaine do not lie, those who have used them to demonize cocaine have not told the whole truth. When the literature on animal drug taking is considered as a whole, the study results take on a nearly opposite meaning. These early studies were surprising not for the toxic results they inflicted on the animals but for the extreme conditions that were created to encourage animals to administer cocaine and other drugs. Not only were they provided in unlimited intravenous quantities, but the environment was stripped of all that was meaningful to the animals, including the presence of social companions and other healthy activities. High levels of drug usage followed, which was hardly surprising given the stimulant nature of the drugs.

Later studies showed that enriching the environment prior to making a drug available not only decreased drug consumption but actually reduced the number of animals that acquired the habit of drug taking in the first place.[74] In a series of studies that took place in "Rat Park," opiate usage significantly decreased when the context was changed from isolated to social.[75] Another series of studies found that whether intravenous cocaine was preferred by the monkeys depended on the number of sweet treats that were available as an alternative.[76] Still other studies showed the powerful effects of even modest changes to the experimental setting; making the drug available every other hour, rather than continuously, for example, changed cocaine usage from highly compulsive and toxic to highly regulated and benign.[77] Furthermore, despite the rhetoric that cocaine "is the most powerful reinforcer known," the same toxic effects that occurred in the original studies also occurred for stimulants other than cocaine. One study reported, for instance, that while two monkeys died from cocaine self-administration, six monkeys died after being provided with unlimited access to d-amphetamine or d-methamphetamine, the latter two being synthetic drugs later prescribed to children.[78]

Thus, rather than proving that cocaine is inherently addictive and destructive, initial animal studies examining cocaine self-administration revealed that drug usage is actually sensitive to the context in which it occurs; environments that are stripped of all meaningful activities promote drug seeking and elevate the significance of the drug experience to the point of obsession. Thus, even in laboratory animals, what goes on in the name of drugs appears to involve much more than just the pharmacological actions of the drug.

Unfortunately, this conclusion also had no place in America's evolving culture of differential prohibition. As with the WHO/UNICRI study, accepting this finding meant acknowledging that a drug's virtues were uncertain and changing and that various elements of society and culture may ultimately be responsible for society's drugs problems. Such a perspective makes irrelevant a rigid black-and-white system of drug policy — the differential prohibition of drugs — which must give way to a system that focuses not on drugs per se but on the contexts of drug use that transform pharmacological substances into "drugs" in the first place. Some European countries adopted this approach in the 1980s and 1990s, often to positive effect.[79] But that was not the American way; instead, differential prohibition reigned supreme across the nation, ordained within a cult of pharmacology.

As with Ritalin, many of the psychoactive drugs prescribed as "medicines" during the latter half of the twentieth century turned out to have pharmacological actions, or at least liabilities for misuse, that were comparable to the "drugs" that were being demonized as a societal menace. But there was one real difference: the later "medicines" were not organic substances that originated from outside the country — as were cocaine, heroin, and marijuana — but artificial commodities, synthesized within an esteemed pharmaceutical industry.

The distinction made between opiates and the barbiturates is an example of the differential prohibition of "drugs" and "medicines," and it is at least as dramatic as that made between Ritalin and cocaine. As depressants, the barbiturates were also addictive for those most possessed by their mood- and mind-altering effects. As a result, they quickly acquired much the same status in domestic American life as had the opiates late in the nineteenth century. Indeed, by 1972 the U.S. Bureau of Narcotic and Dangerous Drugs had proposed that greater restrictions be placed on the barbiturates, concluding that they "are more dangerous than heroin."[80]

Another example is of the prescribing of fentanyl, a synthetic form of heroin sold on the street as "China White," which was approved by the Food and Drug Administration in 1994 as a prescription drug for children.[81] Heroin could not be given to adults, even in a medical setting, yet a synthetic, patented, and medicalized version of it could be given to children in the form of a lollipop.

Perhaps the most striking example of differential prohibition, though, was methamphetamine, a drug that acquired a double life as both an angel and demon in the twentieth century. While street "meth" was considered "a potent, highly addictive form of amphetamine," the same drug, when prescribed in pill form, was considered a useful medicine for reducing hyperactivity in children (sold under the brand names Desoxyn, Desoxyn Gradumet, and Methedrine).[82] While serving as drug czar, Barry McCaffrey called methamphetamine "the worst drug that has ever hit America," and the *New York Times* opined that it was "feeding an epidemic of addiction that . . . rivals that of heroin and cocaine over the past few decades."[83] Taken as a medication, "meth" was seen in a quite different light: "I've reviewed some other ADHD treatments here rather poorly (i.e. Ritalin and Adderall), but this is a true wonder-drug for the disorder," wrote one user about Desoxyn. "It has all the qualities you could possibly want in an ADHD med — it doesn't cause anxiety, it barely raises heart rate or blood pressure, it totally wipes out depression and fatigue, and it lasts a full twelve hours — not 3–6 hours like those 'other' drugs. My ADHD symptoms have been completely relieved by using this drug." Similarly, a physician notes about prescribed methamphetamine, "For many of my clients this medication has helped them to function at work, school, and in relationships, in ways they have never been able to before."[84]

Methamphetamine illustrates the multiple worlds, myths, and histories that the same psychoactive substance can inhabit. Used for different reasons, taken in different forms, and at different doses, the same drug can serve dramatically different ends — ends that in the era of differential prohibition could lead to radically different social and legal consequences.

Consider the case of Anne Mea Urrutia.

Thirty-six years old and a resident of Rubidoux, California, Ms. Urrutia was arrested in November 1999 after her son was found walking the streets of Riverside County. A deputy sheriff stopped the nine year old, suspecting him of being truant, and found him to be carrying a crack pipe. When the authorities brought him home, they found the house was beyond squalid: the water and electricity had been shut off, and the cupboards were barer than Old Mother Hubbard's. What they also discovered, as Ms. Urrutia later admitted, was that she had been smoking methamphetamine with her son. This had been taking place since he was seven.[85] The local media's response to the Urrutia case was one of abject horror. One report started with the headline, "Boy's Meth Abuse May Haunt His Life," going on to state that the drug is "an addictive stimulant [that] can irreparably fray the brain's wiring. The drug also can permanently prune the nerve cells endings that act as signalling antennae for the brain's chemical messengers, according to the National Institute on Drug Abuse, a federal research agency." The article also noted, "Children who have been exposed to methamphetamine often have difficulty concentrating, sleeping or even eating, said Sharon Dillon, regional manager for Riverside County's Child Protective Services."[86]

Certainly, even under ideal living conditions, "spinning-out" on crystal meth with one's mother is not going to do anything positive for a child or for his or her developing nervous system. Still, no amount of pharmacologicalism can resolve the contradiction of meth as a demon drug and methamphetamine as a prescription angel. Another media report covering the Urrutia case quoted a child-welfare manager who stated that his department "investigates a handful of cases every year involving parents providing drugs to their children."[87] This is quite a narrow use of the word *drug*, since thousands of parents at the time were providing the same drug (or the drug Ritalin) to their children under the guise of medical treatment.

The only real pharmacological difference here is the way in which the drugs were being used: kids receiving their daily doses of pharmacological stimulation in the 1990s did not usually snort, shoot, or smoke it—they swallowed it. As with Ritalin, this route has the effect of slowing down the drug's absorption into the brain, greatly diminishing any possible stimulant rush. As important as this difference may be, it has nothing to do with the inherent pharmacological properties of the drug. The quest for a drug rush from a substance like methamphetamine is as historically specific as the popular prescribing of Ritalin (or the chewing of coca by Colombians), and a molecular science of pharmacology offers little in the way of an explanation for either.

Chapter Two **Cult of the SSRI**

God is dead.
  —Friedrich Nietzsche, *The Gay Science*

Prozac can help.
  —Eli Lilly advertisement

William Forsyth met and married his wife, June, in 1955. After two years of military service in West Germany, Bill and his wife headed to Los Angeles, where he had grown up. Soon after arriving, he bought several Volkswagens and started a rental-car business near the L.A. airport. Times were tough at first, but the business eventually caught on. Bill and June had two kids, Susan and Bill Jr., and their business and other property investments continued to grow. In 1986 they cashed in. Four years later, after more than thirty years in California, Bill and June retired to Maui, where Bill Jr. lived. Bill Forsyth was sixty-one at the time; June was fifty-four.

As is often the case with retirees who leave their home for the romance of a new life, the transition was difficult for Bill Forsyth. The Hawaii move did not suit him well, although his wife was content, even thriving. Personal difficulties led to marital difficulties, but marriage counseling seemed to help, and there was a general consensus in the family that Bill was working through his difficulties. Three years after the move to Maui, with Bill still feeling unsettled, a local psychiatrist prescribed Prozac. Despite diagnosing Bill with depression, the psychiatrist, who had been seeing Bill since the previous year, did not believe him to be seriously depressed or suicidal. Indeed, Bill Forsyth had never spoken of nor attempted suicide; nor did he have any history of violence, domestic or otherwise.

After his first day on Prozac, Bill felt as one might expect after having read Peter Kramer's *Listening to Prozac*: he was "better than well." The second day, however, he felt horrible and for the first time put himself under hospital care. After ten days, Bill felt well enough to leave the hospital. He was still taking Prozac. Everyone seemed to agree that he was doing better, and the family scheduled a boat trip for the next day. When his parents failed to show up the following afternoon, Bill Jr. went to their home, where he found his parents lying dead in a pool of blood. After taking Prozac for eleven days, Bill Forsyth had taken a serrated kitchen knife and stabbed his wife fifteen times. Then he had taken the knife, fixed it to a chair, and impaled himself on it.

Depressed people sometimes do desperate things. Yet these were senseless acts that, at least for those who knew Bill Forsyth, were simply unimaginable. For his two grown children the only possible explanation was the drug. And so Bill Jr. and Susan decided to sue its manufacturer. Their lawyers later argued that Prozac can produce a kind of psychological hijacking — a bizarre and nightmarish syndrome, more common with serotonin-related antidepressants, marked by suicidal thoughts, extreme agitation, emotional blunting, and a craving for death. They also argued that the company knew of these risks and, instead of warning doctors to look out for them, had worked vigilantly to sweep them under the rug.

The Forsyth case was not the first wrongful death suit to be brought against Eli Lilly, nor was it the first to make it to trial. The first, known as the Fentress case, concerned the events of an early September morning in 1989 when Joseph Wesbecker, armed with an AK-47 and some handguns, walked into the Louisville printing plant where he had been employed and began shooting. "I'm sorry, Dickie," he told a fellow worker before shooting him five times. When it was over, Wesbecker had shot twenty people, killing eight, and shot and killed himself. Wesbecker had been put on Prozac one month before the shooting. Whether Prozac made him do it one will never know. Certainly, though, it did not make him "better than well."

The Fentress case, named after Joyce Fentress, a widow who was one of several plaintiffs who sued after the Wesbecker rampage, was the first of 160 cases pending against Prozac in the fall of 1994. By that time Prozac already represented about a third of all Eli Lilly's annual income, or some $2 billion. Suits had been filed by families of people who had committed suicide while on Prozac, families of those who had been murdered by persons on the drug, and individuals who had themselves been harmed while taking Prozac, including a woman who worked for Eli Lilly as a sales rep. Many of these cases were dismissed. Others were settled, some for large sums. But Eli Lilly would not settle the Fentress case. Wesbecker was a nut, they believed, and his case would send the right message: don't take Eli Lilly and Prozac to court because you will lose.

And they had a point. At least a year before starting on Prozac, Wesbecker had begun buying guns and ammunition and making threats. He also had a history of psychological problems, which had led him to be placed on several psychiatric drugs before being put on Prozac. Other aspects of the case, however, were curious, if not compelling. After having been on Prozac for a month, Wesbecker returned to his psychiatrist, who found him a changed man. He was agitated, his mood was erratic, and his behavior was even stranger than usual. The psychiatrist tried to persuade Wesbecker to go off the drug, which he felt was responsible for the agitation, and to return to the hospital for further evaluation. Wesbecker went to work instead.

After Wesbecker's rampage and the lawsuit that followed, Eli Lilly also went to work, building a case against Wesbecker that included approximately 400 depositions taken from people who knew him. Lilly's attorneys were determined to show that Wesbecker's madness was the product of a poor childhood environment and abnormal psychological development. In other words, the very company that relies on marketing copy to sell the idea that depression is an internal problem of biochemistry was turning away from its biochemical theories, blaming the external environment instead. Helped somewhat by their expert witness, antipsychiatry hell-raiser Peter Breggin, the plaintiffs' lawyers pointed out the contradiction: if Lilly's drug worked by chemically altering mood and behavior, why might it not also be possible that their drug caused the disastrous mood and behavior changes noted by Wesbecker's psychiatrist just prior to the rampage?

The plaintiffs' lawyers also wanted the jury to know that Lilly had a history of concealing bad news about its drugs, a history that suggested a pattern of placing company profits ahead of public safety. In 1985 Lilly and a chief medical officer had pleaded guilty to twenty-five criminal counts of failing to report adverse reactions for its anti-inflammatory drug Oraflex, including four deaths, to the FDA (eventually, the FDA linked the drug to several dozen deaths in the United States and several hundred deaths abroad). The judge in the Fentress case, John Potter, refused the plaintiffs' request; the material was unfairly prejudicial, he ruled, and would not be allowed in. But Lilly's lawyers blundered by repeatedly introducing testimony that suggested that the company had always taken the reporting of adverse drug effects seriously, which opened the door to rebuttal, the plaintiffs' lawyers argued, and Judge Potter finally agreed.

The jury never heard the evidence. During the recess that followed Potter's reversal, Lilly's lawyers met with plaintiffs' lawyers and made a secret deal. The plaintiffs would allow the case to go forward without presenting the damaging Oraflex evidence, and Lilly would in turn pay to the plaintiffs in the case what was later described as a sum that "boggles the mind." And this is just what happened. The evidence was not presented, the jury returned a verdict in favor of Lilly, Judge Potter dismissed the case, and Lilly and its lawyers claimed total victory. "We are pleased—although not surprised—by the decision," Randall L. Tobias, Lilly's then chairman and CEO, told the *New York Times*. "We have proven in a court of law, just as we have to more than 70 scientific and regulatory bodies all over the world, that Prozac is safe and effective. Our hearts go out to the victims of the terrible tragedy. . . . But the members of the jury . . . came to the only logical conclusion—that Prozac had nothing to do with Joseph Wesbecker's actions."[1]

Still, Judge Potter came to suspect something was amiss. While the jury was deliberating the case, a juror had come forward to say that she had overheard settlement negotiations going on in the hallway. Some months later, during the course of a divorce hearing involving one of the plaintiffs in the case, it was revealed that he was expecting a substantial payment from Eli Lilly. Judge Potter drew his own conclusion and in April 1995 filed a motion to amend his post-trial order, declaring that the case had not been won by Eli Lilly but settled. Lawyers on both sides filed their objections with Kentucky's appeals court. Two months later, the appeals court ruled against Potter, arguing that he no longer had jurisdiction over the case. The case was then appealed to the Kentucky Supreme Court. This raised the stakes too high, and lawyers from both sides finally capitulated and acknowledged that they had conspired to settle without settling. On 23 May 1996, the Kentucky Supreme Court decided unanimously in favor of Judge Potter. Eli Lilly had settled the case, not won it.

The Fentress case revealed much about the back-alley tactics of Eli Lilly. "The history of Prozac litigation reads like a mystery thriller," wrote Michael Grinfeld in *California Lawyer*, "filled with allegations of backroom deals, hidden agendas, and unethical behavior."[2] The trial did not, however, answer the central questions of the case: would Wesbecker have committed his rampage had he never been put on the synthetic substance? Might the rampage been avoided altogether had the drug company warned doctors like Wesbecker's to be on the lookout for signs of drug-induced agitation that can precipitate violence? The case against the Prozac family of antidepressants, known as the SSRIs, was not coming to an end. It was only just beginning.

In March 1999 the Eli Lilly case involving the William Forsyth deaths finally made it to trial, in U.S. District Court in Honolulu. "I know that with all their power and money I don't have much of a chance," said the daughter, Susan Forsyth, "but I feel like I have to try."[3] There was some hope, however, as Prozac's manufacturer was facing a different legal team than it had in the Fentress case, as well as a new expert witness: David Healy.

Healy is an internationally renowned psychiatrist as well as a historian of psychiatric medicine. Author of several books, including *The Antidepressant Era* and *The Creation of Psychopharmacology*, both published by Harvard University Press, Healy has the American equivalent of both an M.D. and a Ph.D. Prior to his involvement in any litigation involving the pharmaceutical industry, Healy had already raised a number of questions about Prozac and other selective serotonin reuptake inhibitors, asking, among other things, whether they were best classified as antidepressants or as anti-anxiety drugs, and whether they produced agitation and other problems with unusual frequency. Most important, Healy wasn't a radical, nor was he an outsider of the pharmaceutical or psychiatric establishment. Healy had a record of conducting research and consulting for various drug companies, and he was not opposed to prescribing Prozac or other psychiatric drugs. Drug companies, unlike tobacco companies, do not place an importance on keeping executives and scientists in the fold, and many CEOs come from outside the industry. As a result, there is a high rate of turnover and a continual loss of institutional knowledge in the industry. Thus, with pretrial discovery laws forcing Lilly — and later Pfizer and SmithKline — to allow Healy into their archives, he would be as close to an industry insider as the public was going to get. And he had plenty to say.

Pointing to Lilly's own internal documents, Healy showed that the company was well aware that Prozac would, in a small minority of cases, produce a psychological state like the one that overwhelmed William Forsyth, a key ingredient of which is a bizarre form of inner torture known as akathisia, a sensation of inner restlessness that in its most intense form can lead to an indescribable sense of terror and doom, even to suicidal behavior. Moreover, Healy argued that the company not only knew of this potentially catastrophic reaction prior to seeking FDA approval but that they had gone to great lengths to conceal it. In 1978, ten years before fluoxetine was branded as Prozac and brought to market in the United States, clinical trials began. Minutes from meetings of Lilly's Prozac project team in July and August of that year noted, "Some patients have converted from severe depression to agitation within a few days; in one case the agitation was marked and the patient had to be taken off [the] drug. . . . There have been a fairly large number of reports of adverse reactions. . . . Another depressed patient developed psychosis. . . . Akathisia and restlessness were reported in some patients. . . . In future studies the use of benzodiazepines to control the agitation will be permitted."[4]

This use of benzodiazepines — anti-anxiety drugs like Librium, Valium, and Xanax — greased the rails for Prozac's approval. The FDA relied only on a handful of studies submitted by Lilly, which the FDA has since described as "adequate and well-controlled trials which provided evidence of [Prozac's] efficacy."[5] Most of these studies permitted the simultaneous use of benzodiazepines and similar drugs, and about a quarter of the patients took them. As psychopharmacologists have since established, benzodiazepines are effective in reducing the Prozac-induced agitation that can lead to violence.[6] If Prozac could cause self-mutilation, suicide, or even murder in some users, these studies would never have revealed it.

But other studies did. Lilly's own internal records show a letter it received from the British Committee on Safety of Medicines, the British equivalent of the FDA, in May 1984, expressing concerns over clinical trial data they had seen: "During the treatment with the preparation [Prozac] 16 suicide attempts were made, two of these with success. As patients with a risk of suicide were excluded from the studies, it is probable that this high proportion can be attributed to an action of the preparation." Similar concern was expressed by the Bundes Gesundheit Amt, the German equivalent of the FDA, in 1985. By this time Lilly was well aware that they had a problem, summed up nicely by the FDA scientist Martin Brecher, who, after noticing Lilly's effort to obscure the problem, wrote to Lilly saying, "I am skeptical whether dichotomizing on the basis of the presence or absence of poisoning with an antidepressant will provide any insight. . . . Most of the fluoxetine

[Prozac] suicides have not been by overdose, but rather by gunshot, jumping, hanging or drowning."[7]

By 1986, clinical-trial studies comparing Prozac with other antidepressants showed a rate of 12.5 suicides per 1,000 participants on Prozac compared to only 3.8 per 1,000 on older, non-SSRI antidepressants and 2.5 per 1,000 on placebo.[8] An internal Lilly document dated 29 March 1985 also quantified the problem: "The incidence rate [of suicide] under fluoxetine therefore purely mathematically is 5.6 times higher than under the other active medication imipramine [a non-SSRI antidepressant]. . . . The benefits vs. risks considerations for fluoxetine currently does not fall clearly in favor of the benefits. Therefore, it is of the greatest importance that it be determined whether there is a particular subgroup of patients who respond better to fluoxetine than to imipramine, so that the higher incidence of suicide attempts may be tolerable."[9]

After Prozac's entry into the market in 1988, reports quickly surfaced, confirming that the beast Lilly had seen in the laboratory had, without warning, been unleashed on the public. In 1990, three years before Bill Forsyth killed his wife and himself, a report appeared in the *American Journal of Psychiatry* entitled "Emergence of Intense Suicidal Preoccupation During Fluoxetine Treatment." Two Harvard psychiatrists, Martin Teicher and Jonathan Cole, and a registered nurse, Carol Gold, described cases in which patients developed serious preoccupations with suicide soon after being given Prozac.[10]

> We were especially surprised to witness the emergence of intense, obsessive, and violent suicidal thoughts in these patients. . . . No patient was actively suicidal at the time fluoxetine treatment began. Rather, all were hopeful and optimistic. . . . Their suicidal thoughts appear to have been obsessive, as they were recurrent, persistent, and intrusive. . . . It was also remarkable how violent these thoughts were. Two patients fantasized, for the first time, about killing themselves with a gun (cases 4 and 5), and one patient (case 6) actually placed a loaded gun to her head. One patient (case 3) needed to be physically restrained to prevent self-mutilation. Patient 2, who had no prior suicidal thoughts, fantasized about killing himself in a gas explosion or a car crash.[11]

This report prompted responses from clinicians describing similar cases. That Teicher and colleagues might be on to something held considerable weight, as these were not the findings of amateurs. Jonathan Cole, the coauthor of the study, had a career that dated back to the 1950s; he has been described by Pfizer, the maker of the SSRI Zoloft, as a "pioneer" in the field of psychopharmacology. Referring to Teicher's and Cole's report during the Forsyth trial, David Healy told the court, "[Cole] is a man who has seen suicidal ideation and yet he and his colleagues were saying that what they witnessed in this instance was something different. These are not investigators who would have easily been deceived by the ordinary kind of suicidal ideation that occurs in depression."[12]

In July 1992 another article appeared, this time in the more prestigious *Archives of General Psychiatry*. Like the Harvard report, this article had two senior researchers among its authors, William Wirshing and Theodore Van Putten, the latter of whom was a leading expert on akathisia. They emphasized in the report that, prior to going on Prozac, none of their patients "had a history of significant suicidal behavior; all described their distress [while on Prozac] as an intense and novel somatic-emotional state; all reported an urge to pace that paralleled the intensity of the distress; all experienced suicidal thoughts at the peak of their restless agitation; and all experienced a remission of their agitation, restlessness, pacing urge, and suicidality after the fluoxetine [Prozac] was discontinued."[13]

The finding that these problems would emerge soon after a selective-serotonin drug was taken and disappear soon after the drug was withdrawn provided compelling evidence, David Healy came to believe, that the problem was often the drug and not the "disease" for which it was taken. Anthony Rothschild and Carol Locke, also of Harvard Medical School, reported three such cases in the *Journal of Clinical Psychiatry* in December 1991. All three patients, the authors noted, were reexposed to Prozac after having made a suicide attempt during earlier fluoxetine treatment.[14]

The first case involved a twenty-five-year-old woman with a three-year history of depression. Two weeks after starting Prozac, and three days after having her dose increased from 20 to 40 mg, she escaped from the hospital and jumped off the roof of a building. She hit a landing, fracturing both arms and legs. With the patient now in a wheelchair, the psychiatrists tried Prozac on her a second time. Eleven days later she noted that she was having the same adverse effects as when she had previously been given Prozac, stating "I tried to kill myself because of these anxiety symptoms. It was not so much the depression." All adverse reactions disappeared within three days after the drug was terminated a second time.

The second case involved a forty-seven-year-old man with an eight-year history of depression. Within two weeks of starting Prozac, he began to experience severe restlessness and anxiety, from which he said death would be a welcome relief. He jumped from a cliff, but his fall was broken by a tree. Put in psychiatric care, he was put on Prozac a second time. And when his dose was increased from 20 to 40 mg, the adverse reaction returned, prompting him to comment, "This is exactly what happened the last time I was on fluoxetine, and I feel like jumping off a cliff again." All adverse reactions disappeared twenty-four hours after he was put on an additional drug.

The third patient was a thirty-four-year-old woman with a fourteen-year history of depression. About a week after her Prozac dosage was increased from 40 to 60 mg, she jumped off the roof of a tall building, landed on a balcony, and fractured her femur. Back in psychiatric care, she was put on Prozac again and, after having her dose increased from 20 to 40 mg, she stated that the restlessness produced by the drug was making her feel "crazy" and that she was feeling just like she had before her last suicide attempt.

Reflecting on these cases, Rothschild and Locke stated, "Patients need to be reassured that the overwhelming symptoms being experienced are the side effects of medication and are treatable. . . . Our patients had concluded their illness had taken such a dramatic turn for the worse that life was no longer worth living." Not only had Prozac suicides and homicides become a hidden reality, the agitation and violent thoughts that preceded them were being misinterpreted as a sign of the very problems the drug was said to treat. Lilly had learned to exploit this tragic irony with earlier drugs, always repeating the claim that it was not the drug but the disease. "Prozac tends to be used by people with psychiatric problems," commented a Lilly executive. "Some people with psychiatric problems happen to be violent."[15]

Doing what Lilly and the other manufacturers of SSRI antidepressants have failed to do all along—that is, warn physicians to watch for agitation and increased suicidality soon after starting patients on an SSRI (or upping its dose)—is crucial, as physicians are not otherwise likely to monitor them during the first weeks of drug use, Joseph Wesbecker being a case in point. Paradoxically, this was in part why Lilly worked so stubbornly to avoid having to issue a warning in the United States and United Kingdom, fearing that the extra burden would reduce physicians' willingness to prescribe the drug. After all, a major factor in Prozac's immediate success was that it needed to be taken only one time daily, "the safe and effective new medication, easy for both prescriber and patient."[16] Instead of issuing a proper warning, and instead of simply remaining quiet on the subject, Lilly actually fought in the other direction, declaring that Prozac's side effects were in fact proof of the existence of the disease the drug was used to treat.

A case described in Teicher's and Cole's report illustrates the results of Lilly's efforts. A nineteen-year-old college student had developed "disturbing and self-destructive thoughts" two weeks after starting Prozac. When the dose was increased from 20 to 40 mg, her problems became worse, and then worse again after the dose was increased from 40 to 60 mg. Still convinced that it was "not the drug but the disease," the doctors increased the young woman's dose yet another time, from 60 to 80 mg, at which point she began violently banging her head and mutilating herself.

Growing reports suggesting that Prozac might be unsafe at any dosage had Lilly running scared. One executive stated in an internal memo in 1990 that if Prozac were taken off the market, the company could "go down the tubes."[17] Responding to concerns expressed by the FDA, Lilly agreed to conduct a study examining the question of whether Prozac induced aggression and suicidal thoughts. The result, known as the Beasley study, appeared in the 21 September 1991 issue of the *British Medical Journal*.[18]

The study, which was authored by Lilly employees and included psychiatrist Charles Beasley, looked and sounded like good science. On the surface, it represented the data pooled to date comparing Prozac with either older non-SSRI antidepressants or placebo. In fact, the data had been handpicked to favor the company.[19] The analysis dealt with only 3,065 patients, less than 12 percent of the total data available from clinical-trial studies at the time. Among those left out was the very population most likely to become suicidal — the roughly 5 percent of patients who dropped out of the clinical trials because they experienced unpleasant side effects after taking Prozac. The report also made no mention of the dozen or so suicides that had already occurred in Prozac's clinical trials, a number that, given the population being studied — primary-care outpatients rather than severe depressives — would be expected to be near zero.

The Beasley study was submitted first to the *New England Journal of Medicine*, where it was rejected. Publication in the *British Medical Journal* was not as high profile, but it would have to do. And it did. In September

1991, after seeing the report and after receiving continued assurances from Lilly that Prozac did not lead to extreme acts of violence, the FDA's Psychopharmacological Drugs Advisory Committee gave the drug a new lease on life. To a great sigh of relief at Lilly, the committee's report stated that there was "no credible evidence of a causal link between the use of antidepressant drugs, including Prozac, and suicidality or violent behavior." From that moment on, instead of having to defend the safety of its antidepressant, Lilly could simply stand behind the "independent" conclusions of the FDA: "Our experience with Prozac does not show a cause-and-effect relationship between it and suicidal thoughts or acts. Our safety track record has been well established," noted the Eli Lilly spokesperson Edward West. Prozac was saved.

Not until the Fentress and Forsyth trials did Lilly's internal documents surface, revealing the depth of the deception. These documents included the statements from the Prozac working group in 1978, acknowledging problems with akathisia and drug-induced psychosis. Also among the documents was evidence that the company had gone so far as to draft wording for a Prozac package insert that stated, "Mania and psychosis may be precipitated in susceptible patients by antidepressant therapy."[20] While this warning never made it into the final package insert, a similar warning was required before Lilly was allowed to sell Prozac in Germany, where it was renamed Fluctin. In Lilly's documents there was also a memo dated 2 October 1990, which referenced an upcoming Prozac symposium in which the issue of suicidality was to be discussed. One Lilly employee queried another: "Then the question is what to do with the 'big' numbers on suicidality. If the report numbers are shown next to those for nausea, they seem small."[21]

There was also a series of Lilly memos concerning two Taiwanese doctors who had completed a study entitled "Suicidal Attempts and Fluoxetine (Prozac) Treatment"; one memo, dated 8 April 1992, reported, "Mission accomplished. Professor Lu will not present or publish his fluoxetine vs. maprotiline suicidality data."[22] A similar case involved Robert Bourguignon, a Belgian doctor who was sued by Lilly after soliciting his colleagues' experiences regarding suicidality and other side effects concerning Prozac. A cease-and-desist order was issued, but Bourguignon eventually prevailed, and the result of his survey, "Dangers of Fluoxetine," appeared in the *Lancet* in 1997. In it Bourguignon cites eleven serious events, including severe nervousness, suicidal thoughts, and "paranoid psychosis."[23] Lilly had also canceled a clinical trial being conducted at a hospital in Indianapolis, Lilly's hometown. While researchers doing trials for Lilly often obscured problems with akathisia by coding it as simple nervousness or anxiety, the chief researcher in the trial, Joyce Small, was actually coding akathisia as akathisia. Furthermore, she was finding the problem in almost one out of ten patients taking Prozac.[24]

Still another finding revealed that, although rates of suicide were four times higher for men than women throughout the second half of the twentieth century, men and women taking SSRI antidepressants had the same suicide rates. Whether Prozac and other SSRIs produced agitation and suicidal obsessions more often in women was not clear, since women were more than twice as likely to be taking SSRIs at any given time. What was clear was that women taking SSRIs not only did not lower their suicide risk, but in fact increased it to the same degree of risk as men.[25]

In the face of all the case reports and epidemiological statistics, and in the face of more than 200 lawsuits claiming a link between Prozac and violence, Lilly continued throughout the 1990s to promote the view that their drug actually lowered suicide risk. "The over 10,000 patients who have been on clinical trials where people have looked at suicidality, suicidal ideation," commented a vice president of clinical investigations at Lilly on the ABC news program *20–20*, "have shown without a doubt that these drugs do not increase suicidal ideation or suicide potential. In fact, they do just the opposite: They reduce it."[26] Prior to the introduction of SSRIs, the suicide rate for those using antidepressants on an outpatient basis was about 30 suicides per 100,000 years of patient use, roughly the same suicide rate as the general population.[27] A 1995 study published in the *British Medical Journal* looked at ten antidepressants used by a total of 170,000 people in the United Kingdom and showed that the suicide rate among Prozac users was 189 suicides per 100,000 years of use. In contrast to the claims of Lilly executives, this suggests a sixfold increase in suicide risk for Prozac relative to non-SSRI antidepressants, a number that is close to Lilly's own internal assessment from 1985, which acknowledged a risk "5.6 times higher than under the other active medication imipramine."[28]

There was, meanwhile, a way to test directly the industry's theory that it was not the drug but the disease, which was to give the drugs to people who had no history of depression or violence. Evidence of just this kind came ultimately from David Healy himself.[29]

Back at his medical practice in North Wales, Healy conducted what is called a healthy-volunteer study. Twenty volunteers were recruited, half of whom were given the SSRI Zoloft for two weeks, the other half of whom were given the non-SSRI antidepressant Edronax for two weeks. Afterward, following a two-week "washout" period, each group was given the other drug for an additional two weeks.[30] Both drugs were administered under double-blind conditions, such that neither patients nor staff knew in what order each individual received the drugs. Healy had designed the study simply to compare the clinical effects of each drug, but two healthy volunteers quickly became dangerously agitated and suicidal—both were taking the SSRI Zoloft. Healy was surprised, but he would not stay surprised. Months later he discovered an unpublished study Pfizer had conducted in the 1980s in which healthy female volunteers were given either Zoloft or a placebo. The study was cancelled after four days because all those receiving Zoloft were complaining of problems of agitation and apprehension. Although Healy's study was not as dire overall—in fact, some of the healthy volunteers rated the Zoloft experience positively—one of the participants, a thirty-year-old woman, began having nightmares about having her throat slit one week after starting Zoloft and within two weeks was suicidal. Obsessed with the idea that she should throw herself in front of a car, an idea that had struck other SSRI users as well, she felt "it was as if there was nothing out there apart from the car, which she was going to throw herself under. She didn't think of her partner or child."[31]

Given the study population, such adverse reactions could not easily be blamed on psychiatric instability, and an agitation rate of 10 percent indicated that such results were not so rare as to be at all negligible. Nevertheless, these were normal, healthy volunteers, and their experiences would not resolve the ambiguity that remained in psychiatric cases like William Forsyth's. Did the drug cause him to do it in the sense that the violence would not have occurred had he not been prescribed the drug? Did the drug simply precipitate the inevitable? Or did it have no bearing whatsoever on the events of 3 March 1993? This ambiguity perhaps explains in part why, despite David Healy's testimony and the surfacing of the Lilly papers in the Forsyth trial, the jury once again found in favor of Eli Lilly.

The challenges plaintiffs' lawyers face in cases like William Forsyth's are considerable. There may be overwhelming statistical and clinical evidence against a "medicine" and its manufacturer, but such evidence may not overcome the uncertainties specific to the case at hand. This ambiguity is especially strong in the case of psychiatric medications, since suicides and homicides occur unexpectedly even when no drugs are involved. A pair of dice that comes up with double sixes on half of all rolls is clearly biased, but how does one know, on any particular roll, whether two sixes might not have come up anyway?

Drugs, their users, and the context of use all come together to produce drug outcomes. Whether it is cocaine or Prozac, a drug can produce a diversity of effects, even in the same individual at different times or in different situations. Certainly the public imagination can absorb the idea of a drug causing its user to become agitated, violent, or suicidal; similar claims have successfully been made of marijuana, alcohol, stimulants, and opiates. But in the scheme of differential prohibition, Prozac was classified as an angel, and thus it was protected by the assumption that, since the chemistry and pharmacology of a drug constitute its essence, Prozac, like Ritalin, could not possibly be as bad as all that. Indeed, pharmacologicalism — the myth that pharmacological potentialities contained within the drug's chemical structure overwhelmingly determine drug outcomes — offers no explanation for how the same drug might coexist as both good and evil.

Still, not all cases involving the SSRIs were overwhelmed by ambiguity. The Australian David Hawkins was freed from prison in May 2001 after a supreme-court judge concluded that his actions, which included killing his wife, were wholly out of character. Two days after going on Zoloft, the seventy-four-year-old Hawkins had strangled his wife, then attempted but failed to kill himself by carbon-monoxide poisoning. "But for the Zoloft," said the judge, "which [Hawkins] took on the morning of August 1, 1999, it is overwhelmingly probable that Mrs. Hawkins would not have been killed on that morning."[32]

A month after Hawkins's release, a federal court in Cheyenne, Wyoming, found against the SSRI manufacturer SmithKline Beecham (now GlaxoSmithKline) in the case of Donald Schell. After complaining of anxiety, stress, and possible depression, the sixty-year-old Schell was diagnosed with mild depression and, like most SSRI users, was prescribed an SSRI by his family doctor. Two days after he was given promotional samples of Paxil — the same duration of SSRI use that preceded David Hawkins's murder of his wife — Schell committed the most violent act in recent Wyoming history.

The jury in the case concluded that the SSRI can cause some individuals to commit suicide and homicide and that it did just that in the case of Donald Schell, who, on 13 February 1998, shot to death his wife, his adult daughter, his infant granddaughter, and then himself.

The $6.4 million decision against SmithKline Beecham represented the first court case to be lost by any SSRI manufacturer. Known as the Tobin case — Tim Tobin was the husband of Donald Schell's deceased daughter — the trial lasted for only two weeks, with the jury reaching a unanimous verdict in three-and-a-half hours. During the trial, SmithKline Beecham faced an experienced legal team — with the same core members as in the Forsyth case, including the expert witness David Healy — and a different and apparently more effective legal strategy: in the Forsyth case the plaintiff's lawyers focused on the man, William Forsyth, but in the Tobin case they focused on the company. Also, as Healy revealed in the trial, there was much in SmithKline's records to warrant concern about the company's behavior and their drug. SmithKline had carefully researched Paxil and in the process had produced extensive evidence that the drug posed the same kind of dangers as Prozac, yet the company had done nothing to mitigate those dangers. Among SmithKline's internal files were thirty-four healthy-volunteer studies involving company employees. These studies showed that, though the participants had had no noted history of depression or anxiety, 25 percent of them experienced some degree of agitation after taking Paxil.[33] These studies were not conducted by psychiatrists, however, and those that had been were unaccountably missing from the company archive, although Healy did find a note that made reference to one of the latter; on it the investigating psychiatrist had written that he had never seen such a high incidence of problems in a healthy-volunteer study.[34]

Healy also discovered other problems, problems that spoke to the various other adverse reactions one can experience when taking an SSRI. In addition to agitation, akathisia, suicidal thoughts, and violence, the SSRIs also came to be known for the physical dependence they produced in many users.[35] As a class action complaint against the maker of Paxil summarized,

Currently, on one website alone there are thousands of electronic signatures of persons complaining to GlaxoSmithKline Corporation about withdrawal reactions they have suffered from Paxil. Given that the signatures provide the full name of each person, many of whom provided their e-mail addresses and lengthy commentary, this is a reliable example of the numerosity of the persons suffering from Paxil withdrawal. Over the past two years, approximately 500 Paxil withdrawal victims have individually contacted plaintiffs' attorneys. The pain and suffering experienced by each of these individuals is the direct result of GlaxoSmithKline Corporation's failure to warn users of Paxil's addictive nature, the drug's inducement of physical or psychologic dependency, and its infliction of dependency/withdrawal syndrome when the patient's Paxil dosage is reduced or terminated.[36]

This accounting is consistent with what David Healy found when researching the SmithKline archives. In one healthy-volunteer study conducted within the company, researchers reported that, on drug discontinuation, nearly 85 percent of the volunteers suffered agitation, bizarre dreams, insomnia, and other adverse effects. Healy noted that as many as half of the volunteers showed symptoms that suggested the onset of physical dependence on the drug. One of the volunteers, Lisa, wrote in an on-line chat session on antidepressants, "I was addicted to Effexor. Was horrified of the thought of going without it — and for good reason!! I don't think the physical/mental dichotomy makes sense. If you can't get by without the stuff, you're addicted. Effexor IS addictive, I'm off the stuff, but I've never been so physically sick in my life as when I was in withdrawal."[37]

Sexual side effects also pose a substantial problem with the SSRI antidepressants, with perhaps as many as 70 to 80 percent of users experiencing lowered sex drive and impotence.[38] Beyond this are a variety of more minor side effects, including nausea, insomnia, nightmares, fatigue, drowsiness, weakness, loss of appetite, tremors, dry mouth, sweating, and even yawning. The one advantage that SSRIs have over the older, tricyclic antidepressants is that it is more difficult to overdose on the SSRIs. Of course this hardly matters when the drug itself precipitates suicide and other forms of violence in an unprecedented manner, as the following cases show.

Fifteen days after starting Prozac, the fifty-six-year-old singer known as Del Shannon died after he shot himself in the head with a .22 caliber rifle.

Ten days after starting Prozac, a forty-one-year-old woman began experiencing a longing for pain, which she satisfied by mutilating her legs, stomach, thighs, arms, and torso, along with six suicide attempts, all of which ended abruptly after she was taken off the drug.

Three days after starting Prozac, a fifty-eight-year-old man began having suicidal thoughts and tried to hang himself with a rope, prompting a discontinuation of the drug and, four days later, a complete disappearance of his suicidal ideation.

Within a week after having her dose of Prozac gradually increased from 20 to 60mg, a twenty-eight-year-old woman began to suffer akathisia and started fantasizing about jumping out of the hospital window, which prompted the discontinuation of Prozac and, in about a week, the elimination of all adverse effects.

Twenty-four hours after accidentally increasing his dose of Prozac from 60 to 80mg, a forty-four-year-old man began making superficial cuts to his throat, wrist, and abdomen while driving, a behavior which disappeared twenty-four hours after decreasing his dose.

Two weeks after starting Prozac, a thirty-two-year-old woman felt better except that she began experiencing restless and out of control feelings, which led her to state that "I feel like I need to hold onto my chair or else I'll jump out the window," all of which disappeared several days after discontinuing Prozac.

Eleven days after starting Prozac, a sixty-three-year-old Englishman suffocated his wife and then jumped off a 200-foot cliff.

Several weeks after starting Zoloft, a thirty-five-year-old man stabbed his wife and two children in their home, then killed himself with a .22-caliber rifle.

Six days after starting Prozac, a sixty-year-old woman stabbed and slashed herself more than sixty times as her husband ate breakfast in the kitchen. She died the next day.

One week after a mom and dad were told of, and started their thirteen-year-old son on, a "terrific" new medicine called Zoloft, the boy went into his bedroom closet and, while his family slept, killed himself by hanging.

Almost three months after her dose of Prozac was doubled, a woman living in Randolph, Vermont, took a .22-caliber pistol, shot and killed her eight-year-old son and her four-year-old daughter, then shot and killed herself.

Several days after Brynn Hartman was given Zoloft samples by her child's psychiatrist, she shot and killed her husband, Phil Hartman, while he slept. Four hours later, she shot and killed herself.

Two weeks after being prescribed Prozac, a forty-six-year-old man cleaned out the milking parlor on his farm, returned to his house, and shot himself in the forehead with a .22-caliber rifle.

A few days after starting on Prozac, a seventeen-year-old boy complained that the drug was "messing with [his] mind." A few days later, he hanged himself in his bedroom.

By the end of the 1990s, tragic events tied to the SSRIs littered the communities and countrysides of North America and Europe. Few of them ever made the headlines, however, buried instead behind the confusion and secrecy that so often marks sudden family tragedies. Before the Forsyth case made it to trial, in March 1999, two-thousand Prozac-associated suicides had been reported to the FDA and recorded on their "adverse event system." At least a quarter of these records included explicit references to agitation and akathisia. Based on estimates derived from decades of drug monitoring, the FDA has concluded that only about 1 percent of serious and fatal adverse drug events are ever reported on the system. This suggests that, as David Healy concluded, tens of thousands of Prozac-related suicides had taken place by the end of the twentieth century, many of which would have been precipitated by an extreme state of agitation. And those were the numbers only for Prozac. The total number of suicides for all SSRIs, including Paxil, would be considerably larger.

Still, these cases were relatively rare. They were exceptional cases and had therefore to be weighed against the millions of others living happily in Prozac nation. There was, however, another, more chilling possibility. If most everything Lilly claimed to be false about Prozac turned out to be true, what if most everything they claimed to be true about Prozac turned out to be false? What if, counter to the media hype that ushered in the Prozac revolution, the SSRIs actually offered few real benefits over older, typically akathisia-free antidepressants? Might all this death and destruction have been for naught? From the outside, this seemed a certain impossibility; from the inside, however, it looked all too likely. Prozac would turn out to be no more a perfect angel than cocaine would turn out to be a perfect demon.

The true story of the SSRIs began in the 1950s, when the use of antidepressants was confined almost exclusively to cases of clinical depression. Although there was some suggestion at the time that the new antidepressant imipramine (Tofranil) might actually make some patients feel "better than well," it was equally true that, as David Healy pointed out in *The Antidepressant Era*, no one was interested in imipramine in the 1950s. Neither was anyone interested in feeling better than well, especially if it required pouring a regular regimen of powerful chemicals into one's brain.

Although difficult to imagine today, depression was understood to be a rare condition in the 1950s and earlier, and there was a commonsense distinction between depression and general states of unhappiness. The rate of depression in the 1950s was estimated at about 50 people per million, an estimate that grew to 100,000 per million by the end of the twentieth century—a 2,000-fold increase in an ostensibly hereditary disease.[39] What happened during these years was not the discovery of a disease or its cure. What happened was that, because of ongoing changes in the drug marketplace, the pharmaceutical industry began taking a new interest in depression.[40]

Ever since the patent-medicine days of the nineteenth century, when drugs of any kind were sold over the counter with almost any claim, drug companies have viewed the general population as a huge legal market for mind-altering drugs. The decades immediately prior to the rise of the SSRIs were no different, although the psychiatric-drug market centered not on depression and antidepressants but on anxiety and anti-anxiety drugs (anxiolytics). When the benzodiazepines were introduced in the 1960s, drug makers declared them to be powerful yet nonaddictive. The market for barbiturates—Nembutal, Seconal, and the like—was collapsing at the time, as the earlier claim that they, too, were powerful but nonaddictive was no longer tenable. These factors combined to encourage widespread promotion of the benzodiazepines, with drugs like Valium becoming the most popular medicines of all time. As long as millions of Americans were taking benzodiazepines, there was no popular market for the antidepressants.

Beginning in the 1980s, however, things began to change. Fewer and fewer doctors were willing to prescribe benzodiazepines to treat every psychological whim and woe, waking up to the fact that, as with the barbiturates, those most interested in staying on the drugs were also likely to develop a stubborn dependence on them. A 1983 study noted, "In the past 3 years there has been a dramatic change in medical attitudes to the prescribing of benzodiazepines. Before 1980 these drugs were regarded as not only safe and effective anti-anxiety drugs and hypnotics (for getting to sleep), but were also said to be free of unwanted side effects. Growing concern about the risks of pharmacological dependence after regular consumption of these drugs soon followed."[41] The peak year for benzodiazepine use in the United States was 1973, when over eighty million prescriptions were filled. By 1986, this number had fallen to sixty-one million. As the number continued to decline, a hole in the domestic drug market began to widen. And the SSRIs were just the drugs to fill it.

Synthesized in the early 1970s, Prozac was in fact the fourth SSRI to come on the market (not the first, as Lilly once claimed).[42] The first was the drug zimelidine (Zelmid), developed by the European drug company Astra. Lilly scientists David Wong, Bryan Molloy, and Ray Fuller began the search for a 5-hydroxytryptamine (serotonin) reuptake inhibitor on 8 May 1972.[43] Although the goal at the time was to produce a drug that acted more selectively on serotonin in the brain (and could be patented accordingly), it was less clear what the drug would be useful for.[44] Shortly thereafter, Lilly's drug 110140 — a.k.a. fluoxetine or Prozac — was born.

After the drug succeeded in not killing laboratory animals in initial exploratory studies — although it turned cats from friendly to growling and hissing — Lilly began to inquire into what possible market might exist for their new compound. At a meeting in England, psychopharmacologist Alec Coppen suggested to the company that it might be useful as an antidepressant.[45] Lilly responded that, of all the drug's possible uses, this was not one of them.[46] Lilly had its eye on Prozac not as an antidepressant drug, nor as a drug for premenstrual syndrome, obsessive-compulsive disorder, smoking cessation, shyness, or anxiety, but as an antihypertensive drug.[47]

Within a decade, however, attitudes at Lilly reversed, although not because of any breakthrough in science or medicine. Astra's zimelidine had appeared on the market as a new, patented antidepressant, joined shortly thereafter by two other SSRIs. With the benzodiazepine market collapsing, Lilly also began to view the "treatment of depression" in a new light, realizing that antidepressants could be the new panacea for those who had been taking benzodiazepines. "The emergence of depression in this sense coincides with the development of the SSRIs," wrote David Healy in *The Creation of Psychopharmacology*, "which in the mid-1980s appeared capable of being developed as either anxiolytics or antidepressants. After the benzodiazepine crisis, the industry had a new set of compounds to sell, but its new offerings did not meet the demand from the marketplace. And indeed since their initial launch as antidepressants, various SSRIs have been licensed for the treatment of panic disorder, social phobia, post-traumatic stress disorder, OCD, and other anxiety-based conditions. Yet for some of the SSRIs, contrary to popular perceptions, it has simply not been possible to show that they are effective in treating classic depressive disorders."[48]

The turning of Prozac into an antidepressant was mirrored in the case of Paxil, which had come under development in the 1970s. Paxil did not make it to market until 1993, however, delayed by a prevailing attitude at Smith-

Kline that although new, patented antidepressants were entering the market (the SSRIs), they were not as effective as those that already existed (the tricyclics).[49] When SmithKline eventually came to the same conclusion as Eli Lilly, Paxil gained importance. The SSRI went on to become a popular drug in the antidepressant market in the 1990s, just as it became an effective backdoor for reentering the anxiety market. "From the beach-head of depression," wrote David Healy, "raids can subsequently be launched on the hinterlands of anxiety."[50] Or, as SmithKline put it in 2001, "Millions suffer from chronic anxiety. Millions could be helped by Paxil."[51]

With benzodiazepine sales a shadow of what they once had been, the number of prescriptions filled for antidepressants in the United States more than doubled by 1989. Less than two years after its release, sales for Prozac nearly tripled, from $125 million in its first year to $350 million, which was more than the total annual U.S. sales for all other antidepressants combined. By 1990, when the cover of *Newsweek* announced "A Breakthrough Drug for Depression," Prozac had become the most frequently prescribed antidepressant of all time. And the antidepressant market continued to grow. Annual Prozac sales reached the $1 billion mark in 1993, and by 1999 Prozac had become the third bestselling drug in the entire market of prescription pharmaceuticals. More than three billion doses of SSRIs were consumed in America in 1999. In 2000 annual antidepressant sales reached the $10 billion mark, with the United States making up 70 percent of all world sales for the drug.

Meanwhile, in Japan, the Prozac revolution laid in wait. Because the Japanese had experienced fewer problems with benzodiazepines, their sales remained strong, which left little market in which to engineer a Prozac revolution.

It was not at Eli Lilly but rather at SmithKline that the concept of the selective serotonin reuptake inhibitor was minted, although all SSRI manufacturers quickly embraced it to promote their new serotonin drugs. Like the Pentium concept used to sell Dell, Sony, and other personal computers, the selective-serotonin-reuptake-inhibitor concept was a brilliant marketing device for products of a similar class. However successful as a marketing device, though, the concept never had much substance to back it up. Paxil, Zoloft, Prozac, Celexa, and Luvox are all considered SSRIs, but the "selective" aspect of the name acquired a popular significance that went far beyond the one initially intended. The SSRIs are not selective in what they treat, or even in what they are claimed to treat (they have been hailed as cure-alls for everything from premenstrual syndrome to panic attacks to smoking to shyness). Nor are they selective in their biochemical actions in the brain. On the one hand, while the older tricyclics act on two neurotransmitter chemicals in the brain—serotonin and norepinephrine—the SSRIs act directly only on the former. However, while the SSRIs may not target norepinephrine, they do affect other biochemical systems, including direct effects on dopamine, after which they produce a cascade of secondary and tertiary biochemical and cellular effects, all of which remain poorly understood. For example, initial doses of Prozac have been shown to increase serotonin activity in an area of the brain known as the substantia nigra, but long-term use has been shown to produce the opposite effect. Aman Khan, a psychiatrist, summarized the problem: "Stimulation or inhibition of one neurotransmitter system by a drug would ultimately produce changes in several other neurotransmitter systems, and may actually involve the entire central nervous system. These mutual interactions extend the scope of a drug's influence far beyond its initial pharmacological action. In a complex dynamic system such as the brain, it is almost impossible to know which of the numerous changes produced by a drug are responsible for its therapeutic effects."[52]

As the science of psychopharmacology became successful in identifying and manipulating the acute, first-order pharmacological actions of drugs and classifying them accordingly, the media and the public came to believe that this meant scientists and physicians understood the drug's brain-altering effects. However, as in the field of human genetics, where it is similarly claimed that mapping the human genome is tantamount to understanding human genetics, the universe of the human brain is not so simple.

Consider cocaine, a drug whose actions in the brain are simple relative to those of the SSRIs. In a series of revealing studies, laboratory animals were grouped into pairs. One animal in each pair was given the opportunity to respond for cocaine. Afterward the other rat received the same pattern of drug administration established by the first, but involuntarily.[53] A basic pharmacological model would predict cocaine to have the same acute and chronic pharmacological effects for each group, since the pattern and volume of drug intake was identical for both animals in each pair. In reality, however, studies that used this methodology reported something quite different: while the first group showed stable and nontoxic patterns of cocaine use, the same patterns often proved fatal for the "involuntary" rats.

Acting on these results, researchers have also employed neurophysiological techniques to show that different environmental conditions actually mediate the drug's actions in the brain.[54] Using the same method of voluntary and involuntary administration of cocaine, these researchers reported that the location and magnitude of the biochemical actions associated with the drug differed significantly across the two contexts of use. In one key area of the brain, for example, the differences between the effects of voluntary and involuntary administration of cocaine on the brain were as great as the differences between the physiological effects of involuntary cocaine versus involuntary saline.

With SSRIs, which are taken chronically for months or even years, even greater complexity arises. As suggested by Lilly's initial idea of marketing Prozac as an antihypertensive drug, there is no reason to believe that one drug is destined to have one, and only one, primary effect. Mental agitation and the lifting of mood may both be potential effects of the drug when taken by different individuals or even by the same person at different doses.[55] What is, or should be, equally clear about the SSRIs, moreover, is that people do not experience unhappiness or depression simply because they suffer a chemical imbalance of serotonin in the brain. While some SSRIs are more selective in their serotonin specificity (Celexa) and some are more potent in causing serotonin release (Luvox), these differences do not result in one SSRI being more effective than another. Furthermore, drugs like Prozac raise serotonin levels almost immediately, so it is hard to see how this can explain their putative therapeutic effects, which can take days or weeks to be achieved.

Despite these pharmacological realities, Lilly and other SSRI makers succeeded in the 1990s in convincing the media and the public that a breakthrough had taken place in brain science, with the SSRIs designed specifically to correct a biochemical imbalance said to be the central cause of depression. "To help bring serotonin levels closer to normal," Lilly claimed in ads in popular magazines in the 1990s, "the medicine doctors now prescribe most often is Prozac." Suddenly anyone feeling down and depressed was confronted with the possibility that perhaps they, too, suffered from low levels of serotonin. As Peter Kramer tells it in *Listening to Prozac*, imipramine, the mainstay of antidepressants before the SSRIs, "is 'dirty' in its main effects and its side effects because it affects both norepinephrine and serotonin. Once imipramine's mechanism of action was understood, pharmacologists set out to synthesize a 'clean' antidepressant."[56]

Relying on a cult of pharmacology, meanwhile, SSRI makers orchestrated a barrage of promotional activity, readily absorbed by physicians, the media, and ultimately the public.[57] In 1990 *Newsweek* put a picture of Prozac on its cover and announced, "A Breakthrough Drug for Depression." *Newsweek* followed up with another Prozac cover story in 1991. In 1994, when 160 product liability cases had piled up against Prozac and Eli Lilly, *Newsweek* did another cover story entitled "Beyond Prozac." On the cover of that issue, the magazine stated, "How science will let you change your personality with a pill," and went on to pose the rhetorical question, "Want to boost your self-esteem, focus better on your work, tame the impulse to shop until you drop, shrug off your spouse's habit of littering the floor with underwear, overcome your shyness or keep yourself from blurting out your deepest secrets to the first stranger who comes along? . . . Now the same scientific insights into the brain that led to the development of Prozac are raising the prospect of nothing less than made-to-order, off-the-shelf personalities."[58]

The frequency of the claim that a revolution had taken place in psychiatric science was proportional to the lack of evidence supporting it. Consider, for instance, the scientific claims made in two popular-magazine articles. "Beyond Prozac," for example, claimed, "Research that once mapped the frontiers of disease — identifying the brain chemistry involved in depression, paranoia and schizophrenia — is today closing in on the chemistry of normal personality."[59] Three years later, "The Mood Molecule," an article in *Time*, stated that such aspects of the brain were in fact not at all understood: "For depression, bulimia, obesity and the rest of the serotonin-related disorders, however, no one knows for sure what part of the brain is involved or exactly why the drugs work. . . . The entire history of serotonin and of drugs that affect it has been largely a process of trial and error marked by chance discoveries, surprise connections and unanticipated therapeutic effects. . . . The tools used to manipulate serotonin in the brain are more like pharmacological machetes than they are like scalpels."[60]

"The Mood Molecule" nevertheless affirmed the notion that SSRIs offer something positively unique: "In the 1960s, a second class of antidepressants emerged. . . . [They] had major side effects, though, including profound drowsiness and heart palpitations. The reason, scientists generally agreed, was that they affected brain chemistry too broadly. The research seemed to point to serotonin as the most important mood-enhancing chemical, though not the only one, and so neurochemists set about looking for a drug that would boost the influence of serotonin alone. In 1974, after a decade of work, Eli Lilly came up with Prozac, first of the so-called selective serotonin reuptake inhibitors, or SSRIs, and the FDA finally approved it in 1987."[61]

This article contradicted itself, however, when it suggested that a new antidepressant had arrived on the market that acted not on serotonin but on the very neurochemical said to be irrelevant to depression, norepinephrine: "Psychiatrists in Europe are buzzing about a new drug, reboxetine, that has just been approved for use in Britain and seems to be even more effective than Prozac for severely depressed patients. Marketed under the brand name Edronax, it totally ignores serotonin and targets another brain chemical, norepinephrine, which is also known to have a powerful effect on mood."[62]

The *Newsweek* article came full circle, pointing out that a new drug entering the market, Effexor, worked even more effectively than the SSRIs, which it did by acting on both norepinephrine and serotonin: "Effexor . . . enhances both serotonin and norepinephrine, a second chemical messenger affecting mood. With its broader effect, Effexor should help some depressed patients who don't respond to Prozac."[63]

While selectively targeting the reuptake of serotonin may have been key to producing akathisia, self-mutilation, suicide, and murder, it appeared that serotonin was not key to raising people's moods. Antidepressants like Edronax showed that direct actions on serotonin might not even be necessary to produce an antidepressant effect. In fact, the trend early in the twenty-first century was away from SSRIs and back to new (or at least newly patented) compounds that acted directly on both norepinephrine and serotonin (or only on the former).[64]

Even Lilly eventually abandoned the SSRI club: after losing its patent on Prozac, the company announced late in 2001 that it would market a new and putatively more effective antidepressant than Prozac late in 2002.[65] Lilly's follow-up drug, duloxetine, finally appeared on the market late in 2004 and was quickly labeled a "dual-action" agent. As noted in Lilly's press releases, duloxetine "enhances levels of two important brain chemicals," serotonin and norepinephrine.[66] A presentation on the drug by Lilly scientists at a meeting at the National Institute of Mental Health similarly noted,

"The increased extracellular levels of serotonin and norepinephrine produced by duloxetine administration suggests it would enhance serotonin and norepinephrine neurotransmission and is expected to be efficacious in the treatment of major depression."[67]

So much for Prozac being a breakthrough antidepressant tailored to fit the latest scientific knowledge about serotonin and depression. Fortunately for Eli Lilly, however, the media once again proved to have a poor memory. In December 2001 the *Boston Globe* hailed the prospects of Lilly's future drug, stating, "While Prozac and drugs like it increase the amount of the chemical serotonin in the brain, duloxetine and Effexor enrich the supply of two important mood-boosting chemicals: serotonin and norepinephrine. Because these drugs have two different mechanisms of action, rather than one, doctors believe they may be more effective than Prozac-like drugs at improving patients' moods and might help more seriously depressed people."[68]

By the twentieth century's end, the SSRIs appeared to be on their way out, although the cult of the SSRI was still going strong. The public continued to believe that SSRIs were magic bullets, and any suggestion to the contrary was met with a rash of cries and complaints. In 1999, for example, the science writer John Horgan published an op-ed piece called "Placebo Nation" in the *New York Times*, implying that individuals taking Prozac and other antidepressants might be benefiting not just from the package — the pharmacological ingredients — but from the handling — that is, the experience of being treated. Letters of protest poured in, arguing that antidepressants like Prozac had helped millions of people and improved countless lives.[69] That Horgan's message provoked a sharp response was hardly surprising. For those who have seen their mood brighten after taking Prozac, Paxil, Zoloft, or any other antidepressant, such a suggestion often comes as a slap in the face. Prozac is not a placebo: it is a selective serotonin reuptake inhibitor, an SSRI!

Indeed it is. But this was not Horgan's point. Like any other psychoactive drug, including cocaine and Ritalin, Prozac's antidepressant effects are inseparably bound up with the same psychosomatics that swamp all drug use. A placebo response might be taking place, Horgan suggested, with the act of taking the drug setting into motion a powerful psychological shift from hopelessness to hopefulness.[70] Prozac has real effects, and in some users these effects may very well produce "fantastic results," "a blessed relief," "a brighter, more cheerful mood," or other "awesome results."[71] But placebo effects are every bit as real as pharmacological ones, and the two effects are indistinguishable during drug use; therefore, knowing what is and is not an effect of the latest mood molecule is nowhere as easy to discern as one might hope.

A case in point involved MK-869, a compound synthesized by Merck pharmaceuticals. In the realm of psychiatric medicine, concern over placebo effects looms large, for in order to obtain FDA approval, drug companies must demonstrate that their drugs outperform the placebo. As recounted in a *Science* article entitled "Can the Placebo Be the Cure?" early clinical trials suggested to Merck that MK-869 had great promise as an antidepressant, with fewer side effects than other antidepressants, including Prozac.[72] On 22 January 1999, however, Merck announced that they would not seek FDA approval for their new compound. The reason? While the latest data suggested that the drug was indeed effective in treating depression, studies showed it was no more effective than the placebo. "A novel compound — a Merck invention known as MK-869 — then in several clinical trials, seemed set to become a new millennium drug for millions of people who take antidepressant medication every day," noted the *Science* article. "The news [that MK-869 would be shelved] was a downer for Merck and Wall Street: the price of the company's stock dropped 5% on the day Merck broke the news."[73]

A report in the *Archives of General Psychiatry* published several decades earlier illustrated the degree to which a "drug effect" may actually be due, at least in part, to a placebo effect. Lee Park and Lino Covi, two young psychiatrists at Johns Hopkins University, asked what would happen if their patients were both given a placebo and told as much. To answer the question, they took fifteen newly admitted anxious and depressed patients and told them the following: "Many people with your kind of condition have been helped by what are sometimes called 'sugar pills,' and we feel that a so called sugar pill may help you, too. . . . A sugar pill is a pill with no medicine it at all. . . . Are you willing to try this pill?"[74] Of the fourteen individuals who said yes to this question, all kept their second appointment, and all but one reported taking at least two-thirds of the prescribed pills. To their surprise, Park and Covi found that each individual taking the sugar pills experienced a reduction in psychological distress. The average "distress score" was reduced by 43 percent, meaning that a majority of them felt "quite a bit" better after a week of taking sugar pills. When asked to explain why they might be feeling better, nine of the participants pointed to the pill, five of whom actually suspected or insisted that they were given an active medicine rather than a placebo. Of the remaining five, two attributed their improvements to the doctor's care rather than the pills, and three pointed to self-improvement.

Among the former group, one was a forty-five-year-old man, described as rigid, resistant to influence, and suffering from "agitated depression." According to the 1965 report, the man had suffered from severe insomnia, loss of appetite, feelings of despair, death wishes, and some somatic symptoms. During the interview he testified to a reduction in all symptoms, except for his lack of appetite. At the start of the interview he immediately declared, "It wasn't a sugar pill, it was medicine!"[75] He also noted that on taking the pills he was able to think more clearly, which led to a positive change in his attitude about his problems and the future. In addition to positive psychological effects, the man also reported clear side effects of the pills, including dry mouth and butterflies in the stomach. When asked about his improvement, he implied that perhaps he was falsely told he was being given a placebo so that he would attribute the improvement to himself rather than the medication.

Another participant, a twenty-four-year-old woman with three children, was clearly depressed and complained of insomnia, anorexia, irritability, and tension. After a week of taking sugar pills, she also testified, "They're not sugar pills . . . because they worked."[76] This woman was highly skeptical that a placebo could be effective for anyone and stated that the pills she received were actually more effective than other medications she had taken. She noted that she was feeling better than she had in the past twenty years and was pleased with the idea of continuing with the same doctor and pills.

As these cases suggest, the testimonials the public offers in favor of a drug do not have to be accurate to be strong. Determining what is and is not a drug effect requires extracting that effect from a whole range of ongoing experiences, which will not necessarily be easy; it may even be theoretically and practically impossible, as these pharmacological and nonpharmacological effects do not occur side by side in two separate realms of consciousness and behavior, but rather are experienced in combination in the brain—a whole greater than the sum of its parts.

According to reviewers of antidepressant literature, most users of SSRIs are in fact active placebo responders, a finding that further complicates the matter. As the *New York Times* summarized, "A [1998] review of placebo-controlled studies of modern antidepressant drugs found that placebos and genuine drugs worked about as well."[77] Much of the credit given to the SSRIS, then, should in fact be attributed to the placebo effect. The report cited by the *Times* was one of three meta-analyses of the antidepressant literature that appeared in the 1990s, each of which independently concluded that placebo effects account for much of the effectiveness of the antidepressants.[78] Overall, about two-thirds of the effectiveness attributed to the SSRIS appears to stem from the placebo effect.[79]

Admittedly, this is confounding. Because one often associates a placebo effect with a placebo, one also tends to think of drug effects and placebo effects as mutually exclusive. How can a drug effect really turn out to be partly a placebo effect? Yet placebo effects require no placebo per se, as they are just another reflection that nonpharmacological factors are contributing to what is deemed a drug effect, whether the drug is cocaine, Paxil, or sugar pills. If placebo effects are mobilized by beliefs and expectations, then what could be better than an active drug for launching the placebo effect? While some individuals will respond positively to SSRIS and not at all to placebos, the vast majority of individuals will experience the blessings of both pharmacological and nonpharmacological factors working in combination. Thus, when considering the cult of the SSRI, a larger question lingers: Can anyone really be so sure that the therapeutic effect they experience is due to the drug? Might it also be partly due to the placebo effect?[80] In one sense, this is the same question asked of juries in civil actions like the one involving William Forsyth: are these effects really attributable to the SSRI? There is one substantial difference, however: while treatment effects may be all or partly of a placebo nature, placebo effects rarely, if ever, include negative reactions like self-mutilation, suicide, or murder.

The claim that SSRIS may sometimes function merely as placebos might even sound like an outright contradiction: How can the SSRIS be linked to suicides and homicides, yet for many users be effective only as a placebo? In fact, there is no contradiction. The very creation of the FDA, as well as the passage of the Food, Drug, and Cosmetic Act in 1938, were motivated by just such a scenario, where a patent medicine was found to be unquestionably powerful, but not very powerful in doing what it was claimed to do. While a variety of the patent medicines of the nineteenth century had little hope of ever working as advertised except as placebos, their active ingredients nevertheless posed a clear hazard to the public health.

A century later, the same was true of the SSRIS. While they may have been more effective "medicines" than were most "patent medicines," they were not the angels the American public believed them to be. The spell of pharmacological magicalism was cast, Prozac was promoted as the latest panacea for easing the malaise of modern life, and millions of people were exposed to a group of drugs that were more toxic, more expensive, and less effective than drugs that already existed. Given the powers of the prescription marketing machine, and given the subsequent trend back to drugs that target neurochemicals other than serotonin, Prozac may not have even been necessary for the "Prozac revolution" to occur. Any number of non-SSRI antidepressants could have been fashioned for the revolution, just as they would be for the next one. Shrink-wrapped with the same promise of helping users become "better than well," such new wonder drugs could have given the people just what they wanted — and without all the wreckage.

Chapter Three **The Emperor's New Smokes**

*The entire matter of addiction is the most potent weapon
a prosecuting attorney can have in a lung cancer/cigarette
case. We can't defend continued smoking as "free choice"
if the person was "addicted."*

—Tobacco Institute memo, 9 September 1980

A t about the time Eli Lilly had completed its promised study for the Food and Drug Administration, in 1991, claiming no positive link between Prozac and suicide, the commissioner of the FDA held a historic meeting at agency headquarters in Rockville, Maryland, just outside Washington. A select group of FDA scientists, lawyers, and administrators met with Commissioner David Kessler in the fourteenth-floor conference room. The subject was not Big Pharma, Prozac, and suicide, however, but rather Big Tobacco, cigarettes, and addiction.

David Kessler had become the fifteenth commissioner of the FDA seven months earlier in October 1990, when he was only thirty-nine years old. That he was so young a commissioner was hardly an accident. Kessler had followed his private liberal-arts education at Amherst College, where he graduated with honors, with a medical degree from Harvard and then a law degree from the University of Chicago. At the time of his appointment to the FDA, Kessler was already teaching courses in food-and-drug law at Columbia Law School and had already served as medical director of the Albert Einstein Medical Hospital in the Bronx. Appointed by President George H. W. Bush, he served under both the Bush and Clinton administrations before stepping down in 1997.

Kessler arrived at the FDA in the wake of two terms of deregulation under Ronald Reagan, a time, Kessler later remarked, when the agency had become "a slow-moving target that bleeds profusely when hit." A few early successes gave Kessler greater confidence, however, as well as a clearer sense of what the regulatory agency could do. These successes also bought the agency a bit of much-needed respectability within the Washington beltway.

One of these successes involved the FDA's Center for Foods, which included a compliance office responsible for ensuring that marketing claims made by food producers were in fact true. When Kessler first visited the center, he was made aware of a variety of ongoing compliance problems, including use of the word *fresh* in the labeling of such things as reconstituted spaghetti sauce and concentrated orange juice. Such claims were misleading, which was enough for Kessler to send the FDA's Office of Compliance into action, even if it had been more-or-less out of action for a decade. Unilever, the maker of Ragu products, responded immediately by adding a clarification to their label. Procter and Gamble, however, which made the Citrus Hill brand of concentrated orange juice and which splashed the phrase "Fresh Choice" on its label in huge lettering, dismissed the FDA's warning, arguing that such labeling was standard industry practice. After further negotiations failed to get Procter and Gamble's attention, the FDA followed up on their ultimatum, seizing 24,000 half-gallon cartons of their juice. The action sent a message throughout the food industry: a sleeping dog was awakening, and they had better wake up as well.

Kessler followed up this early action with another success that involved the issue of nutritional labeling—a victory that was especially foretelling. Congress had passed the Nutritional Labelling and Education Act, and the FDA was responsible for writing the regulations that would govern it, including what constituted a healthy serving size and what the dietary information was for any given product. Congress also ordained that the same labeling system be used for meat and meat products, so while the FDA was to write the regulations, the U.S. Department of Agriculture would have to give its stamp of approval. However, the USDA wanted only basic, or raw, information on the packaging, leaving the consumer to calculate, say, the amount of fat per serving, which was contrary to Kessler's goal of giving the people the dietary information they needed to make educated decisions about the foods they would eat. The USDA, Kessler realized, was protecting the interests not of the public but of the meat industry. "They didn't want full disclosure," Kessler later remarked.[1] Although he eventually prevailed over the USDA, he took with him an important lesson: any battle against an American industry, even in the name of public health, would also be a battle against those in Washington who protected that industry, regardless of the public health.

Kessler's historic 1991 meeting with FDA scientists, lawyers, and administrators put this lesson to the test, with the question on the table being whether or not the FDA had the power to regulate cigarettes as drugs. Although Kessler called many meetings on the subject, he had not initiated the idea of going after Big Tobacco. A pediatrician by training, Kessler had not arrived at the FDA an anti-tobacco crusader. In fact, he at first agreed with the many longtime FDA staffers who believed that taking on the industry would place too great a strain on an already beleaguered agency and that raising the ire of Congress could also jeopardize the agency's budget, a budget wholly determined by Congress, as had occurred with other controversial campaigns.

Still, forces both inside and outside the agency compelled Kessler if not to act on the idea of regulating cigarettes, then at least to discuss it. One of these was the regular delivery of citizen petitions asking the FDA why it refused to take action against an industry whose product killed many and physically harmed most of those who used it. A second and more immediate push came from an FDA staffer named Jeff Nesbit. As associate commissioner of public affairs at the FDA, Nesbit had access to Kessler and used it to encourage his boss to go after Big Tobacco.[2] Cigarettes were a political hot potato, Nesbit conceded, but something had to be done. At least in principle, Kessler agreed. The subsequent events were chronicled in *A Question of Intent*, a book Kessler wrote soon after leaving the FDA, while serving as dean of the Yale School of Medicine.

Beginning with the 1991 meeting, the two primary questions posed by Kessler were, could it be done and should it be done? Did the FDA have the authority to exert regulatory control over tobacco products? If so, should they use it? As Kessler pointed out in *A Question of Intent*, it was easy for people to interpret "Food and Drug Administration" to mean that the agency regulated all foods and drugs. But as the case involving the USDA illustrated, the FDA hardly had carte blanche jurisdiction over all food and drug products. Moreover, cigarettes were not a food, nor were they established as a drug. A similar example: Coca-Cola contains a psychoactive quantity of caffeine, enough in fact to produce caffeine withdrawal in regular users, yet few consider Coca-Cola a drug, and few believe it should be regulated as such by the FDA. The same paradox had long served cigarette makers. In fact, because cigarettes were neither food nor drug, they had slipped through the regulatory cracks from the start, and stayed there.

The problem Kessler faced was reflected in an incident involving Donald Kennedy, a prior FDA commissioner. In May 1977 the public-interest group Action on Smoking and Health (ASH) had petitioned Kennedy's FDA to exert jurisdiction over cigarettes as a drug. When Kennedy denied the petition, ASH filed suit in U.S. district court. In his hearing, when asked how he could propose a ban of the artificial sweetener saccharin yet do nothing about the much more dangerous product of cigarettes, Kennedy responded, "Senator, I'll be glad to go to work on the cigarette ban as soon as you give me the legislative authority to do so."[3] Kessler used the same excuse to embrace inaction.

Kessler had told this story to his Columbia Law School students years before he came to the FDA, reminding them of the law as it was written. The amended Food, Drug, and Cosmetic Act of 1938 gave the FDA jurisdiction over a substance or device only if it was "intended for use in the cure, mitigation, treatment or prevention of disease," including "articles (other than food) intended to affect the structure and function of the body." The law clearly indicated that the act was to apply only to substances "intended" by the maker to serve a therapeutic function as a health product, where such intention could be discerned from what was written on the packaging. Since a U.S. court of appeals had ruled that cigarette packaging made no health claims, Kessler concluded, as had previous FDA commissioners, that although cigarettes were the nation's number one cause of death, the FDA had never been legislated the power to regulate them.

Kessler also knew why no government agency had ever been given regulatory control over tobacco products: once it happened, cigarette sales would have to be banned. Many years of research and many millions of dollars spent had all but proven that cigarettes were a dangerous product that could not be made safe. Few could imagine the total prohibition of cigarettes, however, so the question of regulating tobacco struck many as moot.

In the months following the 1991 meeting, although Kessler himself maintained only a curiosity about the tobacco issue, he did allow the formation of an informal working group of FDA staffers, with the mission of quietly researching the tobacco question and preparing responses to the petitions received from advocacy groups, including the Coalition on Smoking or Health. The working group was made up of FDA staffers from a variety of departments and was headed by a doctor of pharmacology at the agency, Ilisa Bernstein. While Kessler focused on other matters, the working group compiled research papers and held meetings with scientists. Gradually, a small number of quasi-experts emerged within the group, and in the fall of 1992 the group met with Kessler to discuss options for handling citizen petitions that demanded regulatory action against cigarette makers. While the meeting proved that much had been learned on the issue, Kessler recalled, there was as yet no breakthrough that would have compelled him to act. FDA regulation of cigarettes remained on indefinite hold.

That Kessler's FDA did not remain stuck in a perpetual holding pattern, circling the tobacco issue but never landing, was largely the result of another public-health advocate in the agency, David Adams. An FDA lawyer in the Office of Policy, Adams had been attending the meetings of the tobacco working group. Living up to his reputation as an independent thinker, however, he kept a low profile in the group. And once he had arrived at his own conclusions about how best to approach the problem, he brought them to Kessler alone. It was commonly believed, Adams told Kessler after finding him in his office undisturbed, that the primary pharmacological ingredient in tobacco, nicotine, was an "immutable constituent" in cigarettes. In fact, Adams pointed out, this really was not so, or at least it wasn't any longer.[4] Like caffeine in the coffee bean, nicotine occurs naturally in tobacco and thus also in cigarettes. For various reasons, however, cigarette makers had developed and employed methods of extracting nicotine from tobacco and then adding it back in, thereby allowing greater control over nicotine levels. The implications of this development were immediately clear to Kessler: if the cigarette industry was manipulating nicotine, it could no longer argue that nicotine was a natural constituent of their product and therefore could no longer claim that selling the drug was an inevitable result of being in the centuries-old business of selling tobacco; they had inadvertently turned tobacco into a drug. The evidence Adams brought to Kessler's office provided him with the kind of breakthrough that he'd been looking for. "From that moment," Kessler wrote, "and for the first time, I began to focus on tobacco."[5]

Armed with this new insight and eager to test it out, Kessler scheduled a meeting with the assistant secretary of health, James Mason, who was in effect his boss. The intention, Kessler told Mason, was simply to reflect on the issue of tobacco regulation, not to propose any new action. In the meeting that followed Kessler freely admitted that FDA regulation was guided by safety and efficacy and that cigarettes could not be made safe. And yet "with some 50 million smokers in the United States," noted Kessler, "a total ban was out of the question."[6] To overcome this bind, Kessler added that he was not interested in an outright ban, a comment that opened the way to David Adams's sharing in the meeting the idea he had brought to Kessler: if nicotine was a drug and if Big Tobacco had shown a clear intent to manipulate it as such, perhaps the FDA could regulate the industry not by regulating cigarettes per se but by regulating the nicotine that the industry put in them. It was a trial balloon that took immediate flight: the assistant secretary, taken by Adam's new strategy, concluded the meeting by suggesting that they pursue the matter further. They were to meet at the Department of Health and Human Services in six weeks.

Although the green light had been given, Kessler knew that it could revert back to red at any moment, so he put his tobacco group into action immediately. The goal was to build a case against the cigarette makers, proving that Big Tobacco intended cigarettes to contain nicotine and did so in order first to create an addiction, then to profit by satisfying it. This was a new line of attack, and Kessler was excited about its prospects. For more than a century, death and disease had been common themes in public discussions of tobacco and smoking. But the theme of addiction brought new life to the issue. Indeed, it had considerable implications not just for government regulation but also for civil actions being brought against the industry.

The reason for this was simple. It was common knowledge that cigarette smoking was habit forming and that nicotine was the psychoactive drug in tobacco, which suggested that cigarettes were addictive because of nicotine. Kessler embraced this viewpoint, as had Ronald Reagan's surgeon general, C. Everett Koop. In his 1988 report, *Nicotine Addiction: The Health Consequences of Smoking*, Koop had concluded that cigarettes were indeed addictive and that the drug nicotine was the source of the addiction.[7] With a new emphasis on addiction, Kessler believed it might be possible to show that cigarette makers had brought regulation on themselves by manipulating with scientific precision an addictive drug. If nicotine was no longer an intrinsic attribute of cigarettes and cigarette smoking, it became possible to demonstrate "intent" in the tobacco industry, and intent to treat tobacco as a drug product had been the determining factor in establishing regulatory authority in the past.

The subject of addiction was also gaining attention in civil actions. Government regulators — namely, the Federal Trade Commission (FTC) — had required since 1966 that cigarette makers place health warnings on each pack of cigarettes. The 1966 warning read "Caution: Cigarette Smoking May Be Hazardous to Your Health." This was changed to slightly stronger wording in 1970: "Warning: The Surgeon General Has Determined that Cigarette Smoking Is Dangerous to Your Health." In 1985 this warning became still more specific, explicitly stating that smoking caused cancer and other health problems. Ironically, the tobacco industry used these warnings to have their cake and eat it, too: without ever having themselves to admit that smoking was a health risk, they were still able to warn users about such risks, since they were compelled to do so by the FTC. As a result, the industry could deny product liability in civil court, especially in cases involving persons harmed by smoking that occurred after package warnings were posted in 1966. How could people blame Big Tobacco for a choice they made consciously, the industry argued, with full knowledge of the risks?

It was at that juncture that the issue of addiction gained importance. To counter the industry's argument that smokers had been fully warned about the dangers of cigarettes, plaintiffs' attorneys began in the 1980s to argue that, regardless of the warnings about the health hazards of smoking, smokers could not quit because they were addicted to the nicotine in the cigarettes. The industry was therefore liable, plaintiffs argued, since it had known but failed to inform users that cigarettes were inherently addictive. According to this theory, smokers who did not fail to quit smoking after 1966, as well as smokers who had begun after that date, could also blame the industry, testifying that they had planned to stop smoking well before ever becoming ill but had found that they could not once they tried.

With growing emphasis on the addictiveness of nicotine and growing evidence that the industry could manipulate the amount of the drug at will, the issue of addiction became part of a new legal strategy. A 1980 document from the Tobacco Institute, a research group the cigarette industry formed in Washington in 1958 with an eye toward public relations, expressed the industry's vulnerability: "The entire matter of addiction is the most potent weapon a prosecuting attorney can have in a lung cancer/cigarette case. We can't defend continued smoking as 'free choice' if the person was 'addicted.'"[8] Thus, while plaintiffs' lawyers and the FDA had different goals in mind, both went to work on the same problem, that is, proving that Big Tobacco had long known that nicotine was addictive and that they had knowingly manipulated it in their cigarettes to ensure addiction.

Becoming commissioner of the FDA requires a presidential appointment, and thus it is common to see a turnover in agency leadership following a change in the office of the presidency. In November 1992 George Bush lost the White House to Bill Clinton. Instead of finding himself out of work, however, FDA Commissioner Kessler found himself in a political environment more favorable to regulatory action, especially when taken in the name of public health.

Soon after the Clinton administration took office, however, Kessler ran aground. He had wanted to place greater restrictions on the sale of body tissues coming from foreign sources, but he suffered resistance from above. The Department of Health and Human Services (HHS), which ultimately determined much of what Kessler could and could not do, was full of new political appointees, and Kessler had already failed to gain his superiors' support. To win it Kessler employed a tactic so successful it would later be applied in building the case against the cigarette industry.

When Kessler attempted to restrict the sale of body tissues, HHS told Kessler that there was insufficient evidence of bad practices in the industry to warrant regulation. To get the evidence Kessler turned to Jack Mitchell in the FDA's new Office of Special Investigations, which Kessler had set up in 1991 with the primary mission of anticipating emerging problems facing the agency. (Kessler did not like surprises and had experienced too many of them after first being appointed.) Kessler now asked Mitchell to conduct an undercover operation to learn more about the buying and selling of body parts.

Having made contact with a Russian-born "tissue broker," the undercover Mitchell was informed that his "company" would have to pay $5,000 per body but was offered a discount if he would take one that had tested positive for hepatitis B — evidence of an industry that casually trafficked in diseased tissues. Kessler took the evidence to HHS. When HHS officials continued to resist, Kessler clarified the issue: "We can go to the press with a story about contaminated body parts coming into the United States for transplantation, or we can go with a story about a regulation that makes this sort of thing illegal. Which do you prefer?"[9] The warning had its intended effect, and the new DHHS secretary, Donna Shalala, signed off on the new regulation shortly thereafter. Putting Mitchell on the case had paid off.

As Kessler built rapport with Clinton's people at HHS, he began broaching the subject of tobacco regulation, finding some early encouragement. Phil Lee, who had replaced James Mason as the assistant secretary of health, was a friend of Kessler's who, as Kessler put it, "had little use for the tobacco industry."[10] Meanwhile, advocacy groups petitioning the FDA continued to apply heat. In April 1992 Scott Ballin of the Coalition on Smoking or Health published a letter in the *Wall Street Journal* entitled "When shown tobacco, FDA dog won't hunt." Ballin was among those who doubted Kessler's will to take action. Instead of throwing a bone to advocacy groups by going public with his plans to attack Big Tobacco on grounds of nicotine manipulation, Kessler remained quiet, however, applying the lesson of the body-parts case: don't go forward until all or at least enough evidence is in hand.

The first big opportunity to begin collecting evidence came in the fall of 1993, when the FDA's policy office was made aware of a whistleblower from R. J. Reynolds Tobacco Company (RJR), makers of Winston and Camel cigarettes. The policy office informed Kessler of the whistleblower, code-named "Deep Cough," saying that he could provide them with insider information about RJR's manufacturing process. Kessler saw the opportunity for what it was — the first real break — but wanted the work to be kept quiet and to be conducted by people experienced in dealing with informants of questionable motives and reliability. Thus, instead of turning to the tobacco working group, which continued to grow in size and expertise, Kessler turned to Gary Light in the FDA's Office of Criminal Investigations.

Light knew how to conduct an investigation. Before coming to the FDA, the twenty-year army veteran had conducted undercover narcotics operations as part of the army's Criminal Investigation Division — the very command that had investigated Colonel Hiett in Colombia after his wife had been charged with drug trafficking. Light had also investigated cases of murder, rape, and robbery for the army and was an expert in the use of polygraphs. At his side was another cop, Tom Doyle, who had worked for the New York City police force, the Secret Service, and the CIA. Both Doyle and Light were criminal investigators for the FDA, and on the matter of Big

Tobacco they reported straight to Kessler. "If some headquarters people saw Gary and Tom as cops pure and simple," Kessler later reflected, "the two agents saw others at the FDA as civilians who, while talented and well-meaning, knew nothing about dealing with informants."[11]

Light and Doyle conducted their first interview with the RJR defector by phone on 11 January 1994. After a second phone conversation, Deep Cough agreed to talk with Light and Doyle in person. They met at a seafood restaurant in Virginia Beach on 20 January, and for several hours the former RJR manager told stories of how nicotine had come to be manipulated by the industry. He spoke of how, after being told by in-house counsel that explicit talk of nicotine would put the company at risk for FDA regulation, he and his co-workers cloaked efforts to control nicotine levels in notions of "impact" and "satisfaction." To make sure their cigarettes had impact and produced satisfaction up to the last puff, RJR had developed methods for manipulating their nicotine content. They did this, Deep Cough explained, either by altering the actual nicotine content in the tobacco or by using other chemicals to boost the quantity of nicotine released as a cigarette was smoked. Deep Cough also talked of a cost-saving material called reconstituted tobacco, which was made of inferior parts of the plant, plant scraps, and even tobacco dust. These parts were mulched and mashed and then formed into a kind of tobacco paper, he explained, with nicotine and other "flavors" artificially added in — a process of "fortification" necessitated by the fact that the resulting tobacco had poor flavor and delivered little nicotine when smoked.[12]

Kessler was briefed after each interview. Although it was exactly the kind of information the FDA needed, Kessler knew that, being anecdotal, it was insufficient in itself. However, Deep Cough had suggested that Kessler's team was on the right track, and this encouraged them to keep going. Around the same time, the network ABC was in the process of producing a segment on nicotine and smoking for the program *Day One*, and it was also relying on Deep Cough. After being invited to appear on the program and give their response, RJR went on the defensive. An internal company memo written at the time refers to G7, a code name for reconstituted tobacco, noting, "The nicotine levels were raised by adding KLN [nicotine] extract to the G7 extract. . . . All these materials need to be relabelled."[13] In preparation for ABC's taping, RJR's legal counsel instructed company scientists on how to respond to the most sensitive issues: smoking is not addictive, but rather is a habit or a custom; people freely choose to smoke and give up smoking freely; smoking does not harm or disrupt a person's life the way addictive drugs do; smokers do not show the tolerance and withdrawal that is associated with hard drugs; and so on.

RJR knew that the *Day One* program would reveal a longtime industry-wide conspiracy to manipulate nicotine and perhaps even addiction, but neither they nor the rest of the industry could foresee that once this information was made public, Kessler would get the go-ahead to release his tobacco working group's carefully constructed letter to the Coalition on Smoking or Health. The letter responded to the coalition's petition asking the FDA to regulate tobacco products and showed a marked shift in FDA thinking. With a sharp focus on nicotine and addiction, the FDA's letter suggested that there might indeed be a legal basis for taking jurisdiction over all products containing nicotine as a drug. When the letter was sent out, it was also sent to certain members of the media. On 26 February, a full year after the petition had first been submitted to the FDA, both the *New York Times* and the *Washington Post* ran stories detailing the FDA's shift in thinking. "The letter took the tobacco industry completely by surprise," Kessler later recalled, "and officials quickly scrambled to find out how their intelligence networks had failed so completely."[14]

Kessler had let the cat out of the bag, but as the cigarette makers were well aware, he had yet to take any regulatory action against them. The FDA had only begun to make its case, and Kessler had many a political mind to change before there would be any hope of such action. Kessler knew that he needed to come forward with a case at once so shocking and so credible that policymakers in Washington would have no choice but to go along with it. He also knew that such a case could not be built overnight. Thus, in addition to the tobacco working group, Kessler decided to create a special investigative team on tobacco, headed by Tom Doyle, Gary Light, and Jack Mitchell.

After the FDA letter was sent to the Coalition on Smoking or Health, Kessler outlined a more advanced set of questions to be answered, making it clear that both the working group and the investigative team would need to focus on issues of nicotine and addiction. "We have to find out everything we can about nicotine and its use in cigarettes," Kessler stressed. Some of the most pressing questions: "How are cigarettes made? How is nicotine related to addiction? How addictive is nicotine? Are manufacturers adding nicotine to cigarettes? How does the industry set nicotine levels? Where is the nicotine coming from?"[15]

Guided by these questions, with some prejudice about the answers, the FDA ploughed the fields of Big Tobacco for the next two years. They researched industry archives, met with scientists, and questioned industry insiders. The deeper they tilled, the more dirt they uncovered. The industry had many secrets, and in the 1990s these secrets began rising en masse to the surface.

The first big opportunity for the new investigative team came via another ex-tobacco employee, this time from Philip Morris, the maker of Marlboro cigarettes. Vedpal Singh Malik, a senior scientist at the Richmond, Virginia–based company, had been suddenly let go when his work on genetic engineering was deemed too risky legally for the company to continue. Malik told FDA investigators that he had helped isolate the carcinogenic compounds in smoked tobacco and had helped develop a process for removing them — a process, he said, that Philip Morris had decided to conceal rather than use. Meanwhile, the company was removing nicotine from tobacco, Malik said, which was then used to boost the nicotine levels in their best-selling brand Marlboro. Via a process called supercritical extraction, nicotine was being removed to create nicotine-free tobacco for Philip Morris's experimental "non-nic" cigarettes called Next. Then it was reused by adding it to the tobacco used to make Marlboro cigarettes. Malik also talked of the Institut für Biologische Forschung, a top-secret research laboratory operated by Philip Morris in Cologne, Germany. Malik did not know much beyond the existence of the laboratory and that it was used to house highly sensitive industry documents. Kessler later discovered that the foreign lab was also used to minimize the company's liability for high-risk research on carcinogenesis and on the chemistry and psychopharmacology of nicotine.

Just as important to the FDA were Malik's suggestions of other ex-Philip Morris employees who might be willing to school them on inside industry practices. One of these was William Farone, code-named "Philip," a scientist who for five years had been director of applied research at Philip Morris. In his interviews with the FDA's special investigative team Farone confirmed much of the information that had come from both Deep Cough and Malik, describing in more technical detail the evolved science of cigarette manufacturing. Farone explained, for example, how after the advent of machine-based cigarette production, the technology had remained more or less the same until the 1950s and 1960s, when the industry began investing their massive profits into the development of new cigarette-making technologies. As Deep Cough described it on ABC's *Day One* program, the result was that the cigarette had now become "a complex, scientifically engineered product."[16]

In addition to the use of nicotine extraction and reconstituted tobacco, as well as highly efficient means of manufacturing billions of cigarettes per year, millions per day, and thousands per minute — a century earlier, James Buchanan Duke, the founder of what became the Reynolds Tobacco Company, had been content if his "cigarette girls" could roll four cigarettes per minute — the science of cigarettes also involved sophisticated methods of analyzing cigarette smoke.[17] This advance, Farone explained, allowed the industry to model different aspects of the cigarette and smoking, and to see the combined effect of manipulating these aspects on nicotine delivery. This included such factors as the type of tobacco used, the burn rate of the cigarette, the use of a filter or the type of filter used, and the properties of the cigarette paper. As Kessler later confirmed through industry documents, RJR had concluded long before that nicotine was crucial to the sensory experience of smoking and thus to smoker "satisfaction." In the 1960s, for instance, the industry had concluded that much of the satisfaction provided by nicotine came from its "calming" effect in habituated smokers. With the popularity of mild tranquilizers like Seconal and Valium growing, the industry had begun to worry that such drugs might emerge as an alternative to smoking, decreasing people's desire to smoke. For reasons such as these, studying nicotine delivery and nicotine psychopharmacology became a central activity within the industry, ultimately evolving into a science of nicotine manipulation.

Kessler's challenge, then, was more than just showing that cigarettes were addictive because of nicotine — the 1988 surgeon-general report had already convinced the public of that — it was proving that addiction was an effect *intended* by the industry, which it ensured by turning cigarettes into what antismoking advocates came to refer as "nicotine-delivery devices." The FDA still had not done this. It knew that cigarette makers were manipulating nicotine, but it also knew that the industry always cloaked this work in terms of "flavoring," "acceptability," and "smoker satisfaction," thus providing the defense that, whatever else nicotine might do, it had to be monitored and manipulated to add flavor.

As the FDA continued ploughing, they began looking at patents filed by the industry. One such patent, filed by Philip Morris in 1966, read, "Maintaining the nicotine content at a sufficiently high level to provide the desired physiological activity, taste and odor which this material imparts to the smoke, without raising the nicotine content to an undesirably high level, can thus be seen to be a significant problem in the tobacco art."[18] Another patent discussed the transfer of nicotine from high-nicotine tobacco to the tobacco filter, reconstituted tobacco, and tobacco that was "nicotine deficient."[19] Indeed, a variety of patents suggested that the industry was adding nicotine to different parts of the cigarette to increase the nicotine delivered to the smoker. Other patents went even further. One series suggested that the industry had tried to develop insecticides that had chemical and pharmacological properties similar to those of nicotine, presumably in the hope that they would double as nicotine-like drugs when the tobacco was smoked. (Evolutionarily speaking, nicotine may have evolved in nature as a constituent of tobacco because it acts as an insecticide.) Another patent suggested that the industry was not just concerned with nicotine as a flavor additive; it referred to the use of an acid, levulinic acid, which, by lowering the burning sensation that came from smoking tobacco higher in nicotine content, allowed more nicotine to be added to the product. Why, if cigarette makers were concerned with flavor, why would they want to raise nicotine levels beyond the point at which the taste became too strong?

Malik also referred Victor DeNoble, code-named "Cigarette," a doctor of psychopharmacology who studied the behavioral effects of nicotine in animals while he was at Philip Morris. Among the effects he studied while tucked away in his clandestine lab were the "reinforcing effects" of nicotine; that is, he studied whether nicotine produced a sensory experience positive enough to cause laboratory animals to voluntarily respond to obtain it. In 1983 DeNoble and another ex-Philip Morris scientist, Paul Mele, who the FDA had assigned the alias "Cigarette Jr," had submitted a paper describing their findings of animal self-administration of nicotine to the journal *Psychopharmacology*. For Kessler and the FDA, research like DeNoble's was an important discovery. Reinforcing effects played a role in addiction, and while outside researchers, including Jack Henningfield at the National Institute on Drug Abuse (NIDA), had conducted this type of research, the FDA had until that time been unaware of any such research activity within the industry. The existence of such research suggested that the tobacco industry was in fact well aware of the addiction issue and probably had their own evidence to support it. Before the paper in question could be published, however, Philip Morris forced DeNoble and Mele to withdraw it, and then, some months later, sacked them both. While Philip Morris denied that the two scientists were fired because of the implications of their research, internal documents reveal the company's concern. Philip Morris's legal counsel stressed at the time, "This kind of research is a major tool of our adversaries on the addiction issue. . . . In the final analysis, the performing and publishing of nicotine-related research clearly seems ill-advised from a litigation point of view."[20]

As Kessler worked to track down a copy of the DeNoble and Mele paper, which he eventually received from Jack Henningfield at NIDA — Henningfield had probably been asked years earlier to review the paper — Kessler was sent some interesting data from his own lab in St. Louis. Months earlier the FDA lab had been given the assignment of learning everything they could about cigarette manufacturing by analyzing different brands of commercially available cigarettes. After examining the nicotine content in twenty brands, the lab had discovered something interesting. Since tar and nicotine in tobacco co-vary, low-tar cigarettes should also be low in nicotine. Yet the FDA lab found something quite different in commercial cigarettes. In the Merit line of cigarettes, for example, the brand lowest in tar tested the highest in nicotine, and as the tar levels increased, nicotine levels paradoxically decreased. The implication was clear: the usual link between tar and nicotine had been broken by the industry's manipulation of nicotine, either by adding more nicotine directly to tobacco or by varying the kinds of tobacco, with differing nicotine contents, in different brands. The tobacco industry would not be willing to admit to this, since it might suggest "intent" on their part to produce a pharmacological effect in its users.

Meanwhile, at this same point in the FDA's investigation, Alexander Spears, chief operating officer at Lorillard Tobacco Company, wrote in his prepared remarks for a congressional hearing on smoking and cigarettes, "We do not set levels of nicotine for particular brands of cigarettes. . . . Nicotine levels follow the tar levels."[21]

The data from the St. Louis lab obviously contradicted this statement, as did a report written in 1981 by Alexander Spears himself. Just after the 25 March 1994 hearing held by the House Subcommittee on Health and Environment and chaired by the California representative Henry Waxman, the head of the FDA's tobacco working group, Ilisa Bernstein, discovered Spears's 1981 document. Directed at tobacco chemists, the report noted that current research was focused on how to increase nicotine levels in cigarettes while maintaining lower levels of tar. Contrary to his more recent testimony that nicotine levels "follow the tar levels," Spears had reported "a trend toward increasing nicotine over time" in the lowest-tar cigarettes.[22]

Also at about the time of the March hearing in the House of Representatives, Kessler's team made contact with another industry insider, code-named "Research." The informant's real name was Jeffrey Wigand, and he had formerly been a senior scientist and vice president at the Brown and Williamson Tobacco Company, maker of Kool, Pall Mall, and Lucky Strike cigarettes. Of all the tobacco insiders and informants, Wigand would receive the most public attention. He and his details of industry practices, which included chemical manipulations of tobacco and cigarettes to increase the smoker's exposure to nicotine, were featured on *60 Minutes*, and he was later profiled in the Michael Mann film *The Insider*. The company had fired Wigand after he had resisted the company practice of adding the chemical coumarin to its tobacco. Coumarin was a known carcinogenic, but the company refused to replace it until a suitable alternative was found. Wigand's critical stance against such practices led to his dismissal, and Brown and Williamson frequently reminded their bitter ex-vice president of the confidentiality agreement he had signed when leaving the company. Wigand went public with the information nevertheless, fueling the negative public sentiment that was growing against the industry.

Wigand also told the FDA that Brown and Williamson engaged in an industry-wide practice of impact-boosting nicotine via the use of an ammonia compound called diammonium phosphate. As Wigand explained it, ammonia reacted with the nicotine molecule in tobacco, enhancing the absorption of nicotine into the brain once the cigarette was smoked. He also argued that it was this ingredient in Marlboros, a Philip Morris product, that had led the brand to become the single most popular product in the world. As the St. Louis lab explained to Kessler, ammonia basically allowed cigarette smokers to "freebase" nicotine.

Wigand also reported to Kessler something that led to the agency's most intensive investigation: that in addition to blending tobaccos and chemically manipulating them, Brown and Williamson had developed a strain of genetically modified tobacco called Y-1. This bioengineered plant contained nicotine levels at least twice that of natural tobacco, yet it had a taste that was still acceptable and produced a yield per acre that was financially competitive. Following up on the lead, Kessler's investigators eventually tracked down the creator of Y-1, an agricultural scientist named James Chaplin. Chaplin had worked for the USDA in the 1960s, cultivating new tobacco strains. At first Chaplin denied involvement in engineering Y-1, but as the FDA's investigation grew hotter, he eventually turned witness. When Chaplin finally described the Y-1 work he had done after leaving the USDA, he told of six years of painstaking trial-and-error research that finally led to suitable high-nicotine seeds.

Tobacco producers had long used traditional methods of breeding the best plants, but the practice of genetic engineering, Kessler felt, revealed the lengths to which the industry was willing to go to achieve high nicotine levels in cigarettes. "Why spend a decade developing through genetic breeding high-nicotine tobacco and adding it to cigarettes," Kessler later asked in a congressional hearing, "if you are not interested in controlling and manipulating nicotine?"[23] The behavior of the industry at the time did not contradict Kessler's rhetorical query. According to another industry informant, congressional hearings into tobacco regulation had made Brown and Williamson fearful of being caught with Y-1 on their hands, so they had begun blending millions of pounds of genetically engineered tobacco into any and all of their brands in order to use it up.[24]

That a former director of research at Brown and Williamson, Wigand, was now an informant indicated how deeply Kessler's team had penetrated the industry. Kessler reached even deeper when he received the private papers of another past director of tobacco research, S. J. Green. In addition to having been the director of research for the London-based British American Tobacco company (the parent company of Brown and Williamson), Green had also been on the company's board of directors. Years after leaving the business, however, Green developed a critical attitude toward the industry and began writing and speaking out against it. His private papers told an inside story very similar to those told by Wigand and others. What most interested Kessler about Green's papers were his views on nicotine and addiction, including comments about how "nicotine is the most addictive drug," about how regular smokers "can no longer be said to make an adult choice," and about how "a good part of the cigarette industry is concerned with the administration of nicotine to consumers."[25] Kessler was quick to notice that among Green's three reasons for why people smoked, one was "pharmacological rewards."[26]

The private papers of S. J. Green represented the rush of insider information that became public in the 1990s. Drawn from the internal documents of the three largest American tobacco companies — RJR, Philip Morris, Brown and Williamson — this information confirmed most FDA suspicions about what Big Tobacco knew, what they had done, and why they had conspired to do it. The documentation included a collection of highly sensitive papers smuggled out of Brown and Williamson, which the FDA received word of just prior to the spring hearings in 1994. The whistleblower was Merrell Williams, a paralegal at a Kentucky law firm that represented Brown and Williamson, who had been given the unlikely task of going through thousands of Brown and Williamson documents and classifying them in terms of their significance for pending civil actions. As a longtime smoker of Brown and Williamson cigarettes, Williams was struck by what he read — so struck in fact that he decided to smuggle out the most outrageous documents, make copies of them, and create his own set of duplicate files at home.

Williams, who broke the news of their existence after falling seriously ill with a heart condition, eventually made the stolen copies public. The documents were leaked repeatedly and eventually showed up at the *New York Times*. On 7 May 1994, "Tobacco Company Was Silent on Hazards," the first of any articles to discuss the documents, described overwhelming evidence that the company had taken an interest in the addictive properties of nicotine since the early 1960s and that a common attitude within the industry was "We are, then, in the business of selling nicotine, an addictive drug effective in the release of stress mechanisms."[27] One document, dated 1 July 1965, contained a directive by the head of research at Brown and Williamson: "find ways of obtaining maximum nicotine for minimum tar."[28]

The March 1994 congressional hearing on nicotine and addiction was followed by three more hearings in April and June.[29] These were open hearings on the regulation of tobacco products, and they marked the next step in the FDA's march toward regulation. The FDA's public letter sent in February to the Coalition on Smoking or Health had announced the agency's new attitude toward regulation, and the congressional hearings represented the spread of this new attitude to Congress. Meanwhile, Big Tobacco was increasingly panicked. As Wigand reported to Kessler at the time of the April hearing, Brown and Williamson were "going crazy. The lawyers were in [over the Memorial Day holiday]. The research guys were in. The marketing guys were in."

Kessler's testimony revealed to the public why the industry had every reason to panic, just as it revealed the transformation in Kessler's understanding of tobacco-industry practices since the first FDA meeting on tobacco three years earlier. Kessler told the subcommittee that nicotine was so addictive that smokers essentially lost their freedom to choose whether or not to continue smoking, which locked them into a habit that ensured poorer health and a shorter life. He also argued that the industry had developed an array of methods for manipulating nicotine to ensure this habit formed in its customers. Borrowing from the words of S. J. Green and others, Kessler was able to argue his case using phrases, statements, and conclusions that came straight from the industry's mouth. "Whose choice is actually driving the demand for cigarettes in this country?" Kessler began.

> Is it a choice by consumers to continue smoking? Or is it a choice by cigarette companies to maintain addictive levels of nicotine in their cigarettes? . . . The public may think of cigarettes as no more than blended tobacco rolled in paper. But they are more than that. Some of today's cigarettes may in fact qualify as high-technology nicotine delivery systems that deliver nicotine in quantities sufficient to create and sustain addiction in the vast majority of individuals who smoke regularly. . . . Nicotine in tobacco is an addictive substance. It has all the hallmarks of addiction. Nicotine is why people who want to quit smoking can't quit.[30]

Of course it was not David Kessler who first conceived, cultivated, and coveted the idea that cigarettes were nicotine-delivery devices, that repeated exposure to nicotine would create an addiction in many or most users, or that the cigarette industry was in the business of selling a drug called nicotine. Nor was it the surgeon general. It was the tobacco industry itself. Big Tobacco had gone to great lengths to manipulate nicotine in order to ensure that, while cigarette makers worked to develop a putatively healthier cigarette, the "satisfaction" and "impact" of their cigarettes were not lost.

However guilty the industry was in their efforts to manipulate smokers' experience of the habit, one question ran far deeper than the question of intent, a question that neither Kessler's FDA nor Big Tobacco seem ever to have considered: what exactly was the link between nicotine and the habit of smoking? Despite the strength of the industry's convictions, and despite the depth of their conspiracy to manipulate nicotine for ill purpose, were cigarette makers in fact correct in concluding that cigarettes lead to an addiction because of the drug nicotine? By the end of the twentieth century the belief that cigarettes were addictive and that this was due to a single pharmacological agent was so widely held, and by advocates on both sides of the issue, that it is hard to imagine it could possibly be wrong. Yet there are reasons — indeed, some very compelling reasons — to believe that those conclusions were not just wrong, but profoundly wrong.

Cocaine comes from coca, heroin from poppies, and nicotine from tobacco. The logic is as clear as it is compelling: behind each addiction stands a drug, a pharmacological agent whose physiological effects inflict a dependence on the habitual user. Yet the idea of reducing all drug habits and drug effects down to a single chemical explanation — pharmacologicalism — actually has little evidence to recommend it, even in the case of drugs far more substantial than nicotine. From heroin-using Vietnam vets to coca chewers in Peru to marijuana users in America, most regular consumers of naturally occurring substances either never developed addictions or matured out of them as they and their life circumstances changed. Could the social history of tobacco really be any different? With addiction capturing the public imagination regarding the cigarette habit late in the twentieth century, this was exactly the argument offered: smoking and nicotine do indeed stand apart from other forms of drug use and addiction, given the fact that a greater percentage of those who smoke cigarettes form a habitual attachment to the activity than do users of any other drug substance, including heroin and cocaine. Impressive. Still, the question lingers. Is the high rate of habitual use of cigarettes really determined by the pharmacological actions of nicotine, or might there be a whole other story, a hidden story, behind the rise of the cigarette habit in the twentieth century?

Koop's 1988 surgeon-general report on nicotine addiction concluded with three points: that "cigarettes and other forms of tobacco are addictive," that "nicotine is the drug in tobacco that causes addiction," and that "the pharmacologic and behavioral processes that determine nicotine addiction are similar to those that determine addiction to drugs such as heroin and cocaine."[31] That smokers have at least as much difficulty breaking their "drug habit" as do habitual heroin and cocaine users seems to support the assumption that "the pharmacologic and behavioral processes [of] nicotine . . . are similar to those [of] heroin and cocaine," thus explaining why "nicotine is the drug in tobacco that causes addiction." Under scrutiny, however, this logic leads to a pharmacological puzzle. If nicotine is at least as addictive as heroin and cocaine are said to be, why is it that people do not seek nicotine for casual use? Yes, cocaine comes from coca, heroin from poppies, and nicotine from tobacco, but nicotine is not extracted from tobacco to be bought and sold on the street, nor is it used independently as a recreational drug. Never has a drug deemed so highly addictive by society and science had no history of recreational use in a distilled or natural form. For this reason alone one should be suspicious. Can nicotine really explain why many smokers who would like to quit smoking find that they cannot?

A number of other curious facts encourage further suspicion. For instance, at the very time when smoking began to be redefined in terms of nicotine addiction, during the 1980s and 1990s, smoking-cessation aids containing nicotine became widely available. The nicotine transdermal patch, first approved by the FDA as a prescription drug in 1991, was approved by Kessler's FDA for over-the-counter sale in 1996, as was nicotine gum. This was a peculiar policy decision for an agency that deemed nicotine a highly addictive substance, meaning as it did that anyone wanting to consume nicotine as a drug could now buy it easily and cheaply — and legally — in a purer form. Why didn't nicotine use become a new drug phenomenon, separate from cigarette smoking?

This pharmacological puzzle is clarified somewhat by what happens when people who want to quit smoking are provided a tobacco-free source of nicotine like the nicotine patch. If smokers are dependent on nicotine and the cigarette is simply a way of administering it, one should expect the nicotine patch to free smokers of their urge to light up. What researchers have found, however, is that most smokers who use the nicotine patch to help break the habit do not succeed in breaking it. A study on the effectiveness of "nicotine replacement therapy," published in the journal *Psychopharmacology* in 1992, concluded that the "overall lack of effect [of the patch] on cigarette consumption is perhaps surprising and suggests that in regular smokers the lighting up of a cigarette is generally triggered by cues other than low plasma nicotine levels."[32] Contradicting the notion that the habit is driven by the drug, most patch users in the study continued to smoke while using it, not to mention afterward, thus continuing to consume the carcinogens in cigarette smoke while also obtaining higher body levels of nicotine. Another 1992 study, published in the *Lancet*, used a nicotine nasal spray, a method of drug administration that was predicted to produce better results than the patch or gum because, like smoking, it leads to fast absorption of nicotine into the brain. Nevertheless, only 26 percent of the would-be quitters successfully abstained from smoking while using the spray.[33] Similar results were reported in a review of all the existing studies, published in 2000 by the Office of the Surgeon General.[34] The overall percentage of smokers who successfully abstained was 17.7 for the patch, 22.8 for the nicotine inhaler, 23.7 for nicotine gum, and 30.5 for the nicotine nasal spray.[35]

Even with the most efficacious of methods for nicotine replacement, less than one-third of smokers successfully abstained from smoking even though they were already receiving more than enough nicotine to compensate for their usual smoking. These were individuals, moreover, who wanted to quit smoking and who received other social supports as an adjunct to their external nicotine fix. This further undermines the theory that the smoking habit can be explained solely, or even largely, in terms of the drug nicotine. High levels of nicotine intake, even when administered with fast-acting methods, have not been found to eliminate the desire to smoke.[36] When stripped of the act and experience of smoking tobacco, then, nicotine does not seem to offer effects that would make it a recreational drug of choice. And when administered independent of cigarettes, nicotine does not lead smokers to stop thinking about smoking. Both these findings suggest that non-pharmacological factors must be involved.

Research that looks into what happens when smokers engage in the ritual of smoking with cigarettes that contain little or no nicotine casts further doubt on nicotine's exclusive role in the smoking habit. If the habit is everything and the drug is nothing, one would expect that, at least under blind conditions, smokers would not even notice the absence of the nicotine. By contrast, if the drug is everything and the habit is nothing, smokers should easily discriminate the absence of the drug. For "The role of nicotine in the cigarette habit," a study conducted at the Medical College of Virginia and published in 1945 in *Science*, researchers used a special strain of tobacco that contained very small amounts of nicotine to create two seemingly identical sets of cigarettes.[37] One set contained unadulterated, low-nicotine tobacco; the other contained the same tobacco with nicotine added in, which gave it a level comparable to cigarettes today. Twenty-four smokers received the cigarettes in cartons, starting with cigarettes that contained the raised (or normal) level of nicotine. After some weeks they were unknowingly switched to the low-nicotine cigarettes, then switched back after a month.

Not surprisingly, the smokers showed varying results. A quarter of the smokers experienced no physical or mental change whatsoever; that is, they did not discriminate the near absence of nicotine. Another quarter experienced what was described as a "vague lack in the satisfaction they normally derived from smoking." Only a third experienced a significant loss of satisfaction that persisted the entire time they smoked the low-nicotine cigarettes, an experience that was coupled with withdrawal symptoms, including increased irritability and lowered concentration.

These results suggest that nicotine did play some role in the experience of smoking: some smokers seemed to need it, and some even cheated by smoking some of their own cigarettes. However, these results also indicate that the habit of smoking, independent of nicotine, also played a role in why people found it difficult to quit. Under blind conditions, fifteen of the twenty-four smokers in the study adapted to smoking very-low-nicotine cigarettes, and most of them did so with very little difficulty. Viewed in terms of who might cope better, smokers given cigarettes containing little or no nicotine (like those in the 1945 study) or smokers given nicotine but no cigarettes (like those using the patch), the weight of the evidence falls squarely on the side of the former.

In *The Gentle Art of Smoking*, published in 1954, Alfred Dunhill began by noting, "People smoke more now than ever before; but all too often they only acquire an unthinking habit, and neglect the subtleties of an art both ancient and universal."[38] As Dunhill seemed to suggest, rather than being inherently addictive, cigarettes became nearly so because of how they came to be consumed. They were used in an "unthinking way," Dunhill suggested, assimilated into the ritual activities that connect one day to the next, and to the next. And there was a reason for this: early in the 1900s, the nicotine levels in the tobacco of cigarettes were dramatically higher; as these levels were reduced, cigarettes became milder, and it was largely due to the lower nicotine levels that they came to be smoked in an "unthinking way."

In fact, historically, the idea of boosting nicotine levels actually made little sense. The typical smoker at the end of the twentieth century would have been overwhelmed, if not incapacitated, by the tobacco smoked in the early twentieth, as it had almost three times more nicotine than did the tobacco that filled the average cigarette a century later. This fact hints at an ironic and most extraordinary possibility: the industry's greatest achievement in the twentieth century was not its creation of a potent, nicotine-spiked cigarette, but its earlier and forgotten achievement of producing a very mild one. The creation of a mild and inexpensive cigarette, artificially flavored and sweetened, packaged in a uniform and highly stylized manner — this was the great conspiracy of the tobacco industry in the twentieth century. Or at least it would have been had Big Tobacco fully understood the impact the creation of mild cigarettes would have on the cultivation of the smoking habit.

The German author Wolfgang Schivelbusch described this moment in history in *Tastes of Paradise*, noting that the modern cigarette, as well as the stubborn habit that came with it, was most certainly a product of modernity itself.

In the history of tobacco use the act of smoking accelerates as the smoking process becomes simpler and shorter. Pipe smoking still needs an arsenal of equipment and manipulations before the pipe is already smoked. A small, self-contained procedure is always necessary: cutting the tobacco leaves, filling the pipe, etc. . . .

    With the advent of the cigar at the beginning of the nineteenth century, this elaborate operation fell by the wayside. The product came fully prepared for consumption, needing only to be cut and placed in the mouth, an event that shortened and accelerated the process, and was comparable to the later invention of the wooden match, which reduced the laborious process of striking up a spark to a single instantaneous gesture. . . .

    Half a century after the appearance of the cigar, the acceleration process advanced still further with the cigarette. Like the cigar, it came ready for consumption, yet the time required to finish smoking it was even briefer — quite a substantial innovation. The cigarette was light, short, and quick, in the physical as well as the temporal and pharmacological sense of the word. A "smoke," as this new informal unit of time is called, is as different from the time it takes to smoke a cigar as the velocity of a mail coach is from that of an automobile. The cigarette embodied a concept of time utterly different from that of the cigar.[39]

The modern cigarette was designed not for occasional use, the way cigars and pipe tobacco were (and are) typically experienced, but for regular use throughout the day. About one billion cigarettes were sold in the United States in 1885; a century later, when the U.S. population was five times larger, 600 times as many cigarettes were sold annually. (In 1981, 4.5 trillion cigarettes were sold worldwide. In the same year U.S. cigarette makers spent $1 billion on advertising).[40] The mass-produced cigarette also led to smokes cheap enough that smoking spread beyond the leisure class, a universality that lasted until nearly the end of the twentieth century, when, like other fallen angels of the twentieth century, smoking became a phenomenon involving primarily the young and the lower classes. Cigarettes became an integral part of twentieth-century America as well. They were viewed as instrumental in the world wars, for example, and granted honors of which they would be stripped later on. "The cigarette is every soldier's best friend, for the solace it brings, for the relief from hunger and fatigue it provides, for the relaxation it encourages, for the courage it summons when the fighting gets thick and hard," wrote Richard Klein in *Cigarettes Are Sublime*.[41]

The strength or potency of tobacco having been negatively correlated in the twentieth century with the rise of the smoking habit suggests that the habit involves more than just the drug nicotine. The problem appears to be not so much pharmacological as one of how, as smoking filters into the activities of daily life, it becomes part of it. Once this happens, giving up smoking results, at least for a time, in a diminished quality of life. "Smokers smoke to relax, to concentrate, to handle anxiety, stress and difficult interpersonal situations, as a way of taking a break during the day, as a social lubricant, etc.," wrote Daniel Shapiro in *Public Affairs Quarterly* in 1994.

> Smoking is thus linked with a lot of different situations, moods and emotional states. Furthermore, smoking is well *integrated* into smokers' lives. Though most smokers smoke on a fairly continual basis, smokers aren't, for the most part, prevented from carrying out normal life activities: rather, they weave smoking into those activities. This is partly for social reasons . . . and perhaps partly for pharmacological reasons — the effects of nicotine are mild and subtle enough that it can be used nondisruptively in many situations. Now because smoking is so well-integrated into smokers' lives, it will be difficult to give up: no central change in people's lives is easily achieved.[42]

Commissioner Kessler had noted S. J. Green's outline of the three reasons why people smoked — sensory rewards, psychosocial rewards, and pharmacological rewards—but he ignored the first two. Even the cigarette industry did not believe, at least not prior to their embrace of the nicotine-addiction theory, that a drug was the only factor in why people smoked or had difficulty quitting. Neither did the surgeons general who wrote on tobacco prior to C. Everett Koop and his 1988 report on nicotine addiction.

Although nicotine had been isolated as a drug more than a century before, scientists and public officials did not really begin to characterize nicotine as an addictive drug until the 1980s. *Smoking: A Behavioral Analysis*, a detailed report on the smoking habit published in 1971, did not even include nicotine in its index.[43] Twenty-four years prior to Koop's 1988 report, the Office of the Surgeon General had first attempted to describe the habit of smoking in *Characterization of the Tobacco Habit*. While it declared without reservation that smoking was indeed a health hazard, the 1964 report lacked the focus on nicotine that overtook later surgeon-general reports, instead concluding, "The habitual use of tobacco is related primarily to psychological and social drives." The "pharmacological actions of nicotine on the central nervous system" were said to play only a secondary role, reinforcing the psychological and social aspects of cigarette smoking via "the pharmacological actions of nicotine on the central nervous system." The report also emphasized, "The tobacco habit should be characterized as an habituation rather than an addiction. . . . Nicotine substitutes or supplementary medications have not been proven to be of major benefit in breaking the habit."[44]

The 1964 report did attempt to characterize the pharmacology of nicotine, but continued in the same moderate vein. "The pharmacological effects of nicotine at dosage levels absorbed from smoking (1–2 mg per inhaled cigarette) are comparatively small. . . . The predominant actions are central stimulation and/or tranquilization which vary with the individual, transient hyperpnoea, peripheral vasoconstriction usually associated with a rise in systolic pressure, suppression of appetite, stimulation of peristalsis and, with larger doses, nausea of central origin which may be associated with vomiting."

In 1981 Surgeon General Julius B. Richmond prepared another report on the subject, *The Health Consequences of Smoking: The Changing Cigarette*. Paralleling the changes taking place within the cigarette industry as well as in American attitudes toward drugs and addiction, the report placed greater emphasis on pharmacological factors while deemphasizing nonpharmacological ones. In a chapter on the behavioral aspects of smoking, for example, it stated, "Nicotine appears to be the primary pharmacological reinforcer in tobacco, but other pharmacological and psychosocial factors may also contribute a reinforcing effect." The 1981 report also noted, "Rigorous comparative behavioral studies involving animals are needed to provide comprehensive, experimentally valid results on behavioral aspects of smoking. . . . Laboratory techniques developed for study of opioids and alcohol should be adapted for studies of tolerance and dependence on nicotine."[45]

Kessler and his team took great interest in the subsequent use of animal studies to assess the pharmacological roots of the smoking habit. Contained within this interest, however, was the same prejudice that promoted the idea that the smoking habit flowed from the direct pharmacological impact of a drug. If the "addictiveness" of a drug was determined by its chemistry and pharmacology, in other words, then the addictiveness of a drug like nicotine could be isolated once and for all in the laboratory. Accordingly, studies in which lab animals were provided the opportunity to self-administer a drug were of special interest in addiction research, since they offered a pure context in which to assess such raw addictiveness. As Kessler wrote in *A Question of Intent*, "Self administration is a classic characteristic of an addictive substance."[46] This assumption also explains why the nicotine self-administration studies by the two Philip Morris researchers, DeNoble and Mele, were of such significance to Kessler, suggesting as they did that the company had measured and thus was aware of nicotine's "addictiveness." After he read the article DeNoble and Mele had submitted to *Psychopharmacology* (later suppressed by Philip Morris), Kessler recalled, "I knew we had a bombshell."[47]

In his 1994 testimony to the House Subcommittee on the Regulation of Tobacco Products, as well as in *A Question of Intent*, Kessler insisted that "self-administration studies have shown that nicotine is addictive."[48] Even if animal studies actually were capable of measuring and establishing an inherent addictiveness of a drug that was applicable to most or all people, this statement would still be misguided.[49] Studies examining nicotine did show that laboratory animals would, under certain, contrived laboratory environments, respond for nicotine. The key caveat, ignored by Kessler and other public-health advocates, however, was that animals responded much less vigorously for nicotine than they did for drugs regularly bought and sold on the street and at the pharmacy. The psychostimulants (cocaine, amphetamine, Ritalin), the opiates (morphine, heroin, Oxycontin), and the barbiturates (Seconal) were all more readily administered by animals than was nicotine.

And this was not new information. In a 1973 essay, "Further observations on nicotine as the reinforcing agent in smoking," Murray Jarvik, a prominent psychopharmacologist hailing from the UCLA School of Medicine, had concluded that monkeys in the laboratory were best characterized as reluctant smokers.[50] Furthermore, animals did not typically self-administer nicotine via cigarette smoke unless exposed to an earlier period of forced consumption. Similar results have been reported in studies examining nicotine self-administration independent of smoking. In one of the earliest such studies — "Nicotine self-administration in monkeys," from the 1967 *Annals of the New York Academy of Sciences* — monkeys were given the opportunity to self-administer nicotine intravenously after several days of hourly, involuntary infusions of the drug; while some animals did later respond for nicotine, even they consumed the drug in a manner that was slow and inconsistent.[51] Lab animals that self-administered nicotine in this and later studies were never found to self-administer the drug in a manner as reliable or as robust as for psychostimulants (including Ritalin), opiates, or barbiturates, as well as for various other drugs, foods, and activities.

Laboratory research has revealed much about the nature of addiction, but it has never confirmed that addiction occurs solely or even largely because of the pharmacological actions of a drug. Ironically, the very research that purportedly revealed the pharmacological basis of addiction actually revealed the futility of such a notion, pointing instead to the complexities of drug habits that exist in the real world. If the cigarette habit seemed like a pharmacological puzzle, the answer could be found not in the drug that tobacco contained but in the social and historical contexts in which the puzzle emerged in the twentieth century.

The 1990s, when industry insiders stepped forward and thousands of internal documents were liberated from company files, were clearly a watershed moment in the history of Big Tobacco. By the end of the twentieth century, much had changed in the nation's attitudes toward smoking. Although it remained an act of independence and rebellion for adolescents, it was viewed as a dirty habit by a vast and increasing majority of Americans, a majority that had become defiantly nonsmoking. If not against the law, smoking was at least against the public health and thus was banned in more and more public places and in the workplace. Meanwhile, with car ashtrays being replaced with giant cupholders, America began changing from a nation of habitual smokers to a nation of habitual overeaters. In 2001 the Office of the Surgeon General released a damning report, not on smoking, but on the growing problem of obesity in America.[52] From 1980 to 1999, as smoking declined, obesity among adults doubled. The report also noted that obesity would rival tobacco in the twenty-first century as the leading cause of illness and death; already in 1999, about 300,000 American deaths per year could be attributed to overeating and obesity, while about 400,000 deaths per year were attributed to cigarette smoking. Fortunately for McDonald's, hamburger does not contain a psychoactive drug.

Not all adult smokers stopped smoking during the 1990s, however, although fewer people were starting to smoke and many millions had quit. Even cigarette makers showed a marked change in their public behavior, admitting late in the 1990s to much of what they had steadfastly denied throughout the century. These confessions began in 1997 when the Liggett Group, the smallest of the six American tobacco companies, announced, "We at Liggett . . . know and acknowledge that, as the Surgeon General, the Food and Drug Administration, and respected medical researchers have found, nicotine is addictive." What had been known privately was now said publicly, and the industry found it could no longer stand in denial. And, as suggested by the subtitle of Kessler's book—"A Great American Battle with a Deadly Industry"—the battle over smoking came to be viewed as a classic fight between good and evil.

As a result, smokers found themselves caught in the middle, left literally out in the cold. In the quest to pin the smoking habit on a drug manipulated by a "nicotine industry," few had paused to ask not only whether depicting nicotine as highly addictive was justified but also whether it was wise. Redefining smoking not as a behavioral habit but as a pharmacological addiction may sound like good public policy, but it works against the public health when it teaches people that it is impossible to quit. Indeed, instead of having the intended effect of steering potential smokers—that is, children—away from cigarettes, demonizing cigarettes via nicotine reinforced smokers' feelings of pharmacological enslavement and undermined their will to quit. "Should we be surprised that a theory like this has social effects?" asked John Leo in *U.S. News and World Report*.[53] Probably not. Smokers repeatedly testify that giving up the habit depends greatly on their will to quit, and it is hard to imagine how the will of smokers is strengthened by images of overpowering addiction. "If Dr. Kessler wants people to try to quit smoking," a Philip Morris attorney once remarked, "he ought to tell them to try, because they can quit, and not characterize them as addicts doomed to fail."[54] Coming from Big Tobacco, this sounds like a typical industry smokescreen — but it is most certainly true. As unpleasant as the experience of quitting might be, smoking does not appear to be the irreversible habit it was made out to be.

At the end of the twentieth century there were about fifty million living Americans who had once smoked but no longer did, and at least half of all Americans who had ever smoked no longer did. A 1994 survey of "drug abuse" conducted by the National Institute on Drug Abuse (NIDA) showed that although 73 percent of respondents reported smoking cigarettes at some time, only 29 percent reported that they still smoked (that is, had smoked in the previous month).[55] It thus seems a bit duplicitous to complain, as Jeffrey Klein did in *Mother Jones*, that nicotine is irreversibly addictive, on the one hand, and that Big Tobacco works vigilantly to recruit young smokers to replace "the 1.3 million Americans" who quit smoking each year, on the other.[56] If nicotine is so addictive, even so addictive that it is best characterized as a disease of addiction, how is it that most smokers eventually found it within themselves to quit, about 90 percent of whom did so without any form of pharmacological aid?[57]

Furthermore, if nicotine produces an addiction disease, how can it be that a larger percentage of smokers have quit in recent decades? A survey in 1975 showed that most smokers wanted to quit and that about a third succeeded in doing so for at least one full year. By the end of the twentieth century this number had reached 50 percent.[58] This period of growing success in giving up the habit can be explained by a variety of factors, from new restrictions on smoking, to concerns over second-hand smoke, to higher cigarette prices, to growing social stigmas, to a greater awareness of smoking's effects on one's health. The notion that chronic exposure to nicotine creates a brain disease that makes the habit nearly impossible to break, by contrast, explains very little. For both Kessler and Big Tobacco, the relationship between smoking and addiction should not be a moveable feast; yet, that is exactly what it had become in late-twentieth-century America.

The concept of addiction received a lot of wear and tear in the twentieth century and was rather ragged by century's end.[59] As a result, the medical and scientific community embraced a new term, *dependence*, as a substitute for *addiction*. The concept of addiction was considered a loose and ambiguous term of lay culture, while dependence was introduced as a more satisfactory concept, defined increasingly in biological terms.[60] The fourth edition of the American Psychiatric Association's *Diagnostic and Statistical Manual of Mental Disorders*, for example, defined drug habits as "substance dependence," with various criteria for making a diagnosis, including continued use of the drug despite its harm, tolerance to the drug, withdrawal, and a persistent desire to use the drug.[61] A quote from Steven Hyman, a director of the National Institute of Mental Health, illustrates the concept in use: "Repeated doses of addictive drugs — opiates, cocaine, and amphetamines — cause drug dependence and, afterwards, withdrawal. . . . Dependence on drugs of abuse develops only when the drug is administered in sufficiently large doses, at high enough frequencies, and over a long enough period of time."[62]

Cigarette smoking in the 1980s and 1990s thus came to be defined in psychopharmacology and medicine as a matter of drug dependence rather than drug addiction. Substituting one word for another hardly clarified the situation. In terms of cigarette smoking, addiction was a useful concept, as was dependence. What was needed was not the substitution of one concept for the other, but a clarification of how each concept could be used effectively. Jerome Jaffe, a past director of NIDA, suggested just such a system of classification, maintaining both the concept of addiction and dependence, as well as several others. Canadian addiction researcher Bruce Alexander later elaborated on this system.[63]

Both Jaffe and Alexander began with the idea that, for different individuals or for individuals at different points in their lives, drug use varies along "a continuum of involvement." Placing "abstinence" at one end and full-blown "addiction" at the other, Alexander outlined a total of seven levels of involvement. At the second level, after abstinence, is experimental use, which he defined as any fleeting relationship with a drug taken to experience its effects. Many individuals have experimented with drugs like LSD and marijuana, for example, wanting to know what it is like. Researchers have found this to be a useful category, demonstrating for instance that adolescents who have experimented with marijuana are, on average, better adjusted psychologically and socially than those who have never smoked it, while those who used heavily are less well adjusted.[64]

At the third level of involvement is circumstantial use, which, according to Alexander, differs from experimental use in that it applies to the instrumental use of a drug from time to time, such as taking opiate analgesics for an injury or taking Valium occasionally for anxiety. Circumstantial use is sporadic but ongoing, and thus represents a greater involvement with a drug than would experimental use. The fourth level of involvement is casual use, a good example of which is alcohol consumption in contemporary America. While some people will experiment with a drug and then never use it again, others will continue to use it for a longer period, if only intermittently. A casual user of cocaine while in college, for example, would used it on occasion, say, during the weekend or at parties.

Based on extensive interviews with college students who were asked to categorize their patterns of drug use, Alexander found it useful to distinguish casual use from a fifth level of involvement that he called regular use. The latter signifies what might be defined as a more predictable or repetitive form of drug use, such as having a drink or joint after work; the tradition of drinking wine with meals falls into this category, although it is often consumed more as a food than a drug. The categories of casual and regular use uphold a meaningful distinction, since not all casual use is frequent enough to be considered regular use. The 1990 NIDA "Household survey of drug abuse," for example, found that of those who had used cocaine in the last year, only about one-third reported using the drug twelve or more times a year, and only about one in ten reported using cocaine once a week or more.[65] The vast majority of users were, in other words, casual users rather than regular users. Denise Kandel and colleagues reported similar findings a few years earlier in Nicholas Kozel's and Edgar Adams's *Cocaine Use in America*: "Cocaine use appears to be experimental in nature and to involve few experiences for a substantial portion of those who report any lifetime experience with the drug. One-half (53 percent) of the male users and two-thirds (67 percent) of the female users have used cocaine less than 10 times in their lives; 34 and 28 percent, respectively, have used 10 to 99 times, 9 and 3 percent have used 100 to 999 times, 3 and 2 percent have used 1,000 or more times."[66]

Still, not all drug involvements are so relaxed. Sometimes people acquire a habitual attachment to a drug or drug-containing substance, so much so that they find it difficult not to use, or to stop. At the same time, however, they might not experience any discomfort or suffer any life difficulties during their use of it. Both Alexander and Jaffe classify this sixth level of involvement as dependence. Many habitual coffee (and tea and cola) drinkers and cigarette smokers fit into this category, as do some habitual marijuana smokers and alcohol drinkers. (Amazonian coca chewers do not fit into this category, but qualify instead as regular users.)

Dependence can apply to almost any drug, as was evident in the case of a physician who for five years injected high-grade opiates three to five times daily.[67] Despite his dependence on the drug, he maintained both a successful medical practice and a marriage, all the while hiding his habit from everyone who knew him. He had no medical problems and was said to have a very supportive family. What he seemed to suffer from most was his shame about the habit, which led him to seek treatment.[68]

A similar case of harmless dependence involved a prim and proper eighty-year-old English woman who regularly used cocaine. As reported in 1989 by two British psychiatrists, her habit first formed after having been prescribed cocaine in solution in 1934. She had been twenty-five-years old at the time and diagnosed with an allergy to horses. After that, she took the nose drops almost every day for fifty-five years, for a grand total of approximately 5.5 kilograms of pure cocaine, with occasional breaks of no more than seven days. Although she had asked for the dosage to be increased over the period of use, "She [denied] any feelings of euphoria or increased energy after taking the cocaine nor any depression or craving for cocaine when her supplies run out, although she [had] taken aspirin as a substitute."[69] In fact, despite her chronic use, the woman showed no signs of physical, social, or psychological problems and had outlived several ear, nose, and throat specialists that she had consulted for the allergy over the years.

A person's dependence can also evolve into an addiction, and vice versa. However, according to both Jaffe and Alexander, for a pattern of drug use to qualify as an addiction there must also be a drama to their drug use — a drama produced by an overwhelming involvement with the drug. That is, for drug use to constitute an addiction, it must become an activity so all-consuming that it disrupts the normal functioning of a person's life. This definition has the virtue of conforming to the everyday meaning of addiction, wherein the label "addict" is applied to someone who has essentially turned their life over to drug use (a definition that would rarely, if ever, apply to the traditional use of coca). Because habitual coffee drinking and tobacco smoking are relatively inexpensive and do not lead to any real degree of intoxication, they are unlikely to evolve into addictions.

Addiction is not just about the individual, however. The physician who injected pharmaceutical-grade opiates for five years and the woman who snorted cocaine nasal drops for fifty-five years were relatively unlikely to become addicts for two important reasons: they had stable and satisfying lives as well as a reliable source of inexpensive drugs. Drug use was less likely to overwhelm their lives, in other words, because their lives were already filled with other meaningful activities. Their drug habits were also not going to push them into criminality, since they had an inexpensive source of drugs.

Furthermore, according to this framework of drug use, addiction is defined as a pattern of drug use, not as a fixed characteristic of the drug user. One is reminded of the Vietnam vets who were habitual opiate users while serving but gave up the habit on returning home. Also noteworthy are longitudinal studies of cocaine use, which have consistently found that most habitual cocaine users eventually develop decreasing involvements with the drug, often ending in abstinence.[70]

With regard to the problem of cigarettes and addiction, both Jaffe's and Alexander's taxonomies of drug-use patterns suggest most smokers would be classified as drug dependent. Because smokers report a compulsive need to smoke, especially in certain situations, and because they report a sense of satisfaction on smoking after a period of abstinence, such as in the morning or after a long flight, they cannot be defined as regular users. But neither are they addicts. As the 1964 surgeon-general report concluded, using the term *habituation* instead of *dependence*, "The tobacco habit should be characterized as an habituation rather than an addiction."[71]

As an example of drug dependence, smoking is, however, tangled up with a ritual that becomes a stubborn habit of its own and is quite difficult to break regardless of nicotine. Although nicotine has been implicated in smoking in an attempt to explain why it was a harder habit to quit than other drugs, might not the stubbornness of the habit simply reflect the manner in which cigarettes are smoked? The regular smoker engages in the activity under a wide array circumstances — when bored, after eating, when driving — and across a variety of settings — when at home, work, or in the car. The environmental cues that elicit the urge are considerably more ubiquitous for smokers than for most other forms of drug use, and thus the degree to which smoking becomes central to one's own identity is considerable. The problem of cigarettes and addiction is thus a question of influence: to what extent is smoking difficult to stop because of a physical dependence, and to what extent is it because of the act — that is, the habit — of smoking itself, regardless of any drug?

The distinction between smoking as an addiction to a psychoactive substance versus smoking as a habitual coping ritual began to be addressed in the 1980s by researchers looking at what factors best predicted whether a smoker would succeed in quitting. A 1998 NIDA report on nicotine addiction stated, "Chronic exposure to nicotine results in addiction. Research is just beginning to document all of the neurological changes that accompany the development and maintenance of nicotine addiction."[72] This implies that smoking is an addiction, that the addiction resides as a biological state in the brain, and that this state is the result of chronic exposure to nicotine. The statement thus suggests three testable hypotheses: Do heavier smokers have greater difficulty quitting? Do people who have smoked for longer periods have more difficulty quitting? And, since nicotine withdrawal and craving for nicotine are symptoms of nicotine dependence, are smokers who experience the most intense withdrawal symptoms less likely to quit successfully?

There is little in the literature on smoking to support any of these hypotheses. In the study in which smokers were blindly given low-nicotine cigarettes, for example, the heaviest smoker of all, a gentleman who smoked three packs daily, was among those in the group who experienced no ill effects while smoking the low-nicotine cigarettes. More recent studies also found that whether the smoker was a light or heavy smoker, or had smoked for the better part of their life, predicted little in terms of success versus relapse. In fact, studies do not even show a link between craving and the likelihood of relapse. For example, relapse among smokers is not predicted by the severity of their physical withdrawal from nicotine.[73] The majority of relapses occur after acute physical withdrawal has come and gone, which usually takes from one to three weeks. As for craving, a 1986 study, coauthored by NIDA's Jack Henningfield, a strong proponent of the nicotine-addiction theory, failed to find a significant link even between craving and smoking. This 1986 study looked at the effect of nicotine gum on smoking, finding that although the gum decreased smoking to some extent, this decrease was not correlated with a decrease in smokers' self-reported craving for cigarettes — a result consistent with the entire body of nicotine-therapy literature.[74]

These results cannot be explained by the theory that habitual smoking alters the brain such that a person becomes literally dependent on nicotine. Whatever differences may be found in certain brain areas of smokers compared to nonsmokers, researchers still need to establish a connection between these differences and meaningful aspects of smoking, including one's ability to quit, which they repeatedly fail to do.[75] Moreover, the neurophysiological changes resulting from nicotine exposure do not differ between those who do and do not successfully quit smoking. Those who have the easiest time quitting are psychologically, not biologically, distinct; that is, psychological characteristics that exist prior to the individual acquiring the habit have proved to be better, if still rather poor, predictors of successful quitting. Even the 1988 surgeon-general report and the American Psychiatric Association concede that the difficulties smokers experience when attempting to quit are specific to the individual's psychological make-up, not the degree to which a person is "physically dependent" on nicotine. These individuals are more likely to show a wide variety of coping skills, they are more secure, they have a greater desire to quit, they have a greater sense of self-determination, and they are more optimistic about their ability to quit.[76]

Note that these personal attributes and attitudes might easily be influenced, albeit negatively, by the message that smoking is a brain disease caused merely by exposure to nicotine. By tearing down people's sense of choice and responsibility for their drug use, public-health advocates like David Kessler risked promoting the very habit they so decried. Moving beyond the good and evil of pharmacologicalism, those interested in smoking and health might have instead looked to the broader context in which smoking acquired such significance in people's lives in the twentieth century, especially in light of Kessler's and the FDA's failure to do what they sought out to do, that is, to obtain jurisdiction over Big Tobacco.

Nicotine is a drug, but not a demon drug. Smoking is a habitual activity that bombards the senses, but this habit is not a disease. Richard Kluger, author of the Pulitzer-Prize–winning history of the cigarette industry, *Ashes to Ashes*, explains it well:

Whatever its utility otherwise, smoking is essentially a physical and highly sensual experience. Among the senses, that of touch is most apparent. Tactility begins with the snug fit of the pack in the palm, followed by all the little rituals of crackling off the wrapper, neatly tearing open the pack, surgically extracting the first snow-white tube, percussively tapping its tobacco end against the wrist or any convenient flat surface, deftly inserting it between barely parted lips, and lighting it with the absolute minimum of pyrotechnics — the quintessence of cool. It is, of course, the perfect plaything for nervous hands that cling to it like an anchor, fondle it, and wave it about as a prop to enhance one's words or dramatize one's feelings. Add, then, its raptures to the taste (bitter-sweet, acrid, tingling), the smell (an autumnal pungence, an organic mellowness), the feel (the small, sharp hit at the back of the throat, teasing raspy and enlivening on the way down, the sudden fullness and completeness deep within, the final swift, satisfying surge of emission), and the sight (the little blue-grey cloud proclaiming one's Lebensraum and, between puffs, the lazy, sinuous ribbon wafting upward, signalling that the smoker exists). Here, for the habitué is the very meaning of instant gratification.[77]

Part Two **Earlier Times**

Nothing that grows from the ground is evil.
—Stephen Gaghan, *Traffik*

I f one stops for a moment to glance back to a time a century or so ago — a time before drugs were the subject of so much confusion and contro-versy — one finds four notable conditions: there was a general absence of drug prohibitions; alcohol, the drug that became the "nondrug" drug of choice in the latter part of the twentieth century, was scapegoated as a menace spirit responsible for most of society's ills; the jailhouse epidemic of the late twentieth century was nonexistent; and the public had embraced many of today's most demonized substances, including those derived from coca, poppies, and cannabis. Morphine, a drug derived from opium sap extracted from living poppy plants, was converted to "Heroin" and mar-keted by Bayer Pharmaceuticals as a cure for morphine addiction; cocaine, a drug concentrate derived from the coca plant, was sold in wines and tonics such as Coca-Cola; and marijuana, derived from the hemp plant, was avail-able as a tincture of cannabis, sold by Parke Davis and Company. Popular patent medicines at the time could contain any of these natural substances, which helps explain their ubiquity at the end of the nineteenth century. In 1885 Parke Davis alone had fifteen coca-related products. One of their ad-vertisements, directed at physicians, hailed: "An enumeration of the diseases in which coca and cocaine have been found of service would include a category of almost all the maladies that flesh is heir to."[1] With claims like these, sales of patent medicines in the United States grew from $3.5 million in 1859 to about $100 million in 1904.[2]

While the public was being convinced that the "unrestricted manufacture and sale of ardent spirits is almost the sole cause of all the suffering, the poverty, and the crime to be found in the country," public sentiment regarding opium, cocaine, and cannabis remained comparably soft at the end of the nineteenth century.[3] These organic substances were not just available and put to regular use, they were also consumed largely by a different crowd than was alcohol. The bourgeoisie had not yet any Seconal, Valium, or Prozac to ease their domestic angst or soothe their psychological woes, but they had their tinctures of opium, cocaine, and cannabis, which could do much the same. "The typical opiate addict [at the end of the nineteenth century] was a 30 to 50-year old white woman who functioned well and was adjusted to her life as a wife and mother," noted one drug scholar. "She bought opium or morphine legally at the local store, used it orally, and caused few, if any, social problems."[4]

As this historical snapshot suggests, the perception of "drugs" in America would go through a radical transformation by the end of the twentieth century. Science and wisdom would prevail over pseudoscience and myth, angels would be sorted out from the demons, and a rational system of drug control would be put into place. Or so the story went.

In fact, at the center of the new scientific wisdom remained a firm belief in the magicalism of millennia past. As a drug ideology derived from the eternal notion that psychoactive compounds contain a unique spirit or essence, the cult of pharmacology legitimized the belief that these spirits bypass all social conditioning of the mind and by themselves transform human thought and action. Unlike other worldly modes of influence on mind and human experience, and despite many real advances in the pharmacological sciences in the twentieth century, psychoactive substances continued to be treated in the main as spirits that could enter into the body and take possession of it. Yes, soul was translated into mind, and spirit was translated into biochemistry, giving the appearance that science and medicine had done away with the myths surrounding what had come to be understood as "drugs." Drugs were not demythologized, however, but rather remythologized. Psychobabble and biobabble replaced magical explanations of drug action, creating what had become by the end of the century a new, molecular pharmacologicalism.[5] These modes of explanation were then used to forge a modern pseudoscience of good and bad drugs, enforced via a differential prohibition of angels (like Ritalin) and demons (like cocaine). The "rational" science of drugs, in other words, carried myth along with it; it was itself framed and motivated by myth — a myth of angels and demons.

At the center of the spirit world of pharmacologicalism, both ancient and modern, lies the poppy. From it comes opium and its alkaloid derivatives, the opiates, including morphine, codeine, and with a bit of extra chemical manipulation, diacetylmorphine (heroin). The poppy plant thus also stands at the center of political pharmacology, with opiate addiction being the classical image of pharmacological possession. In the West it came to be believed that simply by virtue of repeated use, the opiates could and would take possession of a person, leading to the now notorious drug addict. "Because opium is one of the most addictive and debilitating substances on earth," writes Barbara Hodgson in *Opium: A Portrait of the Heavenly Demon*, "the opium addict — that is, the person dependent upon or habituated to opium — has been called slave, fiend and ghost."[6] According to pharmacological science, from which such misleading statements derive, the opiates do not just interact with mind and body, they join with it by mimicking the brain's natural pleasure molecules and then causing the brain to stop producing them. Such pharmacologically based outsourcing of biochemical processes leads inevitably to drug dependence, with only one route of escape: the ingestion of more opiates. In short, consumption of opiates creates a physiological need that, if unmet, causes the addict to experience overwhelming and perhaps life-threatening withdrawal; this withdrawal strips the addict of self-control, forcing him or her to do whatever is necessary to score again. This is the core myth of pharmacologicalism as it applies to addiction, and there is surprising little evidence to support it.

Consider the nineteenth-century physician, William Stewart Halsted.

In 1890 William Halsted was appointed the first surgeon-in-chief at Johns Hopkins Hospital and became one of the first faculty members of the prestigious Johns Hopkins Medical School. An official biography of Halsted offered by Johns Hopkins University summarized his outstanding career: born in New York City, he earned his bachelor degree from Yale University in 1874 and his medical degree from the Columbia University College of Physicians and Surgeons in 1877. He served as a medical intern at Bellevue Hospital from 1876 to 1877 and as a physician at New York Hospital from 1877 to 1878. He then traveled to Europe to study in Austria and Germany, which he did for nearly three years. On returning, Halsted entered private practice in New York, where he held various positions at local hospitals, earning a reputation as a skilled surgeon and diagnostician, as well as a developer of creative, new medical techniques. In 1884, for instance, he described a procedure in which cocaine was injected into a nerve to produce anesthesia in the area sensitized by the nerve, marking the advent of local anesthesia.[7]

In 1886 the physician William Henry Welch, one of the founders of the Johns Hopkins Medical School, invited Halsted to come to Baltimore, home of Johns Hopkins, to do research in a newly established pathological laboratory. Halsted accepted. In collaboration with others, he refined various new surgical techniques, some of which transformed the practice of surgery, making it at once safer and more effective. For example, in 1890, the year he was appointed surgeon-in-chief of the Johns Hopkins Hospital, Halsted introduced the use of rubber gloves. In 1892 he became the first professor of surgery at Johns Hopkins. During his more than thirty-year tenure there, which lasted until his death in 1922, Halsted organized new fields of medicine, including orthopaedics, otolaryngology, and urology. He was also an effective teacher whose students went on to make their own significant advances in medical teaching and practice.

In short, Halsted was one of the greatest of surgeons in American history, perhaps even the father of modern surgery.[8] But the Johns Hopkins biography leaves out one interesting detail: for most of his adult life, William Stewart Halsted was a habitual morphine user.

William Welch, John Shaw Billings, and Daniel Coit Gilman founded Johns Hopkins Hospital in 1889 and the medical school four years later.[9] Halsted was the first of two to be appointed to the new medical institution. The other was William Osler, whose secret history of Johns Hopkins Hospital indicated that both he and Welch knew of Halsted's morphine dependence.

Osler had asked that his little black book containing the "inner history" of the hospital not be opened until the hospital's hundredth anniversary, in 1989. After his death, however, his literary executor decided otherwise, and the history was instead opened fifty years after Osler's death, in 1969, at which time Halsted's dependence on morphine came to light.

It was first acknowledged publicly in a report published in the *Journal of the American Medical Association* (*JAMA*).[10] The article described how Halsted's dependence had its roots in his experimentation with cocaine, which he and a few other physicians had tried on themselves during their surgical research with the drug. Halsted must have taken a liking to the drug's effects, for he quickly developed a stubborn habit. "A confused and unworthy period of medical practice ensued," noted the author of the *JAMA* article, Wilder Penfield. "Finally he vanished from the world he had known. Months later he returned to New York but, somehow, the brilliant and gay extrovert seemed brilliant and gay no longer."[11] To free Halsted of his cocaine use, William Welch, Halsted's closest friend even before his move to Johns Hopkins, convinced him to go on a long sail, casting him off the shores of his drug dependence, or at least his drug supply.

Halsted's early biographers claimed that at that point he was cured of his addiction, having used the same great personal strength to conquer his cocaine habit as he did later to build his overwhelmingly successful career in medicine.[12] In truth, the vacation treatment failed completely: Halsted "cured" his cocaine habit only by replacing it with morphine. Halsted turned to morphine while he was still in New York, at the age of thirty-four, before his departure to Baltimore. Welch's invitation, asking Halsted to come to Baltimore in 1886, was thus a tentative one. Osler wrote in his secret history that it was not until Halsted proved "an immediate success" that he was asked to join formally the hospital staff. "When we recommended him as full surgeon to the Hospital in 1890, I believed, and Welch did too, that he was no longer addicted to morphia. He had worked so well and so energetically that it did not seem possible that he could take the drug and do so much."[13] In fact, Halsted had not stopped his daily morphine injections. "About six months after the full position had been given, I saw him in a severe chill and this was the first intimation I had that he was still taking morphia. Subsequently I had many talks about it and gained his full confidence. He had never been able to reduce the amount to less than three grains daily [1 grain = 60 milligrams]; on this he could do his work comfortably and maintain his excellent physical vigour (for he was a very muscular fellow). I do not think that anyone suspected him, not even Welch."[14]

Everything that is known about Halsted suggests that until the day he died, in 1922, at the age of seventy, he was in good health, still highly esteemed as a surgeon, and "probably addicted, until the end."[15]

According to Bruce Alexander's model, while Halsted remained reliant on morphine into old age, he was not in fact an addict. Like the eighty-year-old English woman who snorted cocaine for fifty-five years yet showed no signs of physical, social, or psychological injury, Halsted also failed to show any evidence that his continuous morphine use harmed his career or family life in any way. Indeed, the very absence of such evidence kept those who worked with Halsted convinced that he was free of pharmacological possession (although his wife of thirty-two years most certainly knew of his continued use). Also analogous to the eighty-year-old cocaine user, Halsted had easy access to an inexpensive source of a high-grade drug, which kept his use of "one of the most addictive and debilitating substances on earth" from being just that.

Cases of dependence like Halsted's are less widely known today not because they are rare but because they are typically concealed. This is due in part to the fact that the label of "addiction" casts a shadow over the individual and his or her family, not to mention employer and friends. But it is also due to the fact that such a life seems paradoxical: it fails to conform to the myth of opiates as inherently addictive and debilitating.[16]

And yet there have been many such cases. Another notable case involving a physician's dependence on morphine was that of "Dr. X," which was first reported in the *Stanford Medical Bulletin* in 1942.[17] At the time of the report, Dr. X was eighty-four years old, had been retired for three years, and had been dependent on opiates for sixty-two years. As a twenty-two-year-old medical student, he had come down with a bad cold that was treated with Scott's Emulsion, a popular medicine of the day that was fortified with a good quantity of morphine. Dr. X took the formula several times daily and was on the mend six months later. When he re-entered medical school, he had only one remaining problem: whenever he failed to take his "medicine," he found he had a craving for it; after a full day without the drug, he would experience nervousness, sleeplessness, and nausea. By contrast, when he took the drug he felt neither high nor drugged, but rather physically and mentally charged, able to "concentrate upon [his] work to a remarkable degree."[18] Facing this situation, Dr. X kept taking morphine twice daily, without worry, and finished medical school among the top students in the class. The author of the 1942 case report, Windsor C. Cutting, noted, "He found that his addiction caused him little inconvenience. . . . Sometimes he went for a few days, or even weeks, without the drug, but then 'suddenly the overpowering desire would come.'"[19] At the time the case report was published, Dr. X was still injecting 150 milligrams of morphine daily. The report concludes, based on physical and mental examinations of the physician, that after sixty-two years of use he was in very good health, especially for an eighty-four-year-old man. "The evidence of damage is surprisingly slight, as regards both physical and mental functions. . . . The morphine has always been obtained without undue economic complications, make the condition one of socially uncomplicated, pure morphinism."[20]

Of course, physicians are not the only individuals to become habituated to opiates while showing few or none of the debilitating effects considered synonymous with their use. In *Opium: A History* Martin Booth reported on various historical cases taken from British literary society. Although Booth was certain that the regular use of opiates necessarily led to addiction, he at least recognized that not all such cases were problematic. One such case involved Thomas Shadwell, "the leading Whig supporter, Restoration dramatist and poet."[21] More specifically, Shadwell was a seventeenth-century playwright who, despite his dependence on opiates, became the nation's poet laureate and historiographer royal. Other notable habitual users of opiates included Sir Robert Clive (1725–1774), a soldier of fortune also known as "Clive of India"; Thomas Wedgwood (1771–1805), who, with the British scientist Sir Humphrey Davy, developed an early form of photography in the late 1790s; the poet Samuel Taylor Coleridge (1772–1834), who from early adulthood was dependent on opium, which had first been used to ease his rheumatism pains; the physician, poet, and priest George Crabbe (1754–1832), whose life and writings are said to have been improved by his opiate habit, which began in 1790; and Wilkie Collins (1824–1889), the author credited with the first full-length detective story, *The Moonstone*, into which he poured his first-hand knowledge of opium's conditioning effects on memory. Perhaps most notorious, though, was Thomas de Quincey (1785–1859), author of the opium classic *Confessions of an English Opium-eater*. "De Quincey's controlled addiction does not seem to have made his life unduly miserable, for he was contentedly married, kept his addiction manageable, and, although he frequently locked himself away for weeks on end with his laudanum and book, he was always a keen and erudite conversationalist. . . . For many addicted writers, opium did little to affect their characters adversely. They lived artistically successful lives, often becoming wealthy from their writings."[22]

These Englishmen represent the better known among many reputable figures, both men and women, who prospered despite their opium habits.

That there were so many is hardly surprising, moreover, given the availability of opium and opium-related products at the time, and given the prevailing social attitudes about such products. As social mores hardened against the opiates, cases of regular but harmless opiate use remained common but were kept secret, as evident in the lives of William Halsted and Dr. X.

In the Consumer Union report *Licit and Illicit Drugs*, published in 1972, Edward Brecher and his colleagues noted two interesting and secret cases from the late 1950s, one of which involved an unnamed congressman familiar to Harry J. Anslinger, commissioner of the Federal Bureau of Narcotics.[23] Anslinger described the man as an "addict" as well as "one of the most influential members of the United States Congress."[24] The congressman died in office, Brecher noted, "still legislating, still addicted, and still unexposed."[25] Anslinger also knew of a graduate of the U.S. Naval Academy who, although dependent on opiates, obtained the rank of commander and wrote many best-selling books.[26]

Cases in which women developed opiate habits have been less frequently remarked on, despite their prevalence. Brecher described a 1950 study that reviewed the records of 142 individuals habituated to opiates who were treated at an expensive private institution. The study found that the most common category of user among this high-income group was "housewives."[27] "Physicians" and "housewives" together accounted for more than two-thirds of those treated (85 patients), with businessmen coming in a distant third (13 patients). Speaking of the group as a whole, the author of the study, Dr. Eugene Morhous, noted, "A great majority of these persons were actively engaged in their chosen livelihoods, and some had even made definite upward gains since they had become addicted to narcotic drugs."[28]

That opiates might not only fail to diminish a person's quality of life but actually improve it was a conclusion also drawn by Thomas Szasz in his pathbreaking 1974 book *Ceremonial Chemistry*. His assessment of the opiates is also applicable to habits like coca chewing and cigarettes smoking, as well as, perhaps, to pill popping drugs like Valium and Prozac: "The . . . evidence clearly justifies the conclusion that addictions are habits; that habits enable us to do some things, and disable us from doing others; and hence, that we may, indeed must, judge addictions as good or bad according to the value we place on what they enable us to do or disable us from doing. Furthermore, what any particular habit enables a person to do, or disables him from doing, may . . . be either a matter of fact or a matter of attribution.

Although this is obvious, it must be re-emphasized because of the ever-present human tendency—now directed especially toward certain pharmacological agents—to make utterly false attributions of harmfulness to scapegoats."[29]

Whatever the possible costs and benefits might have been for being an opiate habitué, it was clear that regular opiate use did not necessarily court disaster: factors other than pharmacological ones seemed to determine the dramatic structure of individual drug stories. Still, there remained in the twentieth century a strong impression that the repeated use of opiates like morphine and heroin necessarily led if not to immediate addiction then to physical dependence, forcing people into lifelong use. If opiates were not in fact inherently "debilitating substances," it was believed, they were at least inherently dependence producing. And yet, if some people become dependent on opiates without showing the untoward signs of addiction, perhaps there are those who, even with chronic, regular opiate use, never show signs even of dependence.

One place to look for such stories is within traditional cultures where opiates have been used regularly for centuries. Just as the coca chewer preceded the cocaine addict historically, the opiate eater preceded the heroin addict. And just as traditional coca chewers showed a pattern of regular coca use that did not involve dependence or addiction, traditional opium-eaters showed an overall pattern of regular, nondependent opium use. Many compelling examples come from the opium-eaters of the Punjab, a region now split between India and Pakistan, but that was under British control late in the nineteenth century.

The Scottish physician Henry Martyn Clark went to the Punjab in 1882, where he directed a medical mission and where he eventually became a noted expert on matters of Indian health.[30] Testifying to the Royal Commission on Opium, formed in 1893, Clark presented his view on the use of opium in India, where it was almost exclusively "eaten" (swallowed) in the form of small opium pills, usually twice daily. (In China, at the time, it was typically smoked.)[31] Clark described a pervasive yet moderate use of opiates by those of different Indian groups (such as Hindus and Sikhs), by those of different economic classes, and by both women and men, and he argued that, regardless of group, class, or sex, such use affected neither health nor productivity, even after several decades of use.[32] "There is no such thing as a murderous opium mania, or a man under its influence assaulting people," Clark reported. "The fact that a man takes moderate doses of opium does not of necessity imply that he forms the opium habit."[33]

A British professor of medicine working in Bombay, Sir George Birdwood, gave a similar report to the commission, distinguishing between Indian use of opium and the use of morphine in the United States. Although he acknowledged that the latter might be harmful, Birdwood asserted that the use of opium in India was not: "The healthiest people I knew, the best people, the wholesomest people, and those you trusted most in their work, were always the opium-eaters; invariably."[34] The royal commission also heard testimony from a retired surgeon general, Sir William Moore, who described the Indian use of opium in a manner one might use to describe the casual use of alcohol in America today, noting its role as a much-needed distraction from everyday boredom, exhaustion, and stress. In terms of addiction and dependence, Henry Waterfield, a high-ranking British military officer who served in India, reported to the commission that 80 percent of the Sikh soldiers were regular but casual users of opium, 15 percent were habitual users, and only 1 percent were excessive users.[35] William Biscoe, another high-ranking military official, testified that among the opium-eaters in his Sikh regiment, 60 percent "took it and left it off as occasion required."[36]

This moderate attitude toward opiates, used without any inevitable escalation toward intensive use (via smoking or injection), suggests the possibility of casual, addiction-free use of opiates. It even suggests that in some cases nondependent use is the rule rather than the exception. Like Amazonian coca chewing, however, Indian opiate use was largely restricted to the oral use of drugs, which raises the prospect that dependence may have been avoided in these peoples and cultures because the drug was taken via a less-direct (slower) route of administration. So concluded Henry Martyn Clark, for he believed that the smoking of opium was responsible for much of the "ruin, harm, and mischief" found in China at the time.[37] While opium eating does not necessarily escalate into more intoxicating modes of drug taking, can individuals smoke or even inject opiates and still remain casual users? If so, are such cases at all common in modern American history?

Not until the second half of the twentieth century was the casual use of opiates in the United States investigated. When it was, researchers were able, with little difficulty, to locate individuals who showed patterns of casual use, patterns later dubbed "chipping." (Casual users were called "chippers," a term subsequently applied to casual, nondependent cigarette smokers.) One of the most in-depth studies to describe these putatively paradoxical cases was conducted by Richard Jacobson and the noted drug scholar Norman Zinberg.[38] Zinberg and Jacobson interviewed "controlled heroin users" who had been using opiates for between two and twenty-three years. The study, published in the *American Journal of Psychiatry* in 1976, characterized five "representative patterns of controlled opiate use," each illustrated by a case report.[39] Somewhat ironically, the Drug Abuse Council of Washington had funded the study, assuming that "controlled use" would prove to be nothing more than a transitional moment before the inevitable onset of addiction. In fact, as Zinberg and Jacobson found, "Occasional or controlled users of heroin . . . are well-known in the street, but have been mentioned rarely in the professional literature."[40]

The subject of the first case study was "Mr. A," a forty-year-old married man with three children. From late adolescence through early adulthood, Mr. A had used a variety of drugs casually, including alcohol, marijuana, psychedelics, and amphetamines. He first tried heroin when he was twenty-four years old, and his use was intermittent for two years but then increased steadily. At the age of twenty-seven, Mr. A recognized he had a heroin habit. Then, after an arrest for drug possession, for which he received a suspended sentence, he began dating a woman who, two years later, became his wife. Because she disapproved of his drug use, especially of injected opiates, Mr. A broke his habit, although he never stopped using. At the time of the interview he had for ten years been engaging in controlled heroin use, which took place on weekends with his drug-using friends, along with the occasional, secret shot during the week, the latter of which had all but stopped in the previous five years.

The second case involved "Dr. B," a fifty-eight-year-old married man with two grown children and one grandchild. After having been in private medical practice for five years, he injected morphine to ease his nerves during a series of extramarital affairs. A year later he was injecting morphine four times daily, except on weekends and family vacations. At that time, federal regulations for monitoring narcotics prescriptions began to tighten, which frightened Dr. B and caused him to scale down his habit to intermittent use. While he experienced minor withdrawal on weekends and at the start of vacations, his controlled use had been ongoing for more than a decade at the time of his interview. In their report, Zinberg and Jacobson remarked, "He feels morphine 'has been a good friend,' and he resents the lack of official and medical understanding that drug use such as his could be very helpful to many people."[41]

The third representative pattern involved "Ms. C," a twenty-year-old woman who used marijuana, psychedelics, and amphetamines regularly after graduating from high school. While studying at an art school in Boston for a year, she tried barbiturates and heroin. After returning home later that year, she began injecting heroin with two friends. Her use thereafter varied from periods of abstinence to periods of regular use, in much the same pattern as her boyfriend's. Increased free time and a certain out-of-town visitor were associated with periods of greater use, which remained casual, rather than habitual, up to the time of the interview.

The fourth case involved "Mr. D," a thirty-six-year-old single man. A hemophiliac, Mr. D had been given opiates since childhood; likewise for his two brothers, who were also hemophiliacs and controlled opiate users. Mr. D was prescribed pharmaceutical opioids for pain (and false complaints of pain), including meperidine (Demerol) and hydromorphone (Dilaudid), which he took orally, although he also occasionally injected opiates. Mr. D had used these drugs daily for more than fifteen years, although he reported having once gone off opiates for two weeks without experiencing any notable withdrawal. In more recent years he had developed a practice of occasionally cutting down on his daily use, either selling what remained or saving it up for occasions on which he wanted to get high.

The final example involved "Mr. E," a thirty-three-year-old married man employed as a mental-health worker. He had used alcohol since adolescence and in early adulthood had begun regularly using marijuana and other substances, including opium, which he injected. At the age of twenty-four, Mr. E got married and stopped injecting opium. He continued his oral use of opiates, however, which he used casually with his friends and wife, usually on weekends.

These five patterns are representative of the fifty-four cases of controlled opiate use identified by Zinberg and Jacobson. While periods of casual use were sometimes intermixed with periods of regular and perhaps even compulsive use, Zinberg and Jacobson saw no evidence of an inevitable out-of-control escalation of opiate use, ending in a pattern of lifelong addiction.

Emphasizing the difficulty of finding either psychological or sociological factors that differentiated dependent users from long-term controlled users (or periods of dependent use from periods of long-term controlled use), Zinberg and Jacobson concluded, "Project data obtained so far have not been able to correlate a particular pattern of use . . . with family background, job classification, degree of education, occupational status, marital status, or even the amount of the drug consumed. Our findings similarly indicate no correlation between chipping and specific personality types."[42] Nor were these results particularly surprising, as nearly all longitudinal studies of drug use have found that there are "multiple pathways" for any given drug user. The factors affecting individuals' patterns of opiate use were often highly contingent, such as developing relationships with significant others who disapproved of opiate use. The problem raised by the existence of modern-day chippers is thus not what distinguishes them from addicts, as though they were two distinct kinds of people — those with and without, say, an "addictive personality" — but rather what factors influence whether opiate use will be casual, dependent, or addictive for a person over any given period of time. Despite the image of the down-and-out street addict, even habitual users of opiates go through periods of abstinence and intermittent use.

The classic image of the lifelong opiate junky is a stereotype that emerged alongside differential prohibition in the twentieth century. Even William S. Burroughs, the most notorious American drug fiend, sometimes promoted the homogeneous view that use equals addiction: "Addiction is an illness of exposure. By and large those who have access to junk become addicts."[43] Noting the tendency of the public to embrace a bogus opiate pharmacologicalism, Brecher and colleagues warned in *Licit and Illicit Drugs* that problems of addiction are historical and cultural phenomena, as well as pharmacological: "In 1962, the United States Supreme Court characterization of the drug addict as 'one of the walking dead' can no doubt be illustrated many times over among addicts living under twentieth-century conditions of high opiate prices, vigorous law enforcement, repeated imprisonment, social ignominy, and periodic unavailability of opiates."[44]

According to statistics, the opiate user as "one of the walking dead" represented a pattern of opiate use no more common in the twentieth century than patterns of nondependent, casual use. Both were points on a continuum of drug involvement, with abstinence on one end and overwhelming, habitual use (addiction) on the other. A 1967 study by medical epidemiologist Lee Robins found that as many as 86 percent of the individuals identified by her team as having once been heroin addicts had not used heroin in the last year.[45] Similarly, in an oft-cited study of opiate use, the *Road to H* (1964), Isidor Chein and colleagues found, "The sheer addictive properties of heroin are certainly not sufficient to account for the change [toward heavier use], for heroin has no universal addictive impact, and certainly not if taken in intervals of more than a day. Furthermore, there is some evidence that many youths go on using heroin on a more-or-less irregular basis — for example, week-end and party use — for several years and eventually stop altogether. In our study of heroin use in gangs, we found that, of the eighty current heroin-users, less than half were using daily or more often and that fourteen boys who had used heroin in the past had stopped completely."[46]

With long-term studies of opiate addiction beginning in the 1960s, a number of other careful investigations were made showing that even so-called addicts typically go through periods of abstinence and moderate use, with investigators using terms like "de-addiction," "remission without treatment," "maturing out," and "natural remission."[47] Among the first to describe this process was Charles Winick, who in 1964 ascribed the maturing out of habitual opiate use to a "varying mix of physiological, psychological, and environmental factors."[48] Robert Scharse drew similar conclusions in 1966 in an investigation that looked at forty-five Mexican Americans who had used opiates for a short period, either casually or habitually, and then quit using altogether. In the course of forty interviews, Scharse found that some users stopped for explicit reasons (e.g., a concern over physical dependence), whereas others simply drifted away from opiate use, often for minor, chance reasons (e.g., the loss of the drug supplier).[49]

The picture of diverse opiate careers that emerged in the 1960s was highlighted in the early 1970s by a natural experiment involving Vietnam veterans.[50] Large numbers of U.S. soldiers in Vietnam used opiates, largely because they were inexpensive, widely available, and helpful. The prospect of thousands of these individuals returning to the United States and creating an epidemic of opiate addiction generated considerable concern for public officials. In the early 1970s Lee Robins received funding to assess opiate use both one year and three years after soldiers returned home.[51] What she found mystified public officials. Although as many as 20 percent of the soldiers reported opiate addiction while in Vietnam, where opiates were smoked, snorted, and swallowed, and although many of them reported opiate use during their first year back in the United States, fewer than 1 percent of them showed any sign of opiate dependence after one year. Of those who reported a subjective sense of being addicted to opiates while in Vietnam, about 33 percent tried opiates after returning home, yet only one in five of them showed any sign of dependence a year later.[52] Equally perplexing to those who viewed drug issues through the lens of pharmacologicalism was Robins's finding that those "addicts" who did not receive treatment after returning home fared as well as those who did, which suggested that addiction in Vietnam was neither an individual or pharmacological problem nor a disease, but purely a situational phenomenon. As Zinberg and Jacobson and Scharse had also concluded, changing the context underlying drug use changed the drug habit as well.

In part because of the Vietnam study and in part because of the persistent myth of opiate addiction, long-term studies of opiate-use patterns continued in the late 1970s and 1980s, and lent further support to the theory that drug habits were often shaped by situational factors.[53] In 1981 David Nurco and colleagues published a study that had followed 238 opiate addicts for ten years and found that only one in three habitual users went the entire ten-year period without a voluntary period of nonaddictive use, with addiction defined as the use of opiates at least four days in each week for a month, a definition that conflates dependence with addiction.[54] As with the Zinberg and Jacobson study, the patterns of opiate use in this group were quite varied. One individual used opiates in an addictive manner for one month and was then abstinent for most of the remaining ten-year period. Nurco and colleagues estimated the average period of ongoing "addiction" to be approximately two years, although this statistic was affected in part by involuntary abstinence (e.g., incarceration). Overall, more than one in five of the white addicts had from three to six periods of voluntary, nonaddictive use; the number for black addicts, who came from consistently poorer backgrounds, was about one in ten.[55]

The sociologist Dan Waldorf and his colleague Patrick Biernacki also conducted in-depth investigations into the matter.[56] Looking at the "natural history" of opiate addiction among specific individuals, they found that a significant number of addicts went on to nonaddictive use or abstinence without the aid of any formal drug treatment. After comparing eighty-four treated "ex-addicts" with fifty untreated "ex-addicts," they found that the concept of multiple pathways aptly characterized drug-use careers, noting again that situational factors strongly influenced people's experiences with addiction and dependence: "The idea to give up opiates usually emerged from feelings of dysfunction with the effects of heroin and the life style of addicts which is expressed in such terms as 'being tired of the life, changes, hassles, junkies and going to jail or prison.' . . . 'Maturing out' of addiction is only one of several ways to overcome an addicted life. Some people move on to other drugs (usually alcohol), some retire from heroin use but maintain the lifestyle, while others are addicted in certain situations and change when the situations change."[57]

Despite the many different realities that described opiate use in the twentieth century, it was with heroin and the other opiates that the myth of pharmacological possession took strongest hold. Modern pharmacologicalism therefore had its roots in the idea of opiate addiction.[58] According to the typical account, regular use of opiates creates a physiological need, this need causes the addict to experience withdrawal, and this withdrawal motivates the desperate "addict" to do whatever is necessary to procure more drugs. The casual use of opiates casts doubt on the metaphor of the vicious cycle of addiction, however, as does the natural history of opiate addicts. Both sets of observations are extensive enough to suggest that nonpharmacological factors are intimately tied up with opiate dependence and addiction, if and when they occur, and that the passage from experimental to casual use and on to withdrawal and then dependence or addiction is just one of many possible pathways for an opiate user.

Alfred Lindesmith, a sociologist at Indiana University, was perhaps the first drug scholar to provide a rigorous, scientific critique of the pharmacologicalism of addiction. Lindesmith began his questioning in a 1938 essay entitled "A Sociological Theory of Drug Addiction," published in the *American Journal of Sociology*.[59] After conducting about fifty in-depth interviews with so-called addicts, he fleshed out his argument, which culminated in his book *Opiate Addictions* in 1947 (republished as *Addiction and Opiates* in 1968). Lindesmith ultimately developed an alternative, nonpharmacological account of opiate addiction, in which he also attempted to resolve the question of why regular users of opiates do not necessarily become dependent or addicted.

What he came to conclude about opiate dependence began with the recognition that although continuous opiate consumption did cause many users to experience physical withdrawal later on, the subsequent move from withdrawal to dependence was hardly an absolute. This observation derived both from Lindesmith's interviews with "addicts" and from general reports by individuals who, despite regular use of opiates, failed to become habitual users. Lindesmith came to view addiction and dependence as contingent products of a dynamic learning process, of which physical withdrawal was but one element. He wrote that his framework had "the advantage of attributing the origin of addiction, not to a single event, but to a series of events, thus implying that addiction is established in a learning process extending over a period of time."[60]

The learning process described by Lindesmith has two parts. First, the opiate user must associate drug withdrawal with his or her use of the drug. Individuals who use a drug as a form of escape from reality, for example, are likely to find that reality returns with a vengeance when the drug escape ends. If this is then interpreted as a form of withdrawal, the conditioned urge for more drugs may be strong. By contrast, a hospitalized patient who receives chronic opiates will, after leaving the hospital, likely fail to associate any physical withdrawal with opiate use, attributing the experience instead to illness or surgery. In fact, because hospital patients often associate opiate analgesia with an illness and/or hospital care, and because the drugs cause sedation and other mind-altering effects, patients rarely experience any withdrawal. They also typically want nothing to do with opiates after being discharged from the hospital.[61]

If and when an opiate user identifies opiate withdrawal as such, still another step must be taken for drug dependence to emerge. Specifically, he or she must complete a ritual activity that is partly physiological, partly cognitive, and partly behavioral. That is to say, the opiate user must experience withdrawal (a physical phenomenon), he or she must develop a concern over the withdrawal experience as such (a cognitive phenomenon), and then he or she must engage in drug use, taking opiates repeatedly to eliminate or avoid opiate withdrawal (a behavioral phenomenon). A breakdown in any part of this biopsychosocial circuit can prevent a pattern of dependent opiate use from emerging. For example, an individual may experience little physical withdrawal following repeated opiate use, or, as found in Scharse's study of Mexican Americans, a person might interpret withdrawal as a sign of impending drug dependence and subsequently reduce or quit his or her drug habit.[62] If, on the other hand, a withdrawal experience causes an individual to become obsessed with the prospect and experience of withdrawal — and to continually use in order to avoid it — the circuit will be completed, with the learning process now occurring repeatedly, thus reinforcing the drug habit at all three levels: physiological, cognitive, and behavioral.[63]

As in other realms of human perception, the saliency and meaning of withdrawal as both a motivating and experiential factor changes depending on the significance it is given, first by the culture and subculture, then by the individual. Lindesmith emphasizes cognitive processes in his account, but such psychological processes are conditioned during one's lifetime according to cultural or subcultural beliefs and expectations.[64] Viewed from an anthropological perspective, this makes perfect sense. The opiate addict of Western culture takes opiates in a radically different societal framework than does the Indian opium-eater; he or she also inhabits a very different myth about opiates and addiction. Internalizing the myth of opiate pharmacologicalism, the twentieth-century American opiate user must confront the bogeyman of drug withdrawal, which for many becomes a source of overwhelming anxiety that encourages compulsive drug use to keep the demons away. Thus, according to Lindesmith, opiate addiction is the product not of an individual's exposure to opiates per se, but of a dramatic perceptual shift in his or her attribution and attention, often with the individual realizing that he or she is hooked, and then behaving accordingly. At this point many users will essentially be hooked — a self-fulfilling, mythical prophecy — since regular opiate users are likely to persist at this stage in ritualistic drug use. The end result is that many opiate users become trapped within the prevailing pharmacologicalism of addiction — a *placebo text*, in essence, that promotes drug dependence by teaching individuals that withdrawal is a pharmacological and physiological fact that cannot be denied.

Placebo text refers to any unwritten cultural script that, like a religious text, informs a group's beliefs and expectations about a given drug, animating the "drug effects" once the substance is taken. If by *placebo effect* one means an outcome produced not by a drug but by beliefs and expectations about a drug, then a placebo text becomes the cultural teachings, however subtle, that inform these beliefs and expectations. According to this view, once a substance is taken, beliefs and expectations join with the first-order pharmacological effects of the substance to mediate or animate the immediate and long-term effects attributed to the drug. Peter Laurie provides some examples in a commonsense booklet called *Drugs*: "Whisky in a pub in the Gorbals excuses hitting your friends with bottles; Bloody Marys at a Chelsea party facilitate sexual advances towards other people's wives. Each society uses alcohol as a key to unlock different forms of behavior."[65]

Craig MacAndrew's and Robert Edgerton's classic study, *Drunken Comportment*, contributes rigorous research along these lines. Appearing two years after Laurie's book, in 1969, the book provided a detailed ethnographic analysis of drinking patterns among Native Americans at the time when European traders introduced alcohol to various tribes. Contrary to the myth that "Indians can't hold their liquor," MacAndrew and Edgerton found, abundant evidence indicates dramatically different behavioral, psychological, and social effects of alcohol intoxication depending on the teachings the Native Americans received (or did not receive) from outsiders.[66] This variability ranged from alcohol's capacity to induce calm reflection in one culture to its seemingly equal capacity to produce uncontrolled hostilities in another. "Persons learn about drunkenness what their societies impart to them," concluded MacAndrew and Edgerton, and "comporting themselves in consonance with these understandings," they become living confirmations "of their societies' teachings." MacAndrew and Edgerton added, "We would propose that this formulation is similarly applicable to our own society, but with this difference: our society lacks a clear and consistent position regarding the scope of the excuse and is thus neither clear nor consistent in its teachings. . . . In such a situation, our formulation would lead us to expect that what people actually do when they are drunk will vary enormously; and this is precisely what we find when we look around us. Thus, paradoxical as it may sound, we would argue that in our society this very unpredictability is the clearest possible confirmation of the essential correctness of our theory."[67]

There are, of course, different placebo texts for different drugs, even for identical or nearly identical ones; consider, for example, cocaine versus Ritalin, or morphine versus heroin. And, as the study by MacAndrew and Edgerton suggests, not every user or group of users is influenced by the same script. The scripts differ for men versus women, younger users versus older; indeed, throughout the long history of drugs, placebo texts have remained highly gendered. With rare exceptions, however, the placebo text does not guarantee any particular drug effect or experience, but only enhances the likelihood of certain drug outcomes. Andrew Weil gives an account of members of a South American tribe who all report having had the same hallucinatory experience after ingesting a prepared psychedelic substance.[68] Such a uniform effect would not be expected of users of mescaline or LSD in the United States late in the twentieth century, since the placebo text for these drugs was far less tightly scripted and was more secular than sacred.

For opiates and addiction, the placebo text identified by Alfred Lindesmith appears not as a universal process applicable to opiate users throughout the world, but as one that originates and unfolds primarily in the West. Fear of withdrawal and the cycle of drug dependence that follows does not happen to the individual who, like the traditional Indian opiate-eater, has no indoctrination into this particular placebo text, or, like the hospital patient who, despite being administered opiates for weeks on end, never realizes that the text is even relevant to him or her.

Although Lindesmith's account was a radical departure from the scientific pharmacologicalism that emerged in the twentieth century, it nevertheless received considerable empirical, if not public, support in the decades that followed. For instance, investigators determined that habitual opiate users were in fact poor discriminators of physical withdrawal,[69] a finding that lent credence to the tenuous link Lindesmith had observed between opiate withdrawal and a habitué's desire for opiates. Just as recreational cocaine users often failed to discriminate between a placebo and cocaine or other stimulants, and just as smokers have failed to discriminate very-low-nicotine cigarettes from normal cigarettes, the discrimination of withdrawal among so-called opiate addicts seems surprisingly unreliable.[70]

When opiate users are led to believe that they are receiving opiates when they are not, they often experience little or no withdrawal; when they are led to believe that they have not been given opiates when in fact they have, opiate users often experience withdrawal, or what is in fact pseudo-withdrawal. Such blind testing has also been accomplished in "reduction-treatment" programs in which habitual opiate users unknowingly receive smaller opiate dosages each day over a period of a few weeks, until, unbeknown to them, the "drug" they inject contains no drug at all.[71] In such cases the habitué often remains certain that he or she is still on the drug and shows no outward signs of withdrawal, even though he or she has not actually injected real opiates in days. On the other hand, habitués who unknowingly receive the same opiate dosage each day over a period of a few weeks but are led to believe that their dosage may be decreasing have been known to complain incessantly that they are experiencing withdrawal, sometimes even displaying physiological signs of withdrawal. In one study, conducted in New York City in the 1930s, individuals were put on either a seven- or fourteen-day reduction treatment, but were left blind as to which one.[72] After one week, individuals in the two-week group, who were still receiving opiates, began to show considerable agitation and a "paranoid, suspicious state."[73]

Lindesmith also wrote of a curious case in which two women went unknowingly for a month without receiving morphine, and another in which a former patient confessed to him that he "had been getting sterile hypodermics for ten days and was feeling quite well until an attendant, whom he had bribed to find out how much morphine he was getting, disclosed the truth."[74]

In such instances it is unlikely that physiological withdrawal has been totally eliminated. What is more likely is that the perceptual circuitry between withdrawal, the withdrawal experience, and withdrawal-elicited drug use has been disconnected, freeing the person from their conviction that every instance of mental and physical discomfort is a sign of impending anguish and doom. This process was nicely captured in the case of one woman who, when facing a painful surgery, pleaded with the medical staff not to be given opiates, even as a matter of life and death. The woman explained that she had once been an addict and was gravely afraid of becoming readdicted to opiates. Unfortunately, her postoperative pain was severe, and the physician had no choice but to administer opiate analgesics. However, suspecting that the women was enslaved to her beliefs and fears more than to any pharmacological substance, the doctor administered the drug in a disguised, liquid form. His approach worked perfectly. On leaving the hospital the patient experienced no withdrawal and thanked the physician for cooperating with her request not to be readdicted.[75] If the drug is a vessel in which to sail on an experiential sea, the placebo text becomes the compass that guides its course.

These cases were reinforced by other, even more bizarre findings, including the discovery that some of the positive relief received from opiates may be provided by the drug administration itself. Such was the implication of D. G. Levine's 1974 report "'Needle freaks': Compulsive self-injection by drug users," which described how, via a process of repeated conditioning, the injection ritual came to elicit its own positive "drug experience," independent of any drug.[76] As Lindesmith wrote, "Knowing that he is addicted, the addict ascribes his mental changes to the drug, not because they are recognizable as such but because they always accompany the shot."[77]

The idea that the injection experience alone can elicit a drug experience may seem impossible, but it dovetails with another such finding, namely, that after being issued inaccurate drug information, opiate habitués have difficulty discriminating not only their inner state of withdrawal but also the purity of opiates bought and sold on the street. If anticipating and injecting the drug become critical elements of the drug experience for habitual opiate users, the purity of drug may become an almost secondary factor, so it follows that habitual opiate users might also be poor discriminators of drug purity. This might explain the fact that, during a period in America in the 1960s, heroin's purity in the black market dropped to as low as one-half of one percent without having any marked affects on drug demand.[78] Lindesmith also cites earlier cases of adolescent heroin users who looked and behaved as if they were addicts, and claimed to be big-time heroin users, yet failed to show the telltale signs of physical withdrawal on drug discontinuation. As it turned out, these youths were being sold heroin of such low purity that it actually failed to produce withdrawal after continuous use. If these youths were in fact "addicts," it is unlikely that it was the drugs that they were addicted to. The ritual of drug use, used in combination with a certain attitude and a certain placebo text, was enough.

The report of the Royal Commission on Opium examined the use of opium in the British Indian empire and inquired into the possibility of prohibiting the drug, except for medical use. When the commission was formed, in 1893, opium had already been a major commodity in international trade for several decades, with exports headed mostly from India to China and Southeast Asia. The commission was composed of nine individuals—seven Brits and two distinguished Indians—and was the product of growing religious pressures in Britain. Protestant groups had long questioned the morality of the opium trade, viewing opium as an inherently destructive, if not demonic, drug. These concerns were addressed when the Liberal Party came to power in 1891 and formed the commission two years later.

The commission's final report, the product of seventy days of public hearings with 723 witnesses from fifteen Indian cities and townships, totaled more than 2,500 pages and was organized into seven volumes.[79] Although religious pressures had been the impetus for the commission, it nevertheless deferred in its report to an abundance of experts who had concluded that opium should be feared or abhorred to no greater degree than alcohol. The Indian public was opposed to a ban on opium, and the commission recognized that, in India at least, opium was not a cause of "extensive moral or physical degradation."[80] Because of the incorporation of opium consumption into the fabric of everyday life and society in India, the commission also concluded that it would be impractical, if not impossible, to separate medical from nonmedical use. The British medical journal *Lancet* supported the anti-opium movement prior to the report of the commission, but reversed its position afterward. An editorial in the April 1895 issue stated that the commission's report had dealt a "crushing blow to the anti-opium faddists," whose claims were found to be "either ridiculously exaggerated or even altogether unfounded."[81]

A somewhat similar situation existed at the time for opium eating in America.[82] While there was indeed concern over the pervasive use of opiates, especially from religious groups and other moral puritans, public alarm at the end of the nineteenth century was focused more on alcohol than on opiates. As of 1885, the year of the Royal Commission on Opium's report, opiates had been widely available in the United States and Britain for more than a century, usually consumed orally in the form of patent medicines and elixirs, sometimes with alcohol in a popular drug combination known as laudanum. Morphine and heroin were isolated from opium in the nineteenth century, in 1804 and 1874 respectively, products of the same Western reductionist attitude that led to the isolation of cocaine from Mama Coca. (The hypodermic needle, a similar step in this direction, was developed in 1853.) Products that contained opiates, like those that contained cocaine and marijuana, were regularly sold over the counter and by mail order in the United States. There was no restriction on the amount of opiates in these products, nor was a label stating that they contained opiates required. Sometimes the makers of these tonics also employed obvious placebo texts, selling them as treatments for opiate withdrawal even though they contained healthy quantities of opiates.[83] Along with their sale in patent medicines, opiates were also widely dispensed by physicians — one of the few medicines on offer that worked in a robust and predictable fashion.

Together, these conditions resulted in a steady and significant increase in opiate use throughout the nineteenth century in America, with opiates being part and parcel of everyday life. As a consequence, the average habitual opiate user of the nineteenth century had almost nothing in common with the stereotypical image of the heroin junky, which emerged several decades later. A survey conducted in Massachusetts in 1889, for example, when opiates were still sold without prescription, asked druggists to describe the economic classes of habitual opiate users: 22 percent of respondents pointed to the upper classes as the principal users, while only 6 percent pointed to the lower classes.[84] This broad spectrum of use meant that opiates were not associated with criminal activity, nor were they associated in the public imagination with crime. In fact, at the time, women were more often habitual users of opiates than men: an 1878 Michigan study found that 62.2 percent of "addicts" were women; a 1914 Tennessee study put the number at 66.9 percent.[85]

When reflecting on this period of American history, some drug historians have interpreted the permissive use of opiates as a time when America was still waking up to the dangers of these drugs. David Musto, for example, wrote in *The American Disease*, "Eventually the medical consensus was that morphine had been overused by the physician, addiction was a substantial possibility, and addition of narcotics to patent medicines should be minimized or stopped. There is reason to emphasize the gradual development of this medical opinion since physicians, as well as everyone else, had what now seems a very delayed realization that dangerously addicting substances were distributed with little worry for their effect."[86] This view runs somewhat counter to reports at the time, however, including those that concerned "Heroin," the brand name for a cough suppressant made by the German pharmaceutical company Bayer.

At the time of the Royal Commission on Opium, heroin was being hailed in the United States as a minimally addictive substance, as well as a substitute for codeine and a new treatment for morphinism. In 1890 James R. L. Daly wrote in the *Boston Medical and Surgical Journal*, Heroin "possesses many advantages over morphine. . . . It is not hypnotic; there is no danger of acquiring the habit."[87] Much the same sentiment was reported in 1900 in the *New York Medical Journal*.

A sufficiently long period having elapsed since the introduction of heroine, the new substitution product for codeine, during which it has been used very extensively, we are now enabled to pass judgment upon its real value, and to definitely determine in what manner this drug has fulfilled the expectations raised in its behalf. . . . Habituation has been noted in a small percentage . . . of the cases. . . . All observers are agreed however that none of the patients suffer in any way from this habituation, and that none of the symptoms which are so characteristic of chronic morphinism have ever been observed. On the other hand, a large number of the reports refer to the fact that the same dose may be used for a long time without any habituation.[88]

Obviously these investigators were unaware that heroin, once taken into the body, is metabolized into morphine. Pointing to this fact, historians have often assumed that it was a lack of pharmacological sophistication that was responsible for the permissive use of opiates prior to the twentieth century, as well as the widespread dependence and addiction that putatively came as a result. Opiates would have never been made so freely available in the nineteenth century, according to this view, if people had known what they were getting themselves into.

There is, however, another interpretation of this period of general naïveté. The lack of knowledge about opiate pharmacology also meant that the myth of opiates as inherently addictive drugs was not fully formed. Indeed, many individuals consumed large quantities of opiates unknowingly, and thus independently of any addiction-related placebo text. When examined according to Lindesmith's model of opiates and addiction, a very different interpretation arises, namely, that the permissive use of opiates prevailed for so long not because of persistent ignorance about the "inherent pharmacological dangers" of the drug, but because of a dramatic difference in the demographics of who used opiates and in the prevailing social and psychological ethos that governed their use.

If the liquid opiates administered to the ex-addict patient described above were not addictive, and if the cocaine-like drug Ritalin was in use in America for decades before reports surfaced of dependence or misuse, perhaps the same was true of heroin and morphine. When administered with a placebo text that viewed them as nonaddictive, were these opiates in fact less addictive? Could the public's ignorance about the basic pharmacology of heroin versus morphine have been more of a blessing than a curse? When American physicians concluded in 1890 that heroin "possesses many advantages over morphine. . . . It is not hypnotic; there is no danger of acquiring the habit," are we to conclude that this was a fraud or a delusion? Or is it more likely that what these Boston and New York physicians actually witnessed was due to a particular attitude about opiate consumption—that is, a momentary shift in the prevailing placebo text that, although concerned with essentially the same drug, governed dramatically different drug attitudes, drug expectations and experiences, and drug outcomes?

While this alternative interpretation may sound speculative, it helps explain why the massive use of opiates in the nineteenth century did not translate into widespread dependence and addiction. Opium consumption increased fivefold from the 1860s to the 1890s, and the consumption of opiate alkaloids, including morphine, increased thirty-four-fold during these years.[89] These increases, however, did not lead to an epidemic of opiate dependence or addiction. In *Dark Paradise: Opiate Addiction in America before 1940* the historian David Courtwright argued that most regular opiate users became dependent on the drug, but he belied this claim with the statistic that there was, at most, a sixfold increase in opiate dependence from 1842 until the end of the century.[90] Courtwright also cited a number of surveys of pharmacists, even though each pharmacy reported only between two and five addicts per store. An 1880 survey of fifty drugstores in Chicago, for example, revealed a total of 235 "addict-customers" (i.e., fewer than five addicts per pharmacy), a number that, considering the massive daily use of opiates, hardly suggests an epidemic of dependence and addiction.[91] By comparison, with drug prohibition running at full pitch in the United States at the end of the twentieth century, there were nearly one million "hard-core heroin addicts" and nearly 40,000 heroin users receiving methadone in New York City alone.[92]

That there was relatively little public concern over opiate use in the nineteenth century was further evidenced by the fact that it was not until the next century that the first federal restrictions were placed on opium—a time, early in the twentieth century, when opiate use was beginning to decline anyway.[93] Drug historians like David Courtwright explain this lack of public concern by suggesting that the individual and social problems associated with opiates, while enormous, were also somehow overlooked. In fact, the ill effects of drugs were well recognized at the time, if not generally overstated: morphine was acknowledged as habit forming well before the end of the century (morphinism), while alcohol was identified by many as an insidious drug, one against which a growing moral minority would soon prevail, beginning with state prohibitions (in the first decade of the nineteeth century) and later with federal prohibition (passed in 1918 and ratified by the individual states in 1920).

If twentieth-century investigators were able to document dependence-free opiate use with ease, this pattern of use was even more common in the nineteenth century, since opiates were consumed daily by people who had little or no risk for dependence or addiction and who had little or no fear of it. The addiction theorist Stanton Peele drew this same conclusion in his book *The Meaning of Addiction*, noting that the vast majority of nineteenth-century opiate use was, like alcohol use today, in fact "moderate use." Peele described how, with the rise of differential prohibition in the twentieth century, the possibility of dependence-free opiate use actually became hidden from public view, only to be perceived, when perceived at all, as an anomaly. An anti-narcotic campaign early in the twentieth century, according to Peele, "changed irrevocably conceptions of the nature of opiate use. In particular, the campaign eradicated the awareness that people could employ opiates moderately or as a part of normal lifestyle."[94]

The addiction-light placebo text was not the only reason habitual opiate use in nineteenth-century America (and Britain) was unlikely to turn users into addicts, junkies, or the "walking dead." Habitual users had access to high-grade opiates via a licit (i.e., white) market and at a relatively low cost. Just as most of the circumstantial and casual use of opiates in the nineteenth century did not escalate into opiate dependence, most cases of dependence did not lead to compulsive, out-of-control addiction. What Henry Martyn Clark had reported about India to the Royal Commission on Opium — "The fact that a man takes moderate doses of opium does not of necessity imply that he forms the opium habit. . . . There is no such thing as a murderous opium mania, or a man under its influence assaulting people" — was equally descriptive of America at the time.

In the first half of the twentieth century, however, things changed dramatically, and for the worse. Prohibitions were enacted, black markets and violent drug syndicates emerged, soft images associated with opium smoking and opiate eating were overshadowed by hard images of heroin-injecting users, and a myth of opiates as inherently addictive drugs acquired almost universal status. The power of the placebo text was still very much intact, but the content of that text had changed. The effects of the new text began appearing early in the twentieth century, with each one unfortunately reinforcing the others. The end result was a harsh regime of differential prohibition that by the end of the twentieth century had turned America into the world's most troubled drug culture.

If the use of opiates and other fallen angels of the twentieth century was already in decline prior to the enactment of drug prohibitions at the end of the nineteenth century, why did a scheme of differential prohibition — of pharmacological angels and demons — emerge? Because drug effects and understandings are historically conditioned, the fall of these drugs, as well as the initial rise of differential prohibition, stemmed not from increases in the absolute quantity of drug use, but from a relative shift in who used them and how they were used — a pattern exemplified by the first drug to be demonized in American history, the demon rum.

The public meaning of alcohol in the late nineteenth century originated within groups that championed its use and among those who consumed it socially and publicly, who included immigrant workers, *mostly men*, and others among the less economically fortunate. Alcohol's reputation suffered, justly or unjustly, from the reputation of those who used it and how they used it, as it benefits today for the same reasons. Thus the "problem" with alcoholic spirits lay not in alcohol per se, but rather in those who predominantly — and publicly — consumed it. "Prohibition was not just a matter of 'wets' versus 'drys,' or a matter of political conviction or health concerns," wrote one drug scholar. "Intricately interwoven with these factors was a middle-class, rural, Protestant, evangelical concern that the good and true life was being undermined by ethnic groups with a different religion and a lower standard of living and morality. One way to strike back at these groups was through prohibition."[95] Another author noted, "Prohibition was in many ways the single most effective political move of [the] century, for its principal goal was to destroy the Irish Catholic-American political clubs."[96]

Although by the early twentieth century cocaine and opiates were increasingly considered to be potentially destructive and habit forming, they provoked little of the hatred directed at alcohol at the time. Why? The former were consumed by individuals, mostly women, of higher social standing and under the guise of patent medicines. The reputations of cocaine and the opiates were protected as long as most or all of those who used them had an upstanding reputation.

But of course things changed. The situation for opiates and alcohol essentially reversed itself during the twentieth century, in part because the medical practice of relying on opiates as panaceas lost its legitimacy. Opiate use in the nineteenth century mirrored alcohol consumption a century later: with drug use shared among such a broad spectrum of people, it was impossible to portray either drug as inherently harmful or addictive. Taking note of this, Alfred Lindesmith pointed out that habitual opiate use was perceived at the time as a misfortune rather than as a form of deviance and that some physicians advocated that alcoholics be converted to what they considered the healthier habit of opiate dependence. "Little emphasis was placed on the effects of evil association, and dope peddlers were not mentioned because they were rare or nonexistent. . . . Narcotics users were pitied rather than loathed as criminals or degenerates."[97]

As the "therapeutic" use of opiates was reigned in, the demographics of opiate use quietly transformed. Prior to the prohibition of over-the-counter opiate sales, the average age of an opiate user was forty, and most were women from the middle and upper classes. By the early 1970s, only about 14 percent of users were forty or older, and the great majority of them came from the margins of society.[98] Before prohibition, most users were opium smokers, but within a decade of prohibition, they were more likely to be morphine or heroin injectors than opium smokers. In her book *Creating the American Junkie*, Caroline Jean Acker described the change using first-person accounts, like that of James Martin: what had cost $4 prior to the ban on opium imports cost $50 afterward, so Martin switched to sniffing heroin; when prohibition and prices escalated further, he began shooting up, realizing that he had "to get a better kick out of it."[99] David Courtwright described this escalation in terms of dependence and addiction: "The net result was that opiate addiction, while declining relative to population, began to assume a new form: it ceased to be concentrated in upper-class and middle-class white females and began to appear more frequently in lower-class urban males, often neophyte members of the underworld."[100]

The shifting form of opiate use that took place outside the realm of "medical" use also influenced drug attitudes and public policies concerning opiates early in the twentieth century. As opium smoking, which was restricted to opium dens and a circumscribed clientele, was replaced by the injecting of morphine and heroin, opium dens closed and the street addict emerged. Nonmedical opiate use thus became a less private and more public activity. The change of venue and the more invasive method of drug administration were deemed objectionable, especially when compared to the predominant practice of earlier decades, opiate eating. Even opium smokers considered the habit of the street addict to be in poor taste, not to mention a threat to the sanctity of their tradition and lifestyle. Lindesmith wrote of an opium smoker who had discovered someone shooting up in the bathroom of a New York City opium den, "He immediately reported to the proprietor that there was a 'God-damned dope fiend in the can.'"[101]

The story of cocaine early in the twentieth century presented a similar picture. Although still widespread, cocaine use was decreasing. As with the opiates, the decline in the over-the-counter market for products containing cocaine shifted the demographics of drug use. The decline in both opium and coca products was due in part to the Pure Food and Drugs Act of 1906, a federal act that required manufacturers of patent medicines to list on their labels the true active ingredients of the products, which essentially meant revealing the "secret" contents that defined them as patent formulas. Meanwhile, as David Musto wrote, "Cocaine was being transformed in the public mind from a tonic to a terror."[102] In 1908, for instance, the *New York Times* wrote that cocaine was becoming a lower-class drug, with the exaggerated claim, typical of the newspaper's embrace of differential prohibition, that it is "destroying its victims more swiftly and surely than opium."[103] A year later, President William Howard Taft sent to Congress a State Department report demonizing cocaine, linking its use to the so-called darker elements of society: "The illicit sale of [cocaine] . . . and the habitual use of it temporarily raises the power of a criminal to a point where in resisting arrest, there is no hesitation to murder. It is more appalling in its effects than any other habit-forming drug used in the United States. . . . [I]t has been authoritatively stated that cocaine is often the direct incentive to the crime of rape by negroes of the South."[104]

The change in cocaine's demographics produced a rapid and lasting change in its public image. "All the elements needed to insure cocaine's outlaw status were present by the first years of the twentieth century," wrote another drug historian. "It had become widely used as a pleasure drug, and doctors warned of the dangers attendant on indiscriminate sale and use; it had become identified with despised or poorly regarded groups—blacks, lower-class whites, and criminals; it had not been long enough established in the culture to insure its survival; and it had not, though used by them, become identified with the elite, thus losing what little chance it had of weathering the storm of criticism."[105]

In short, what people think about a drug depends greatly on who uses it. From this come two other historically relevant points: the fall of such psychoactive derivatives of nature was influenced at least as much by the shift in how they were used as drugs as by their inherent pharmacological properties; the origins of America's drug prohibitions were rooted not in drugs per se—not in their chemical structures or actions in the body, as was steadfastly believed—but in the meanings these drugs acquired once they had fallen into the "wrong" hands and thus became associated with the wrong behavioral, social, and economic practices. The black market itself created an underworld of crime in twentieth-century America, yet crime was typically blamed on the drugs and drug users, either in terms of the "desperate acts" of the drug-enslaved addict seeking to sustain his or her addiction, or in terms of the psychological transformations produced by the drug. The differential prohibition of drugs may have been erected in the name of specific drugs—crack, ecstasy, heroin, LSD, marijuana, methamphetamine, PCP—but was it rooted in their pharmacological actions, or rather in the meaning the drugs acquired as their most visible users and the beliefs about their effects changed?

Full-scale prohibitions did not appear overnight. First came taxation and regulation. While the sale and use of alcohol had been controlled via taxation since early in the history of the republic, such controls over "drugs" came much later. Taxes were not levied against opium imports until the second half of the nineteenth century, for example, and taxes and regulations on other drugs and drug products did not appear until early in the twentieth century. These taxes and regulations were explicitly used to suppress the legal avenues to buying and selling products containing coca, opium, and cannabis—not to mention alcohol, which was banned from 1918 to 1933. Consequently, black markets quickly emerged, followed in turn by an escalating series of prohibitions, first against manufacturing, then distribution, then selling, then possession, and finally against use and users altogether. The Harrison Act of 1914, in particular, served as a foundation for the differential prohibition of drugs for more than a half century, until President Richard Nixon enlisted the nation in a "war on drugs" with the Comprehensive Drug Abuse Prevention and Control Act of 1970.

That drug prohibitions paralleled heightened public awareness of new "drug problems" is hardly a revelation. For it is no surprise that the public would react against any drug deemed by public officials or the media to be a threat to people or society. However, ironically, anti-drug reactions — and the first drug prohibitions they spawned — promoted the very marginalization that created the "problem" in the first place. While the Harrison Act did not prohibit opiate use per se, it did make it impossible for street addicts to obtain opiate narcotics legally. As an almost immediate consequence, a black market emerged, prices skyrocketed, and still use persisted. This led to the passage of the Jones-Miller Act of 1922, which increased the penalties for selling illegal opiates, including severe fines and imprisonment for up to ten years, as well as making possession a potential crime — all of which had little effect except to raise drug prices.[106] Thus was completed one revolution in a vicious cycle of prohibitionist policies against opiates that would continue escalating throughout the century.

None of these side effects had been anticipated. The intent behind the Harrison Act was simply to place formal controls on the selling of opiates (and cocaine), thus restricting use to medical care — the assumption being that once general access to these drugs was cut off, their nonmedical use would fade away. This never happened in part because the government body overseeing the Harrison Act, the Treasury Department, interpreted it so narrowly that nearly all individuals habituated to opiates before 1914 could no longer obtain them through medical channels. Habitual opiate use was deemed outside of the act's definition of "legitimate medical purposes," and the Treasury Department warned physicians that they would "be held accountable if through carelessness or lack of sufficient personal attention the patient secured more narcotic drugs than are necessary for medical treatment, and devote[d] part of his supply to satisfy addiction."[107] In the absence of a legal source of the drug, use among the general population did decrease, so the logic behind the legislation was not totally absurd. However, many if not most of the estimated 200,000 opiate and cocaine habitués did not cease their use, but sought illicit sources of the drugs instead. The sudden creation of the illicit opiate markets early in twentieth-century America, encouraged into existence by a persisting demand, set into motion a cycle of drug prohibition and illicit drug trafficking that was all but impossible to stop. All but impossible, that is, if prohibition was not brought to an end.

The immediate rise of illicit opiate markets in the United States was also unsurprising: while the markets that emerged to meet the existing demand were illegal, they were nevertheless markets; that is, the Harrison Act did not eliminate the nonmedical use of opiates, as policymakers had hoped, but rather encouraged the creation of a secondary market, the construction of which was paid for by the handsome profits received from selling drugs at higher prices, with less purity, and usually of poorer quality. Had the medical establishment been allowed, as it had in Britain, to register and provide opiates (or cocaine) for existing habitués, the initial impetus for the illicit markets and for recruiting new users into them would have been far slower to emerge, as was indeed the case in Britain. Instead, an enormous and powerful institution in the differential prohibition of drugs—the black market for opiates and cocaine—emerged and triggered more prohibitions, more criminal arrests, more convictions, and more state and federal inmates, all of which further reinforced the increasingly negative views of these drugs. Lindesmith, writing in 1947, already sensed the irony, as authoritarian efforts to exert more public control over drug use via the Harrison Act led to a growing loss of control: "While the severe restrictions that are placed upon the handling of drugs prevent a part of the population from being exposed to the possibility of addiction, it should be noted that, at the same time, the illicit traffic, called into being by the same regulations, imports and distributes a vast quantity of the forbidden drugs, thus doubly exposing another portion of the population to addiction. The illegal dealer does not keep records or pay taxes on the supplies he handles, and there is nothing to prevent him from giving or selling the drug to anyone he pleases. As a consequence, the spread of the habit in the underworld is not subject to any public control."[108]

The same process occurred for marijuana, perhaps the most benign of all the drugs demonized in the twentieth century. Marijuana's fall from grace began in the 1930s with Harry J. Anslinger—America's first de facto drug czar—and the Treasury Department's new Federal Bureau of Narcotics and Dangerous Drugs.[109]

Just as the lights were going out on alcohol prohibition in the early 1930s, Anslinger helped focus them on the task of rooting out marijuana as the new public enemy. Along with independent groups of "concerned" citizens, Anslinger was responsible for framing (some might say, destroying) the image of marijuana in America, which he did first by characterizing it, with the help of the media, as an "assassin of youth."[110] A poster advertisement for a film by the same name, sponsored by the Bureau of Narcotics, headlined with the caption "Marihuana — Weed with Roots in Hell." Both the movie and its promotional materials tell of an unknown drug, "marihuana," that can transform even casual users into deviants, murderers, and rapists. Another antimarijuana advertisement at the time read: "This marihuana cigarette may be handed you by the friendly stranger. It contains the killer drug 'marihuana' — a powerful narcotic in which lurks Murder! Insanity! Death!"

The ease with which Anslinger raised public awareness to strike down this benign drug came partly from the fact that media reports had also begun stirring public sentiment against the drug in the 1920s. With individual states beginning to enact anti-marijuana laws, for example, the *New York Times* ran a fantastic drug story, with the headline "Mexican Family Go Insane."

A widow and her four children have been driven insane by eating the marihuana plant, according to doctors, who say that there is no hope of saving the children's lives and that the mother will be insane for the rest of her life. . . . The tragedy occurred while the body of the father, who had been killed, was still in the hospital. . . . The mother was without money to buy other food for the children, whose ages range from 3 to 15, so they gathered some herbs and vegetables growing in the yard for their dinner. Two hours after the mother and children had eaten the plants, they were stricken. Neighbors, hearing outbursts of crazed laughter, rushed to the house to find the entire family insane. Examination revealed that the narcotic marihuana was growing among the garden vegetables.[111]

Marijuana's downfall — like that of alcohol (if temporary), cocaine, and heroin — happened as its use became associated with more marginal elements of society and with special pharmacological powers that purportedly controlled and corrupted users. Less well known than cocaine or opiates, marijuana was easily associated with "undesirable" elements of American society—blacks, Mexicans, and countercultural groups such as jazz musicians. From these users, officials claimed, the dangers spread. By 1936 one could read in *Scientific American*, "Marihuana smoking has spread so rapidly that the drug has become a serious menace. . . . Marihuana produces a wide variety of symptoms in the user, including hilarity, swooning, and sexual excitement. Combined with intoxicants, it often makes the smoker vicious, with a desire to fight and kill. . . . Despite the vicious effects of marihuana, only 17 states have laws against it and its control is not yet included under the federal Harrison narcotic act."[112]

The marijuana story was a harbinger of what was to come later in the twentieth century. The differential prohibition of angels and demons that was emerging would not be rooted in any real evidence of pharmacological activity in the brain. Nor could it have been. As the chemist James Johnston had warned a century earlier in his *Chemistry of Common Life*, drug outcomes vary too greatly across individuals to construct a true pharmacological taxonomy of good and evil drugs.[113] Instead, differential prohibition would be anchored by public perceptions and an age-old cult of pharmacology. Beginning with a shift in the demographics of opiate use, public perceptions of drugs changed and led to the demonization of opiates, cocaine, and marijuana. Demonization itself only accelerated each drug's fall from grace, moreover, encouraging the enactment of even more restrictive drug laws. As illicit drug markets emerged in America, exorbitant prices, fewer quality controls, and the threat of violent crime were instituted to defend what would become, and what would remain, the most lucrative drug market in the world. Visible drug users and dealers were therefore marginalized further, with use itself becoming a crime, which reinforced once again the public perceptions that had prompted initial anti-drug reactions. Meanwhile, a variety of new placebo texts emerged—including the text deconstructed by Alfred Lindesmith—and they governed much of what took place in the name of opiate addiction and withdrawal in twentieth-century America.[114]

Chapter Five **America's Domestic Drug Affair**

*The junkie knows he is hooked; the housewife on
amphetamine and the businessman on meprobamate
hardly ever realize what has gone wrong.*
—Bruce Jackson, "White Collar Pill Party"

A t this point in the story, the most significant drugs consumed at the
turn of the twentieth century — alcohol, opiates, cocaine, and marijuana — had all begun their fall from grace. In the end, only alcohol
survived. It survived in part because it was the one substance indigenous to
America and its economy, and in part because, with the fall of the other
angels, it served a critical societal function: it became the one legally sanctioned public intoxicant available for all adults. Yet, with the stimulants, the
narcotics, and marijuana out of the picture, would alcohol be enough?

Since the stress, the malaise, and general discomforts that made these
fallen angels so popular in the nineteenth century had not themselves
drifted out of the mainstream, new prohibitions were likely to spawn new
illegal markets, as well as a public desire for new angels. Equally unlikely was
the prospect that makers of the popular tonics, elixirs, and other preparations would up and walk away from a patent-medicine industry worth
hundreds of millions — eventually tens of billions — of dollars. And they
didn't. While the emergence of differential prohibition was due in part to
the specific prohibition of a few fallen angels, it was also due to the capacity
of the pharmaceutical industry to manufacture new, artificial ones, which
they succeeded in doing first by developing new, synthetic drugs, and second by navigating, embracing, and eventually reinforcing the same prohibitions that had once seriously threatened their mass market of mood- and
mind-altering substances.

As prohibitions appeared, drug companies adapted in three ways. With the guidance of an increasingly powerful American Medical Association (AMA), drug makers shifted from head-to-head competition with medical practitioners, reflected in "patent medicines" made by an independent industry, to joint cooperation, reflected in the advent of prescription drugs. The industry also synthesized new, artificial angels that could substitute for the organic ones that had fallen from grace (such as barbiturates versus opiates); the artificial angels were then slyly reintroduced, one after the other, into existing medical practices as "safer and more effective" treatments. And finally, in order to legitimize drug use under the guise of medical treatment, drug makers carried the day in redefining the stress and dysfunctions of everyday life in terms of illness and disease, which the new drugs were said to treat.[1] Thus, with millions of individuals still wanting legal access to stimulants (uppers) and sedatives (downers), a new white market of "ethical" drug use was erected side by side with the emerging black markets of illegal drugs.

The prohibition of alcohol, although enacted after the Harrison Act of 1914, presented America with its first full-scale experience of prohibitionist philosophy. It also provided the first example of how medical sanctioning of drug use was employed to safeguard casual, domestic drug use, at least for some.

Prior to the United States' ratification of the Volstead Act, which prohibited the manufacture, sale, and distribution of alcohol, were individual state prohibitions. These surfaced in the 1850s, died down in the 1870s, then sprang up again in the 1880s. At the time that Prohibition was being enacted, about 60 percent of Americans were already living in dry states.[2] Despite their popularity, however, state prohibitions did not curb drinking. More often they simply changed the form that it took. Legal bars were closed, but speakeasies quickly took their place. And for those not wanting to participate in illegal activities, patent medicines were always available; these preparations often contained alcohol and continued to be sold over the counter and via mail order, even in dry states. Anticipating what was to come, *Ladies' Home Journal* reported in 1904 that 75 percent of the members of the Women's Christian Temperance Union "regularly took patent medicines" of up to 60 proof.[3] Temperance Christians even produced one of these preparations — Lydia Pinkham's Vegetable Compound — which was about 20 percent alcohol, or 40 proof. Another such product was Whisko. Contrary to the manufacturer's claim that it was "a nonintoxicating stimulant," and despite the Pure Food and Drugs Act of 1906, which required accurate labeling, Whisko was in fact 55 proof. Golden's Liquid Beef Tonic, sold as a recommended "treatment of alcohol habit," was 53 proof, and Kaufman's Sulfur Bitters, sold as a nonalcoholic preparation, was 40 proof and contained no sulfur.[4]

National Prohibition in 1920 changed this situation very little, although patent medicines continued to lose respectability and decline in sales. At the same time, the American medical profession was acquiring authority over the production and selling of legal drugs, with medical preparations increasingly available only through a doctor's prescription. One result was that as whisky became a federally prohibited substance in the 1920s, it also came to be commonly prescribed as medicine by physicians.

To understand the shift from liquor in over-the-counter patent medicines to liquor as a pseudomedical prescription treatment, one must recall that in the century prior to Prohibition, doctors had acted essentially as their own pharmacists, preparing medicines for patients in much the same way as shamans or medicine men in traditional cultures. An alternative to these individual preparations, available only from physicians, were so-called patent medicines, which were sold over the counter, without a prescription (and not necessarily with a patent). That two-tier system was similar to what existed in pharmacies at the end of the twentieth century, except for two characteristics. First, with no restriction on the kinds of drugs that could be sold as such and no requirement to list active ingredients on the bottle or in packaging, the earlier system was unencumbered by the regulations that later limited the number of over-the-counter medicines available. Second, in the earlier system the selling of patent medicines was in direct competition with the services and prescriptions of individual physicians, whereas by the middle of the twentieth century the two providers had united, with physicians prescribing drugs made by the same companies that also produced the over-the-counter drugs. In other words, instead of two classes of drugs positioned on each side of the pharmacist's counter, drugs such as morphine were available as both patent medicines and doctor-prescribed medicines.

In light of the questionable authority of physicians in the early twentieth century, and in light of the fact that patent medicines were considerably less costly than being treated by a physician — with no less promise of a cure — drug makers were able to compete effectively against the medical industry;

in fact, physicians were sometimes desperate enough to recommend patent medicines to their patients or to hand them out with the labels removed.

This bifurcated market collapsed early in the twentieth century, largely because of the newly acquired strength of the AMA. Among the actions the AMA took to undercut the legitimacy of the patent-medicine industry and assume power over the selling of strong medicines was to subdivide drug substances into "ethical" and "patent" medicines. This marked the beginning of a new era — an era of differential prohibition that would define America's drug scene for the remainder of the century.

Ethical medicines were defined as preparations of known composition advertised exclusively to physicians. Patent medicines were defined as preparations of unknown or secret composition advertised, usually in a shamelessly deceitful manner, directly to the public.[5] Subsequently, patent medicines were banished into the realm of the "unethical," a culture shift with broad implications. By cultivating a public sensibility in which drug use was deemed unethical if not taken for medical purposes and sanctioned accordingly, the AMA became the guardian of pharmaceutical angels. This sensibility was bolstered by legislation like the Harrison Act, which prohibited the dispensing of coca and opiates, save for "legitimate medical purposes." With a differential prohibition of drugs established, suddenly any form of nonmedical drug use was illegitimate. The only exception was alcohol following the repeal of Prohibition, a contradiction that was eventually resolved by separating in the public imagination "alcohol" from "drugs."

The rhetorical attack on patent medicines as unethical might not have been effective, however, were it not for other, related changes. In 1905 the AMA created its own Council on Pharmacy and Chemistry, which evaluated drugs and reported on them in a prototype of the *Physicians' Desk Reference* called *New and Nonofficial Remedies*.[6] This publication quickly acquired almost legal authority, putting further pressure on drug makers to develop medications that had some promise of effectiveness. The media had also begun to raise questions about the dangers of over-the-counter panaceas and to publicize the deceptive business practices of their manufacturers, which helped to safeguard the passage of the Pure Food and Drugs Act of 1906. In the face of growing attacks, drug makers themselves came to realize that their future lay in an alliance with the medical profession, not in competition against it. In rather short order, physicians wrestled control of a drug industry that realized it could no longer operate without the blessings of the medical establishment.

As for medically sanctioned alcohol use during Prohibition, the shift toward "ethical" prescriptions, prepared increasingly by pharmacists, led to fewer opportunities in the 1920s for obtaining alcohol via patent medicines. Whisky and brandy, for example, were dropped from the list of medically approved drugs in 1915.[7] Still, this hardly meant an end to alcohol sold under the guise of a curative. In fact, the consolidated power of physicians to deal in licit mood- and mind-altering substances, along with the financial security such power offered for medical practices, first appeared during this era. The AMA, holding to their notion of ethical use of drugs, condemned the casual use of liquor as a beverage, relying on epidemiological statistics to defend their support for the Volstead Act.[8] The AMA used the same notion, however, to permit, if not encourage, physicians to write prescriptions for liquor, including whisky and brandy. Once in motion, and despite claims by the AMA that it was "discouraging" the use of alcohol as a "therapeutic agent," this black-and-white treatment of drugs generated huge revenues for medical practices across the country.[9] As much as $40 million was made annually just through the writing of whiskey prescriptions alone.[10] Much the same situation simultaneously developed in Canada, which suffered through federal alcohol prohibition as well, from 1917 to 1920. There, physicians wrote as many as 4,000 prescriptions per month.[11] In British Columbia the secretary to the premier painted a picture soon to be reproduced in the United States: "Toward Christmas especially it looked as if an epidemic of colds and colics had struck the country like a plague. In Vancouver queues a quarter of a mile long could be seen waiting their turn to enter the liquor stores to get prescriptions filled. Hindus, Chinese, and Japanese varied the lines of the afflicted of many races. It was a kaleidoscopic procession waiting in the rain for a replenishment that would drive the chills away; and it was alleged that several doctors needed a little alcoholic liniment to soothe their writer's cramp caused by writing their signatures at two dollars per line."[12]

The writing of prescriptions for "medical liquor" was not a bootleg operation nor a deviant medical practice. Prescription forms were even printed by the Bureau of Prohibition of the U.S. Treasury Department, issued under the authority of the National Prohibition Act. Such an obvious back door to obtaining liquor might seem like a contradiction to the prohibitionist philosophy, but it was not. Like other drug prohibitions emerging at the time, including those that began with the Harrison Act in 1914, alcohol's prohibition was directed principally at a certain kind of drug use in America — drinking in taverns — and by a certain kind of people — Irish immigrants. Medical prescriptions for alcohol did not run counter to this intention. Rather, they were a way for "ethical" people to forbid and degrade a practice viewed as corrupting and immoral. They wanted their alcohol banned but wanted to drink it, too, and that is just what they got.

By the time Prohibition was repealed with the Twenty-first Amendment, in 1933, the lesson of prohibition was clear: the solution was worse than the problem. Unfortunately, the lesson was quickly forgotten. Although Prohibition failed to exert public control over drinking, it raised few doubts about the virtues of the same philosophy when applied to opiates and cocaine, which began with the Harrison Act and by 1933 was yielding many of the same pernicious effects for opiates as Prohibition had produced for alcohol.

The Harrison Act restricted the use of both opiates and cocaine to "legitimate medical purposes," and when it failed to suppress their use — prompting the usual "crimes of prohibition" instead — the Jones-Miller Act of 1922 was passed. This act banned all cocaine imports, doubled the maximum penalties for dealing in illegally imported drugs, and included "a fine of not more than $5,000 and imprisonment for not more than ten years for anyone, who fraudulently or knowingly imports or brings any narcotic drug into the United States or any territory under its control or jurisdiction, contrary to law, or assists in so doing, or receives, conceals, buys, sells, or in any manner facilitates the transportation, concealment, or sale of any such narcotic drug."[13] These acts were in place prior to the demise of Prohibition, which suggests that they may have been kept on the books afterward because of institutional momentum. The passage of the Marihuana Tax Act, which occurred not before but after the repeal of Prohibition, raises doubts about this view. Indeed, the Marihuana Tax Act of 1937 did for marijuana what the Harrison Act had done for cocaine and opiates: it took the first step toward complete prohibition by regulating marijuana, imposing a tax for importing, buying, or selling it.

Restrictions placed on the use of opiates, cocaine, and marijuana continued to escalate after the repeal of Prohibition. While black markets were built, the industry that first profited from making and selling mood- and mind-altering drugs also evolved, trying to maintain a parallel, legal drug market by synthesizing new, artificial angels to replace those it had lost. Cocaine would not be allowed back into the kingdom of ethical drugs, but the loss of such a potent stimulant was overcome with the discovery of a group of artificial stimulants called the amphetamines.

In 1932 Smith, Kline and French (SKF) — which later became Smith-Kline Beecham, then GlaxoSmithKline, the maker of Paxil — introduced the Benzedrine Inhaler, to be sold over the counter in drugstores. Benzedrine was SKF's brand name for a product containing leavoamphetamine, one of the three types of amphetamine. Usually referred to simply as amphetamine, leavoamphetamine was first synthesized in 1887. Of the two other forms of amphetamine, classified as such because of their similar chemical structures, one is methamphetamine, which was first synthesized in the West in 1919 and marketed under the brand name Methedrine. The other is dexamphetamine, marketed under the brand name Dexedrine. Although all amphetamines are essentially identical in their actions as central-nervous-system stimulants when taken at comparable doses and via the same route of administration, dexamphetamine is twice as potent per unit dose as amphetamine (i.e., it takes half as much to produce the same effect), and methamphetamine is twice again as potent as dexamphetamine. As a crystalline powder, methamphetamine is soluble in water, making it easy to inject. Toward the end of the twentieth century, when raves appeared on the scene, the term *speed* came to refer not to amphetamine but to the more versatile methamphetamine, which could be swallowed, snorted, smoked, or injected.

The discovery of amphetamine in 1887 by the German chemist L. Edeleano, under the chemical name phenylisopropylamine, had little to do with its eventual appearance as a pharmaceutical drug in the United States, a history that began instead in the 1920s, with a search for a convenient treatment for asthma.

Adrenalin (epinephrine) was an anti-asthmatic, but it could not be taken orally, which constrained its usefulness and profitability. K. K. Chen, a Chinese chemist hired by Eli Lilly in the late 1920s to search for an alternative, started with a traditional Chinese herbal asthma remedy called ma huang.[14] The active substance of ma huang, ephedrine, functions as a natural bronchial dilator that can be taken orally, and following Chen's discovery along these lines in 1928, Lilly quickly marketed it as such.[15] Ephedrine had been isolated once before, in Japan in 1887, the same year that Edeleano first synthesized amphetamine in Germany. The Japanese discovery was made by the pharmacologist Nagayoshi Nagai, who eventually synthesized methamphetamine from ephedrine, in 1893. Neither of these Japanese discoveries, however, appear to have played any role in the appearance of ephedrine or amphetamine on the U.S. market.[16] This seems instead to have begun with Chen's identification of ephedrine while at Eli Lilly.

The search for a new oral treatment for asthma did not end with ephedrine, which had to be imported from China and was therefore potentially exhaustible in its supply. A synthetic version was pursued, most prominently by the chemist Gordon Alles, who in 1927 replicated Edeleano's discovery of amphetamine (leavoamphetamine). The product that first resulted from these developments was SKF's Benzedrine Inhaler, which was marketed to the general public as an over-the-counter nasal decongestant.[17] Contained within the Benzedrine Inhaler was a sizeable quantity of leavoamphetamine — the equivalent of about 50 amphetamine tablets, or 250 milligrams.

Little time passed before the psychoactive effects of Benzedrine and other products containing amphetamine gave way to a new and larger, if not brighter, future for the drug. The medical community immediately seized on amphetamine sold as Benzedrine, in part because it was introduced in tablet form in 1937. Another reason was that it was a potent psychostimulant. The same year amphetamine was introduced in tablet form, the AMA's Council on Pharmacy and Chemistry gave Benzedrine its full backing as a new angel: "A feeling of exhilaration and sense of well-being was a consistent effect, and patients volunteered that there had been a definite increase in mental activity and efficiency."[18] This was the same organization that sought to define "ethical" drugs for the American public. In the context of such praise SKF promoted Benzedrine as a new, effective, and safe panacea, making no mention of any possible risk of abuse or dependence. Indeed, the company joined medical experts and the Council on Pharmacy and Chemistry in behaving as though the naturally derived stimulant that it replaced — cocaine — had never existed.

As with the the SSRIs, which were assigned many new uses after they were first released as antidepressants in the late 1980s and early 1990s, dozens of clinical uses had been identified for amphetamines by the late 1940s. A report issued in 1946, for example, noted thirty-nine different illnesses for which Benzedrine was recommended as the first line of treatment.[19] The amphetamines had become big business, in other words, with physicians prescribing them for everything from depression and opiate dependence to hyperactivity, obesity, impotence, and old age. Some of these indications were practical and reasonably well researched, such as the treatment of narcolepsy; other indications, however, exemplified an emerging pharmaceutical–medical industrial complex that engaged in its own, licit drug trafficking. For example, amphetamines were sold as diet drugs and pick-me-ups, the most common of which was a preparation of methamphetamine called Desoxyn. Although perhaps difficult to imagine today, but very much in keeping with the habits of the patent medicine industry, seniors were also regularly encouraged to use amphetamines — to get an "increase in mental activity and efficiency." Not only did the drug companies promise such an effect, so did the Council on Pharmacy and Chemistry. While Parke Davis could no longer sell a dozen or more cocaine-containing euphoriants directly to the public, it and other drug companies revitalized these markets using amphetamines, still selling them over the counter.

The Harrison and Jones-Miller Acts had established prohibition against cocaine and the opiates, but had achieved nothing in the way of stopping the sanctioned use of stimulants under the guise of "medical treatment." Furthermore, with cocaine no longer available as a legal drug, Benzedrine use quickly drifted out of the sanctioned realm of "medical use" and into the more public realm of nonsanctioned, casual use. Following the path of cocaine in the twentieth century, amphetamine thus strayed into the realm in which public perceptions turn negative, its users being increasingly perceived as those at the margins of society. "Unethical" use took place not just in the United States but also in Britain, Sweden, and Japan.

The creation of the amphetamine subculture in America is said to have its origins in an early human psychopharmacological experiment at the University of Minnesota, in 1936. Examining the performance effects of amphetamine with college students, researchers had failed to anticipate that individuals who experienced the effects of Benzedrine during the study might be impressed enough by the results to seek the drug afterward, which they did. Following the discovery that Benzedrine could be casually purchased at the local pharmacy, amphetamine's use as a party drug and late-night study aid was born. The first published report attributing addiction to the amphetamines appeared in the medical literature one year later.

New amphetamine users and uses evolved as recreational drug takers found that one could break open the Benzedrine Inhaler, remove the paper wadding laced with the 250 milligrams of amphetamine, and extract the drug by plunging it into a drinkable solution (or even chewing it with gum). The jazz artist Charlie Parker was among the many celebrities, including the Beatles, said to have engaged in this practice; he created his own "B-bomb" by soaking the Benzedrine strip in his cup of coffee. In 1946 — the year in which one first heard the ditty "Who Put the Benzedrine in Mrs. Murphy's Ovaltine?" — the article "On a bender with Benzedrine" appeared in the popular magazine *Everybody's Digest*, with a description of the procedure for making the B-bomb: "After I bought an inhaler, Hal worked off the perforated cap and pulled out the medicated paper, folded accordion-wise. . . . Hal took the innocent looking scrap of paper he had torn away and held it between thumb and finger. He alternately dunked and squeezed this paper into his glass of beer."[20]

By 1949 enough of an amphetamine subculture had emerged that, in anticipation of a ban by the FDA, SKF pulled their inhaler from the over-the-counter market. (The FDA did, however, allow a comparable inhaler to remain on the over-the-counter market until 1959.) Still, the amphetamine subculture continued to grow in the 1940s and 1950s, a fact that was hardly surprising given that one could buy speed in bulk in the 1940s without a prescription; indeed, one only paid about seventy-five cents per 1,000 pills.[21]

The prohibition of cocaine had not eliminated the domestic stimulant market, but instead produced a whole new subculture around a drug that, as a synthetic compound, was not tied to foreign imports and could be produced easily and inexpensively.[22]

The amphetamines continued to be available over the counter until the early 1950s, after which they could be obtained legally only by prescription. Nevertheless, both the legal and illegal markets for amphetamines continued to grow. During the Korean War, the intravenous use of amphetamine in combination with heroin ("speedballing") was practiced by American soldiers stationed in Japan and Korea. This initiated a trend toward using drugs in combination — a trend that, oddly enough, the drug companies also seized on. As to the levels of "ethical" amphetamine use, 3.5 billion amphetamine tablets were produced legally in the United States in 1958. By 1970 this number had increased to 10 billion,[23] and by 1971 fifteen different drug companies were manufacturing thirty-one different amphetamine preparations. These drugs were now available only by prescription, however, a hurdle that was overcome by the black market for drugs. During the early 1960s amphetamines had become a valued street commodity, with intravenous amphetamine use found in most urban centers. Methamphetamine labs also began to appear, first in California. Meanwhile, holding to the notion that medically sanctioned use was ethical, regardless of the volume of use, the AMA's Council on Pharmacy and Chemistry reported in 1963, "At this time, compulsive abuse of the amphetamines [is] a small problem."[24]

By 1970 such a view was no longer tenable. With public fear of stimulant mania and addiction reaching new heights, legislation was enacted. The Comprehensive Drug Abuse Prevention and Control Act of 1970, along with changes made to it the following year, grouped together cocaine and the amphetamines as having the same abuse potential, a grouping that also included the stimulant methylphenidate (Ritalin).

By that time beliefs about the pharmacological powers of the amphetamines were almost as efficacious in affecting unusual behavior as the drugs themselves, and not just for those bent on ridding society of them. A study that examined data from five drug-analysis programs in the United States revealed that a potent placebo text now guided the use of amphetamines. Between 1970 and 1974, these programs had analyzed a total of 4,500 samples of various street drugs. Among those samples their owners believed to be speed, a third of them contained no amphetamine whatsoever.[25] Had the *idea* of speed become as psychoactive as its pharmacology, to the point that anticipation and expectations surrounding the drug could all but substitute for the drug itself? That finding was similar to those that showed that experienced users of cocaine, under blind conditions, had considerable difficulty in discriminating between cocaine's effects and the effects of other drugs, including caffeine and placebos; it was also similar to the report of several young self-described "opiate addicts" who had used only trivial doses of opiates.

As the mythical status of the amphetamines as panaceas in medical practice flowed out onto the street, the black market for amphetamines came to rival the scale of the illicit market for opiates, and, beginning in the 1960s, for cocaine. Still, the amphetamines would not be the most dramatic part of the story involving the social history of stimulants in the twentieth century. This accolade would go to Ritalin, a stimulant with pharmacological actions that turned out to be all but identical to cocaine. Ritalin, after all, placed the differential prohibition of drugs in America in the twentieth century in sharpest relief. While historians and drug warriors late in the twentieth century remained steadfast in their belief that cocaine was a demon drug, Ritalin — mother's other little helper — thrived as a mainstream prescription drug, taken by literally millions of children.

In the realm of drug dependence and drug addiction, both in the pharmaceutical marketplace and in the black markets, twentieth-century substances of choice fell into one of two general classes: uppers or downers. The drugs of persistent domestic demand either energized human consciousness or dulled it into oblivion. Being "anywhere but here" had become the chief motivation of America as a drug culture.

Given this pursuit of altered states, and given that nature's most efficacious stimulant had fallen from grace only to return as a "medicine" in the 1930s in the form of the synthetic amphetamines, one might wonder whether an equivalent story also exists for downers and depressants. The loss of heroin as an over-the-counter drug was overcome in part by the development of synthetic opiates, called opioids.[26] Among these are the drugs d-propoxyphene (Darvon), hydromorphone (Dilaudid), meperidine (Demerol), fentanyl (Sublimaze), and oxycodone (Oxycontin). All of them are considered synthetic opiates because they affect the same brain-receptor systems as do natural opiates, which are derived from the poppy plant. The void left by the removal of opiates from the middle- and upper-class drug markets was not filled primarily by the opioids, however, since there was in fact little need for the opioids to take up this role. Not only had alcohol, which is classified as a depressant (or downer), been relegalized in the 1930s, but other synthetic depressants had entered the market first. Although these drugs were not the euphoriants the opioids are, they nevertheless succeeded in filling the void left behind as opium and its derivatives were removed from patent medicines and prohibited from nonmedical use.

Morphine, heroin, and opioids all act as depressants. They can function as euphoriants (making a person blissful), as anxiolytics (making a person less anxious), and as sedative-hypnotics (making a person drowsy). Opiates and opioids are classified medically as analgesics, however, which was the role to which their ethical use was relegated by the medical establishment in the wake of the demonization of opiates. In the meantime, a whole new class of psychoactive drugs became available, variously defined as depressants, sedative-hypnotics, and minor tranquilizers. The primary virtue of these was that they lowered anxiety, created an inner feeling of calm, and with increased dosage, induced sleep. Thus, as the opiates and opioids (not including heroin) remained available as prescription drugs that promised escape from physical pain, new depressant drugs emerged as panaceas that promised escape from its psychological equivalent.

Modern Drugs for the Treatment of Mental Illness summarized the kind of "ethical" argument that legitimized the widespread use of depressants that followed: "Worry and anxiety form the kernel of neurotic and many psychotic conditions and when very intense give rise to psychiatric symptoms amongst which the most important and unpleasant are emotional tension during the day and insomnia at night."[27] Such "emotional tension during the day and insomnia at night" represented of course the same domestic woes that had encouraged the massive use of over-the-counter preparations containing opiates in the nineteenth century.

By 1950 the stage had been set for a reenactment of the story of opiates in the nineteenth century (and the sister act to that of the synthetic stimulants, beginning with Benzedrine). As one writer characterized the mood of the times, "On paper, they didn't seem like such a bad idea. It was all supposed to be so simple: You just turn down the customary stress and static of everyday life by popping a sunny yellow or sky-blue pill three or four times a day, then watch your worries disappear into space. No muss, no fuss, no complicated coping or unnecessary figuring-out of feelings, and certainly no side effects, snide effects, or otherwise-implied effects."[28]

One particular drug lies at the center of America's love affair with downers: meprobamate, the first minor tranquilizer. As with the amphetamines, the discovery of meprobamate as a mind-altering substance began in the laboratory and was likewise the product of serendipitous discovery.

The story begins with the work of the pharmacologist Frank Berger, a Jewish refugee who, while working for the British Drug House in London in 1945, developed drugs whose pharmacological effects occurred outside the central nervous system. This was the age of penicillin, and Berger and his colleagues were attempting to develop new antibiotics that would kill microorganisms that had become resistant to older ones. This involved the testing of phenylglycerol ethers as possible antibiotics, one of which was mephenesin. When Berger tested the toxicity of mephenesin in small laboratory animals, however, he found something interesting: the compound produced muscle relaxation without sedating the animals, an effect described in his first publication on the subject as "tranquilization."[29] This discovery first led to the use of mephenesin in humans as a muscle relaxant in the administration of anesthesia, then was followed by the discovery that mephenesin could also be used as a relaxant in psychiatric populations.

All this had taken place by the late 1940s. The development of meprobamate came about shortly thereafter, as Berger and others attempted to improve on mephenesin, which was limited in its therapeutic use due to its short duration of action. In seeking a better understanding of mephenesin's chemical structure, researchers were able to look for chemical derivatives of the parent compound that were equally effective but acted for longer durations. In collaboration with B. J. Ludwig, Berger, now in the United States, synthesized meprobamate in May 1950. In 1954 he reported on the "unusual" specificity of the drug as a muscle relaxant and sedative, noting a duration of action eightfold that of mephenesin.[30]

Wallace Laboratories brought meprobamate on the market a year later, sold as Miltown, "The Tranquilizer with Muscle Relaxant Action." Miltown was the name of the New Jersey town where Wallace Labs were located, and where Berger now lived. Among the conditions for which it was immediately recommended were anxiety, "tension states," and insomnia, as well as headaches, alcoholism, premenstrual syndrome, depression, and "behavior disorders" — a huge potential market for meprobamate. Soon people were literally lining up at the drugstores to get their dose of the new happiness. In the year of its release, 1955, its monthly sales went from $7,500 in May, when it was introduced, to over $500,000 in December, with the drug receiving the American Psychiatric Association's stamp of approval. The almost immediate popularity of Miltown with America's psychiatric establishment, not to mention the general public, came from the fact that as an anxiolytic it could be targeted not only at the hospitalized psychiatric patient, as was the case with antipsychotics like SKF's Thorazine (chlorpromazine), but also at the domestic market — the same market, incidentally, that roughly 80 percent of the members of the American Psychiatric Association administered to.[31]

In marketing Miltown, Wallace relied on the notion of tranquilization to distinguish it from existing sedative-hypnotics, including another class of depressants known as the barbiturates. As David Healy put it in *The Creation of Psychopharmacology*, "The idea of sedation was not compatible with a treatment that would allow people to get on with their lives, so Miltown became a tranquilizer."[32] The specific claim made by Berger and Wallace Labs was that Miltown reduced anxiety without producing marked sedation, as happened with the barbiturates, and did so without producing a reduction in mental functioning, as happened with alcohol. " 'Miltown' does not 'insulate' the patient from his environment," claimed a Wallace pamphlet, handed out to physicians at the time. "Tranquilization is achieved without loss of alertness, visual acuity or psychomotor coordination."[33] In the end, Miltown was popular for a simple reason: it made many of those who used it feel better.

Miltown was also hailed as being non–habit forming, something that a drug — or anything else that makes people feel better — could never be. Echoing the earlier claim that Bayer's Heroin was not habit forming and was an effective treatment for morphinism, the physician's manual from Wallace Labs reported, "The overwhelming majority of doctors have experienced no habituation problems with meprobamate."[34] As with the consumption of opiates and cocaine as over-the-counter patent medicines, as well as alcohol consumption by the general population, the use of Miltown was indeed habit-free for most people who took the drug occasionally. However, the drug was likely to be a problem for those who felt the greatest relief from it, that is, those who came to rely on the soothing effects of the drug and could find no other escape from their worries, boredom, or stresses. What was more, as an odorless pill, it could also be taken in secret, which gave the drug an advantage — and an increased risk — over alcohol. This was especially true for women: a 1950 study found that the most common category of dependent opiate users among a high-income population was "housewives," and this was true for meprobamate as well.[35]

Meprobamate was not a perfect substitute for opiates, however. In fact, in some ways it was notably worse: with chronic use, it was likely to produce a state of physical dependence more severe and more dangerous than opiate dependence. Even the pamphlet Wallace Labs gave to physicians cited a study published in 1958 in the *American Journal of Psychiatry* in which hospitalized psychiatric patients showed pronounced signs of physical dependence after continued use. Of forty-seven patients given Miltown continuously for forty days, forty-four showed marked withdrawal symptoms, including insomnia, vomiting, and tremors, when the drug was withdrawn. Three of these patients, none of whom had a history of convulsions, developed grand mal seizures.[36] If Miltown was to be the new opiate of the masses, it could hardly be held up as evidence of scientific or medical progress.

Risks of psychological and physical dependence notwithstanding, the ease of access to Miltown ensured the drug's absorption into mainstream popular culture. Combined with the amphetamines as the new uppers, it had the almost immediate effect of turning the legal market of mood- and mind-altering drugs of the 1950s into a mirror image of the legal market of patent medicines of the 1880s. Drug prohibitions, beginning with the Harrison Act of 1914, had curbed the widespread domestic use (and sale) of uppers (coca and cocaine) and downers (opium and heroin), but the effect had not lasted long. Miltown—the "dry martini," as it had come to be known—was being served like one at "Miltown parties" in suburbs across the country.[37] The domestic drug scene of the time was profiled in a 1966 *Atlantic* essay entitled "White-Collar Pill Party," in which Bruce Jackson pointed out, "The publicity goes to the junkies [and] lately to the college kids, but these account for only a small portion of the American drug problem. Far more worrisome are the millions of people who have become dependent on commercial drugs. The junkie knows he is hooked; the housewife on amphetamine and the businessman on meprobamate hardly ever realize what has gone wrong."[38]

Miltown, like Benzedrine, was in the process of spilling out of the sanctioned realm of "ethical" use and falling into "deviant" use within various drug subcultures. As it did, it fell into disrepute even faster than had Benzedrine and the amphetamines. Suddenly Miltown was on the nightly news not as a wonder drug but as a dangerous substance that encouraged both misuse (i.e., nonmedical use by deviants, usually youths), and overuse (i.e., excessive prescribing by physicians to the respectable middle and upper classes). Physicians who prescribed the tranquilizer Equanil overcame this loss of Miltown's reputation to some degree, for it was exactly the same drug sold under a different name (by Wyeth Pharmaceuticals). When Equanil ran into the same troubles as Miltown, however, the problem had to be solved once again—this time with the barbiturates, a class of compounds that had existed prior to the arrival of Miltown.

The barbiturates had not received, when first on the market, as much attention as Miltown did. Not only were they initially viewed as sedatives, rather than anxiolytics, but they were tough to market as safe and nonaddictive drugs. But as Miltown waned in sales, the public demand for downers remained, and so the barbiturates were given a second life.

The initial rise of the barbiturates took place at the end of the nineteenth century. By the 1940s so many barbiturate compounds had been concocted that they could be sorted into four categories: ultrashort-, short-, intermediate-, and long-acting. Ultrashort-acting barbiturates included methohexital (Brevital), thiamylal (Surital), and thiopental (Pentothal). Used for anesthesia, their intravenous administration produced sleep within about one minute. The short- and intermediate-acting barbiturates, however, were to become the most popular domestically and on the street. These included amobarbital (Amytal), pentobarbital (Nembutal), secobarbital (Seconal), a compound of amobarbital and secobarbital (Tuinal), butalbital (Fiorinal, Fioricet), butabarbital (Butisol), talbutal (Lotusate), and aprobarbital (Alurate). When taken orally, these drugs produced sedation within fifteen to forty minutes and lasted for several hours. Long-acting barbiturates, which include phenobarbital (Luminal) and mephobarbital (Mebaral), produced effects that last nearly twelve hours and were used primarily for daytime sedation and the treatment of seizure disorders.

The *barb-* in barbiturate refers not to a chemical structure or a biochemical action, but to the Day of St. Barbara, the patron saint of miners and artillerymen. On that day in 1864, the chemist Adolf von Baeyer, founder of the German pharmaceutical company by the same name, and noted maker of heroin and aspirin, combined urea with malonic acid, thereby synthesizing the compound malonylurea. Malonylurea was renamed barbituric acid in tribute to the day it was synthesized, and it was on this day that von Baeyer celebrated its discovery at a nearby tavern, a tavern frequented by artillery officers. Or so one story goes.[39] Another story claims that von Baeyer named the compound after a woman named Barbara for whom he held affections.

Whatever the story, barbituric acid led to the development of a derivative compound that acted as a depressant on the central nervous system. In 1902 a patent was obtained for barbituric acid, and on 9 July 1903 the German chemists Emil Fischer and Joseph von Mering modified barbituric acid to produce diethyl barbituric acid, or barbital. Immediately recognized as a sedative-hypnotic because it produced sleep in human subjects, barbital was marketed as a replacement for the bromides and chloral hydrate, the two compounds most frequently used as sedatives at the time.

Bromide is a salt. It was first used as an anticonvulsant in 1857 and as a sedative in 1864, the year von Baeyer synthesized barbituric acid. The bromides had an unpleasant taste and odor and, with continued use, could lead to a host of physical problems known collectively as "chronic bromide intoxication."[40] Chloral hydrate, minted in 1832, was credited as the first synthetic sedative-hypnotic and was used as such at least as early as the 1860s. Habitual use of chloral hydrate was identified as early as 1871, when Benjamine Richardson, the physician who had introduced the drug in Britain, noted its use as a "toxical luxury."[41] (In Britain a potent combination known as "knockout drops," or "Mickey Finn," was created by combining chloral hydrate with alcohol.) Chloral hydrate was used throughout the twentieth century, although over-the-counter use ended with the introduction of the barbiturates.[42] The incidence of over-the-counter use of bromides also slowed when the barbiturates appeared, and bromide prescriptions were all but eliminated by the introduction of Miltown. Bromides continued to be sold for a time in some over-the-counter products, however, the most popular of which was a "calmative" agent called Nervine.

In this context the barbiturates were introduced, hailed as a family of new depressant drugs early in the twentieth century. From barbituric acid, more than 2,500 derivatives were eventually produced, although only a small percentage achieved general use. The first of these was barbital, which was marketed under the trade names Veronal and Barbitone. The second was phenobarbital, marketed as Luminal in 1912. Both barbital and phenobarbital were long-acting barbiturates, however, so they did not produce sleep as quickly as one might desire, and their sedative effect could carry over into the next day. Realizing this, pharmaceutical chemists began developing more user-friendly versions, leading to the development of the shorter-acting "barbies," including amobarbital (Amytal, "ammies") in 1923, pentobarbital (Nembutal, "yellow jackets," "nembies") in 1930, and secobarbital (Seconal, "reds," "sekkies") in 1930.[43]

Like the mood- and mind-altering substances that came before them, including cannabis, coca, cocaine, opium, and the opiates, the barbiturates quickly acquired a status as general-purpose drugs, taken as treatment or as a complement to treatment for a wide assortment of ailments, complaints, and diseases. They were in fact the first big commercial success for synthetic drugs of this kind. Like meprobamate, the barbiturates also made many who used them feel better, no doubt in part because the nervousness and stress in their lives made them feel lousy. But the barbiturates were also employed for other, sometimes more substantial reasons: to reduce epileptic seizures; to help individuals experiencing psychoses and depression; to treat arthritis, high blood pressure, and ulcers. Promoted as a possible cure for everything from bedwetting to alcoholism, barbiturate use was now deemed "ethical" for more than seventy medical conditions.

In *Licit and Illicit Drugs*, the straightforward and nonsensational drug text issued by Consumer Reports in 1972, Edward Brecher and colleagues compared the experience of taking moderate doses of the barbiturates to that of another depressant, alcohol, concluding that the barbiturates "resemble alcohol in almost all respects." Specifically, they noted, "You can get drunk on barbiturates (especially the short-acting kinds) as on alcohol. You can become addicted to barbiturates (especially the short-acting kinds) as to alcohol. A barbiturate addict suffers much the same delirium tremens when withdrawn from barbiturates as an alcoholic withdrawn from alcohol. And abrupt withdrawal may in both cases prove fatal. The parallel between the short-acting barbiturates and alcohol is particularly close, for alcohol is also a short-acting drug."[44]

Brecher and his colleagues cite several studies in support of this comparison, one of which had been conducted at the Public Health Service Hospital in Lexington, Kentucky, and reported in 1950.[45] In the study five men serving sentences for narcotic law violations were given a barbiturate. After "volunteering" for the study and undergoing medical and psychological examinations, each was given a consistent sizable dose of a barbiturate.[46] Each one showed, according to the report, a form of intoxication that resembled alcohol intoxication, including disinhibition — that is, they looked and acted drunk. All five individuals showed a reduction in their ability to think coherently and perform normally on cognitive tests. They showed physical signs of alcohol intoxication, including tremors and lack of coordination. Before passing out, two patients "became garrulous, boisterous, and silly," while two others became quiet and depressed (the fifth was less affected). On the next day they all looked and reported feeling hung-over, as though they had consumed alcohol the night before and had become drunk from it.

The barbiturates shared features common not only to alcohol but also to the opiates: they were well tolerated and relatively free of side effects when taken occasionally or if consumed regularly over a short period only. As with Miltown's introduction into the over-the-counter market, such a cheery assessment, while true, also served to conceal the possible risks of dependence posed by chronic use of the barbiturates. As with the opiates, regular barbiturate use could lead to tolerance of the drugs' psychoactive effects, thus requiring that more of the drug be taken to produce the same effect. That this and other risks were ignored in the casual embrace of the barbiturates caused them to fall into trouble, just as Miltown did years later. By 1939 roughly 700 million doses (or one billion grains) of these drugs were taken annually.[47] That same year, Arthur Tatum authored the first detailed report on "the present status of the barbiturate problem," which appeared in the journal *Physiological Reviews*.[48]

As use continued to grow, and as Miltown came and went, signs of a "barbiturate problem" became clearer. In the domestic realm was evidence that the shorter-acting barbiturates produced both psychological and physical dependence in habitual users, as with Miltown, and even that the "barbiturates [were] capable of producing physical dependence that [was] of greater medical consequence than opiate dependency."[49] In *The Drug Hang-up*, Rufus King wrote, "Because barbiturates produce greater mental, emotional and neurological impairment than morphine, informed medical experts expressed the opinion that addiction to them is actually more detrimental to the individual and society than morphine addiction."[50] In 1972, the "year of the barbs," the U.S. Bureau of Narcotic and Dangerous Drugs, which became the DEA in 1973, concluded that greater restrictions needed to be placed on barbiturates as they were "more dangerous than heroin."[51] In 1977 a federal study linked barbiturates to nearly 5,000 deaths a year and about 25,000 visits to emergency rooms and drug-treatment centers.[52]

Gradually, an image of the habitual barbiturate user came into focus in America: "The barbiturate addict is usually unkempt in appearance. With little motor control over gross or fine movements, he may have a staggering gait, and poorly articulated speech. Emotionally he is likely to veer between extremes: one moment warm and friendly and the next erupting into violence. . . . His judgement is impaired and, like the alcoholic, he appears to be indulging in inner fantasies rather than reacting to outer reality. . . . Opiates reduce the primary needs of hunger and sex, whereas barbiturates 'impair the ability of the individual to suppress patterns of behavior which are developed in relation to the active gratification of both primary and secondary needs.' "[53] The opiate habitué and writer William S. Burroughs painted an even grimmer, if exaggerated, picture of the chronic male barbiturate user. In *Naked Lunch* he wrote, "The barbiturate addict presents a shocking spectacle. He cannot coordinate, he staggers, falls off bar stools, goes to sleep in the middle of a sentence, drops food out of his mouth. He is confused, quarrelsome, and stupid. And he almost always uses other drugs, anything he can lay his hands on; alcohol, Benzedrine, opiates, marijuana. . . . It seems to me that barbiturates cause the worst possible form of addiction, unsightly, deteriorating, difficult to treat."[54]

Another aspect of the barbiturate problem sets it apart, one that is independent of any risk of dependence or addiction: the unique risk of accidental overdose, with the concomitant easiness of using barbiturates to commit suicide. For many users, the recommended therapeutic dose for sedation is not terribly far from the minimal dose that produces toxicity and overdose. As one strays beyond the minimal dose for sedation, intoxication occurs, followed by a loss of consciousness, shallow breathing, convulsions, coma, and ultimately death.

Moreover, two factors can—and often did—further narrow the small margin of safety. First, combining barbiturates with other depressants, especially alcohol, but also the opiates, can result in a synergistic (i.e., multiplicative) drug effect; when either is taken with a barbiturate, a lethal overdose can occur with the consumption of fewer than a dozen pills. Second, and not mutually exclusive with the first, tolerance to the desired effects does not yield tolerance to the toxic effects. As more of the drug is taken week after week to maintain an effect such as relaxation or intoxication, the margin of safety narrows. The consequences are rarely good: "This friend of mine was always taking barbs. He also drank whisky a lot. Anyway one night he'd had a skinful of both. He was out in the back garden and his flatmate had started a fire to burn a load of garden rubbish. He collapsed and fell into the fire."[55]

Instead of acquiring opiates from patent medicines, the middle and upper classes were now taking barbiturates, also sold as over-the-counter "medicines." According to the new prohibitionist philosophy, this was progress. But it was an abstract, head-in-the-sand kind of progress, rooted in self-deception. For whatever the risks of dependency and addiction presented by the opiates, and whatever the limited domestic benefits obtained via harsh federal laws against them, all was lost within a few decades with the synthesis, production, and mass marketing of the shorter-acting barbiturates. Even the National Commission on Marijuana and Drug Abuse equated the popularity of barbiturates explicitly with the use of opiates late in the nineteenth century, suggesting that the "overuse" of barbiturates had become America's hidden drug problem.[56]

It was during this long period of barbiturate use that meprobamate (Miltown) made its appearance. Because it had the effect of further popularizing the casual use of depressant drugs prior to its fall, however, barbiturate use actually peaked after rather than before America began its trek down the road to Miltown. In the 1940s the era of the barbiturates appeared to be ending. Popular health magazines, including one published by the AMA, were critical of the casual use of barbiturates; one 1942 article from the AMA's magazine was titled "1,250,000,000 Doses a Year."

But America is a forgetful nation, just as the AMA is a pragmatic organization. The AMA's attitude toward mind-altering drugs had not changed since the creation of the Council on Pharmacy and Chemistry in 1905; while its articles might outline the dangers of some "ethical" drugs, such dangers seemed not to apply as long as the drugs were properly recommended and prescribed by a physician. In fact, because barbiturates could still be obtained without a prescription at the time, the AMA pointed to their dangers specifically in order to emphasize that the safe and ethical use of a barbiturate could be ensured by consulting a physician before taking it. In reality, this did not happen in most cases, and by the time prescriptions were required by law, in the 1960s, this hurdle to legal access would have little effect on the volume of their use. According to one estimate, barbiturate use increased 800 percent from 1942 to 1969, reaching ten billion doses.[57] The FDA reported in 1959 that 819,060 pounds had been produced that year (to be taken along with the eight billion amphetamine tablets produced that year).[58] This explosion was not restricted to the United States, moreover. In Britain over sixteen million prescriptions were handed out for barbiturates in 1966, with a roster listing the names of roughly half a million regular users.

And where the domestic market went, the street market soon followed. In fact, even prior to Miltown parties, the barbiturates were identified as effective party pills and used accordingly. As Brecher and colleagues found,

"By the end of the 1940s, a nation that had for decades used barbiturates sensibly, to go to sleep or to calm the nerves, had been persuaded [by state regulations and newspaper headlines] that the drugs were 'thrill pills.' What might have been anticipated did in fact occur. Some people who would never for the world have taken a sedative or a sleeping pill now began getting drunk on the new 'thrill pills.' For them the warnings served as lures; illicit barbiturate use increased from year to year. Throughout the 1950s and 1960s, the relatively harmless sleeping tablets of the 1930s played their new role as one of the major illicit American drugs."[59]

A drug expert, testifying before Congress in 1971, noted similarly, "For the youngster barbiturates are a more reliable 'high' and less detectable than 'pot.' They are less strenuous than LSD, less 'freaky' than amphetamines, and less expensive than heroin. A school boy can 'drop a red' and spend the day in a dreamy, floating state of awareness untroubled by reality. It is drunkenness without the odor of alcohol. It is escape for the price of one's lunch money."[60]

Once on the street, the patterns of use surrounding the barbiturates also changed accordingly. Barbiturate use merged with existing drug practices, such that barbiturates were not just being popped as party pills but also injected like opiates and amphetamines. When injected, barbiturates produced a feeling of warmth and drowsiness not unlike the euphoric effect of the opiates. Indeed, many street users of opiates found that injecting barbiturates was an acceptable alternative when opiates were unavailable or too expensive.[61] Injection, however, promoted drug tolerance and thus presented a far greater risk of overdose than it ever had for the opiates. Sudden withdrawal from intravenous (or even oral) doses of barbiturates can be fatal as well, which was another difference from the opiates.

By the 1960s, as drug subcultures proliferated in earnest, many of the prescribed barbiturates and amphetamines were finding their way into casual use. The FDA later admitted that "illegal sales of amphetamines and barbiturates occupied more regulatory concern at [the] FDA than all other drug problems combined from the 1940s to the 1960s." This was testament to prohibition's unintended effect of encouraging the pharmaceutical industry to create and market new mind-altering drugs for the general population, and to the success the drug industry had in doing just that.[62]

The effect of these developments—with one drug falling into disgrace, followed by another, then another—did not intimidate drug makers or encourage them to take a more tempered posture in the temptations they sold. Instead, the so-called overuse, misuse, and abuse of depressant pharmaceuticals seemed to have just the opposite effect. Drug makers came to realize how large and lucrative a market existed for mood- and mind-altering drugs in America — a society that wanted to be full of energy all day (uppers), then relax and get some sleep without worry at night (downers). Drug makers also figured out how to nurture and exploit this market by minting ever "newer and safer" synthetic drugs. First came the barbiturates and the amphetamines in the 1930s, and then meprobamate (Miltown) in the 1950s. In the 1960s another new depressant hit the market: methaqualone. As the psychopharmacologist Oakley Ray put it with regard to the latter, "My daddy was right: If you miss a streetcar, don't worry, another one just like it will be along in a little while."[63]

Better known as Quaalude, methaqualone was first synthesized in India as part of a program to develop antimalarial drugs. Although ineffective in that capacity, it did act as a sedative-hypnotic and entered the U.S. market as a depressant in 1965 under a variety of trade names, including Quaalude and Sopor. It entered the British market as Mandrax in 1959 but sold poorly and had to be remarketed in 1965 because of the thalidomide disaster, which created a demand for new and safer sedative-hypnotics. With a huge marketing push in both the United States and the United Kingdom, methaqualone was introduced in 1965 as a new, safe, and nonaddictive substitute for barbiturates (as well as for thalidomide).

By the early 1970s methaqualone had become the depressant of choice, and the idea of "luding out" on the "love drug" had captured the popular imagination in America, which had already happened in Germany and Japan, in the 1960s. It soon became clear that, rather than the drug being a breakthrough substitute for barbiturates, quaaludes were just another depressant drug available to the general public, sought after by both drug-recreating youths and street users. A 1972 *Washington Post* article, "Methaqualone: The 'safe' drug that isn't very," identified a pattern that was hardly unique: "The methaqualone boom should make an interesting case study in future medical textbooks: How skilful public relations and advertising created a best-seller — and helped cause a medical crisis in the process."[64]

An estimated four tons of methaqualone were legally produced and distributed in the decade that followed; estimates of illegal imports and distribution suggest a volume of pills many times greater, including, as reported in

Newsweek in 1981, many counterfeit pills that looked like methaqualone but in fact contained over-the-counter sedatives.[65] At that time, the pharmaceutical market for methaqualone also was expanding because of various "stress clinics" in the eastern United States, whose purpose was to capitalize on the depressant market by providing an easy yet "ethical" means for obtaining methaqualone. The DEA, offended by such a democratic means of obtaining mood-altering pharmaceuticals, later stated, "Investigation of these clinics was complicated by the fact that patients underwent physical examinations so that there was a facade of legitimate medical treatment."[66]

The candle that burns twice as bright burns only half as long, and the market for methaqualone came to a quick and complete close in 1984, with methaqualone prohibited from all domestic use. With the help of the U.S. Congress and the DEA, methaqualone's fall from grace came with the drug's reclassification as a Schedule I drug, that is, a drug deemed to have a high potential for abuse and with no medical value. Like heroin and other demonized drugs before it, including marijuana and LSD, which were made Schedule I drugs in 1970, methaqualone was prohibited from sale, even by prescription. When approved by the FDA twenty years earlier, methaqualone had been classified as a Schedule V drug, assessed as having a low potential for abuse — the FDA approved the drug with the caveat, "addiction potential not established" — and as safe for whatever clinical use a physician deemed appropriate.[67]

Considering how closely the methaqualone parties followed on the heels of the Miltown and Benzedrine parties, and given that all of those drugs rose and fell during the heyday of the barbiturates, it should have been obvious that the FDA was doing little if anything to stop drug makers from bringing new pleasure pills onto the market. The differential prohibition of drugs meant that a gateway had been created, allowing if not encouraging the continued production of escapist, mood- and mind-altering drugs. Labeled as ethical medicines, they were all perfectly legal and inexpensive, marketed and sold with the AMA's and the FDA's stamps of approval.

But that was not the end of the depressant story. Meprobamate and methaqualone did not turn out to be the most striking examples of the freedoms provided to drug makers in the pharmaceutical marketplace in the twentieth century. Nor did that honor go to methamphetamine, or even methylphenidate (Ritalin). In fact, the most striking cases involved neither downers nor uppers, but rather uppers and downers in combination. One such compound was Desbutal, a licit pharmaceutical "speedball" created by joining in a single pill methamphetamine with the short-acting barbiturate pentobarbital (sold individually as Nembutal). Another was Dexamyl, a drug taken by members of the Beatles (along with B-bombs) even before they began to smoke marijuana; Dexamyl was a mixture of d-amphetamine and the short-acting barbiturate amobarbital (sold individually as Amytal). A third was Drinamyl, compounded by SKF, the maker of Benzedrine; Drinamyls, or "Purple Hearts" as they came to be called, had a blue, triangular shape and contained amphetamine and amobarbital.

These new drug cocktails represented the culmination of the industry's efforts to create the largest possible domestic drug market, which it hoped to do by collapsing the pleasures of America's two general drug desires into one. With sales of amphetamines and barbiturates reaching record-breaking highs, the idea of selling a blend of calm stimulation must have seemed immensely attractive and looked immensely profitable. Given that all this was taking place in the context of growing prohibitions on "drugs" and "drug abusers," it was remarkable how drug makers strived toward fulfilling the dream of Orwell's *soma*, a universal panacea that could turn all unpleasantness into a continuous happiness, and without any untoward side effects. The drug subcultures of America continued to grow and proliferate accordingly, as profiled in "White-Collar Pill Party," the 1966 *Atlantic* essay by Bruce Jackson.

Next to the candy dish filled with Dexedrine, Dexamyl, Eskatrol, Desbutal, and a few other products I hadn't yet learned to identify, near the five-pound box of Dexedrine tablets someone had brought, were two bottles. One was filled with Dexedrine Elixir, the other with Dexamyl Elixir. Someone took a long swallow from the latter, and I thought him to be an extremely heavy user, but when the man left the room, a lawyer told me he'd bet the man was new at it. "He has to be. A mouthful is like two pills, and if he was a real head, he'd have a far greater tolerance to the Dexedrine than the amobarbital, and the stuff would make him sleepy. Anyhow, I don't like to mess with barbiturates much anymore. Dorothy Kilgallen died from that." He took a drink from the Dexedrine bottle and said, "And this tastes better. Very tasty stuff, like cherry syrup. Make a nice cherry Coke with it. The Dexamyl Elixir is bitter."

A distractingly pretty girl with dark brown eyes sat at the edge of our group and ignored both the joint making its rounds and the record player belching away just behind her. Between the thumb and middle finger of her left hand she held a pill that was blue on one side and yellow on the other; steadily, with the double-edged razor blade she held in her right hand, she sawed on the seam between the two halves of the pill. Every once in a while she rotated it a few degrees with her index finger. Her skin was smooth, and the light from the fireplace played tricks with it, all of them charming. The right hand sawed on.

I got the Book from the coffee table and looked for the pill in the pages of color pictures, but before I found it, Ed leaned over and said, "They're Desbutal Gradumets. Abbott Labs." I turned to the "Professional Products Information" section [of the PDR] and learned that Desbutal is a combination of Desoxyn (methamphetamine hydrochloride, also marketed as Methedrine) and Nembutal, that the pill the girl sawed contained 15 milligrams of the Desoxyn, that the combination of drugs served "to both stimulate and calm the patient so that feelings of depression are overcome and a sense of well-being and increased energy is produced. Inner tension and anxiety are relieved so that a sense of serenity and ease of mind prevails." . . .

The girl, obviously, was not interested in all of the pill's splendid therapeutic promises; were she, she would not have been so diligently sawing along that seam. She was after the methamphetamine, which like other amphetamines "depresses appetite, elevates the mood, increases the urge to work, imparts a sense of increased efficiency, and counteracts sleepiness and the feeling of fatigue in most persons."

After what seemed a long while the pill split into two round sections. A few scraps of the yellow Nembutal adhered to the Desoxyn side, and she carefully scraped them away. "Wilkinson's the best blade for this sort of thing," she said. I asked if she didn't cut herself on occasion, and she showed me a few nicks in her left thumb. "But a single edge isn't thin enough to do it neatly."

She put the blue disk in one small container, the yellow in another, then from a third took a fresh Desbutal and began sawing. I asked why she kept the Nembutal, since it was the Desoxyn she was after.

"Sometimes I might want to sleep, you know. I might have to sleep because something is coming up the next day. It's not easy for us to sleep, and sometimes we just don't for a couple or three days. But if we have to, we can just take a few of these." She smiled at me tolerantly, then returned to her blade and tablet.

When I saw Ed in New York several weeks later, I asked about her. "Some are like that," he said; "they like to carve on their pills. She'll sit and carve for thirty or forty minutes." . . . "I told her once about the effect of taking a Spansule; you know, one of those big things with sustained release (like Dexamyl, a mixture of dextroamphetamine sulfate and amobarbital designed to be effective over a twelve-hour period). What you do is open the capsule and put it in a little bowl and grind up the little pellets until it's powder, then stuff all the powder back in the pill and take it, and it all goes off at once. I'll be damned if I haven't seen her grinding away like she was making matzo meal. That's a sign of a fairly confirmed head when they reach that ritual stage."[68]

Unlike the dramatic lives of meprobamate (Miltown) and methaqualone (Quaalude), the drama of the barbiturates did not come to a close with the collapse of the legal protections offered them by the institutions of medicine and the FDA. Meprobamate and methaqualone were two attempts to market a substitute for the barbiturates, both of which ultimately failed, with barbiturate use marching on. A still newer family of minor tranquilizers, the benzodiazepines, was another of these attempts, and it was this class of downers that would bring an end to the more-than-forty-year run of the barbiturates.

The benzodiazepines are, like meprobamate, minor tranquilizers. Recall that Frank Berger, a Jewish refugee working for the British Drug House in London in 1945, spearheaded the development of meprobamate in the 1950s, after he relocated to Wallace Labs in New Jersey. After meprobamate, the next minor tranquilizer to appear was from a class of chemically related drugs, the benzodiazepines, and was brought to life after a similar series of events.

What Frank Berger is to the Miltown story, Leo Sternbach is to the story of the benzodiazepines. Born in Abbazia, Austria, in 1908, Sternbach moved around a lot. His father was a pharmacist, and when Leo was still a boy the family relocated to Poland. As an adolescent, he worked in his father's pharmacy, and he later earned a degree in pharmacy from Jagiellonian University in Krakow. During his doctoral work in organic chemistry, Sternbach studied potential dyes by synthesizing substances known as "heptoxdiazines." As anti-Semitism intensified in Poland, Sternbach returned to Austria — to Vienna — and then to Zurich, Switzerland, eventually taking employment with the notable Swiss drug firm, Hoffmann-La Roche in the city of Basel. In 1941, fearing a Nazi invasion of Switzerland,

Hoffmann-La Roche transplanted Sternbach and its other Jewish scientists to the United States. Like Frank Berger, Leo Sternbach suddenly found himself working in a drug company based in New Jersey. Berger was in Miltown and Sternbach was in Nutley, and by the early 1950s both were working on the development of new tranquilizers.

Sternbach began his work in the United States by returning to the earlier work he had done on heptoxdiazines, and in 1954 this led him to studying a class of unexplored compounds called the benzheptoxdiazines. His goal was no longer to develop dyes but to assess the biological activity of these substances with an eye toward finding a new and perhaps better tranquilizer. All forty of the compounds Sternbach derived during this time proved to be biologically inactive, however, and he made no breakthroughs. In 1957 someone cleaning Sternbach's lab asked him about a few compounds that he had left behind during the unproductive period. Sternbach had taken a benzheptoxdiazine derivative and treated it with a substance called methylamine, but he had not completed all the tests. As he later wrote, "This intensive work, of little practical value, finally led, in April 1957, to an almost hopeless situation. The laboratory benches were covered with dishes, flasks, and beakers — all containing various samples and mother liquors. The working area had shrunk almost to zero, and a major spring-cleaning was in order. During this cleanup, my co-worker, Earl Reeder, drew my attention to a few hundred milligrams of two products, a nicely crystalline base and its hydrochloride."[69]

The latter compound had never been tested for pharmacological activity, and the co-worker asked whether it should be thrown away or screened for biological efficacy. Sternbach had been told to abandon his work with benzheptoxdiazine, but on a whim he chose to screen it.[70] When he received word of the results months later, in July 1957, the news came with a jolt of surprise. It stated in part that "the substance has hypnotic, sedative, and antistrychnine effects in mice similar to meprobamate."[71] It was the breakthrough Sternbach had been hoping for — the fortunate discovery that every pharmaceutical chemist prays for should he or she wish to ever make a major advance in the field. The results also stated that the compound was considerably more potent than meprobamate as a muscle relaxant, at least in cats. The chemical was called methaminodiazepoxide, or chlordiazepoxide for short.

Sternbach was not immediately recognized as having almost single-handedly produced a breakthrough drug. Initial clinical trials performed at Hoffmann-La Roche led to the conclusion that the drug was a sedative that had no unique properties. Later, however, the drug was investigated outside of Hoffmann-La Roche. This time it was tested at lower doses and with the population that had so loved meprobamate, namely, the anxious and stressed neurotics and insomniacs of domestic life in America. In this context researchers, including the pharmacologist Lowell Randell, found the drug to be a unique anxiolytic drug.[72] Rather than being a sedative-hypnotic, which was the principle classification of the barbiturates, it could be classified instead as a minor tranquilizer, the category first established for meprobamate. Such a classification was justified, researchers claimed, because it lowered anxiety at doses below what was necessary to produce intoxication and sleep. And they were right. As is now known, the benzodiazepines do indeed act on the brain differently than do the barbiturates, with the latter affecting the brain at a general level (the brain stem) and the former affecting it at a higher and more specific level (the subcortical nuclei).

But what was most important about Sternbach's drug was that, unlike the barbiturates, the toxicity of chlordiazepoxide was low. In fact, it was surprisingly low. For this reason, despite the Miltown parties in the news, the drug was assured FDA approval, which occurred in February 1960. A month later, under the brand name Librium and with extensive praise in the pages of the *JAMA*, it was launched by Hoffmann-La Roche.

According to Robert Dallek's *An Unfinished Life*, President John F. Kennedy was among the first early users of Librium, taking it for the purpose of lowering anxiety.[73] During this period he also took Miltown for anxiety, Ritalin for energy, the opioids Demerol and methadone for pain, and barbiturates for sleep.

What barbital was among the barbiturates, chlordiazepoxide (Librium) was among the benzodiazepines, namely, the first of many of its kind. By 1963 researchers at Hoffmann-La Roche had simplified the chlordiazepoxide molecule to create a second and more potent benzodiazepine called diazepam — branded as Valium. A third benzodiazepine, Serax, was introduced in June 1965, followed thereafter with the synthesis and marketing of dozens of others, including Dalmane (flurazepam), Xanax (alprazolam), Ativan (lorazepam), and Halcion (triazolam). Among the first benzodiazepines, it was Valium that initially achieved celebrity status, even winning an entry in the *Guinness Book of World Records* as the most widely prescribed drug in recorded history. Like early-generation barbiturates, however, these drugs were overtaken in the 1980s by the next-generation benzodiazepines that acted faster and for shorter durations. These newer drugs included triazolam (Halcion) and temazepam (Restoril), the former of which has a half-life of less than three hours.

Safer in overdose than all other depressants, including alcohol, the benzodiazepines nevertheless followed much a familiar trajectory: they were hailed as nonaddictive substitutes for other depressants; they were marketed along with a host of new syndromes for which the drugs were said to be uniquely useful (for those suffering from "battered parent syndrome" and "generalized anxiety disorder," not to mention the mom "who can't get along with her daughter-in-law" or those "who can't make friends"); and finally, when taken chronically by those who were especially anxious, they often led to a hellish syndrome of dependence, partly physical and partly psychological, that kept many chronic users from getting off them.

In 1967, with the benzodiazepines making their debut, Stanley Yolles, director of the National Institute of Mental Health, expressed his concern over what he saw as a tranquilized nation: "To what extent would Western culture be altered by widespread use of tranquilizers? . . . Would Yankee initiative disappear?"[74] That same year, the Rolling Stones released their album *Flowers*, which included the track "Mother's Little Helper," an ode to Valium.

> She goes running for the shelter
> Of a mother's little helper
> And it helps her on her way
> Gets her through her busy day

Two years later, Judy Garland died of a drug overdose after years of chronic dependency on uppers and downers. Jacqueline Susann fictionalized Garland's story in her bestseller, *Valley of the Dolls*, after which the title came to signify the use of tranquilizers as a perilous escape from the doldrums of everyday life.

The popularity of the benzodiazepines nevertheless continued to grow, repeating the same cycle of medical hype, vast nonmedical use, and new and "unexpected" problems of dependency. With the prohibition of cocaine, the opiates, and marijuana in full swing, America now had to confront its drug problems on two fronts, both domestic and illicit. But help was on its way. Because of nagging problems with withdrawal and dependence, physicians were increasingly reluctant to continue prescribing the benzodiazepines, and it was this reluctance that, finally, brought the story of the depressants in the twentieth century to a close. It did not, however, bring an end to the billion-dollar domestic drug market. Something newer, better, even safer was on its way!

Chapter Six **War**

The more fantastic an ideology or theology,
the more fanatic its adherents.

—Edward Abbey, *A Voice Crying in the Wilderness*

The twentieth century ended much as it began, at least in terms of domestic drug use. Despite an ever-expanding mobilization of resources to combat the scourge of "drug abuse," the legal use of powerful, mind-altering — and, for many users, dependence-producing — drugs remained ubiquitous throughout America. Indeed, as powders and tonics were replaced by a technology of the synthetic pill, sanctioned within a medicopharmaceutical industrial complex that stood almost outside the law, domestic drugs acquired even greater standing. Pills came to embody a science of modern medicine, a kind of enlightened self-medicating of an increasingly engineered self, obscuring the new pharmacologicalism while also obscuring the powers of a medical establishment that had seized control over patent medicines to become the official guarantor of the country's pharmacological ups and downs.

By the end of the twentieth century one could not buy psychoactive drugs over the counter. They were still widely available by prescription, however, and in no less efficacious forms. Cocaine was no longer legal, but its close synthetic cousin Ritalin was, and it was taken in the 1980s and 1990s by millions of children and adults with both recreational and medical intent. Even methamphetamine, the drug that the drug czar Barry McCaffrey called "the worst drug that has ever hit America," was dispensed to children by prescription until the end of the century.[1] Heroin was no longer legal in any form or for any purpose, but opioids like Sublimaze (fentanyl) and Oxycontin (oxycodone) had come into popular use, testament to the capacity of the capitalist industry to imitate nature's psychoactive substances and then design right past them. Indeed, all these latter-day substitutes were at least as efficacious and addictive as the natural substances they replaced. In most cases, as with the barbiturates and the benzodiazepines, as well as the SSRI antidepressants that followed, the withdrawal and dependence syndromes these pills produced were at least as debilitating as for any natural drug that came before them.

Many are shocked when they learn that cocaine, heroin, and marijuana were once legal and sold without a prescription. And yet what seems far more impressive is the fact that synthetic drugs of comparable pharmacological efficacy continued to be used under the same pretence throughout the century, and with little public notice. That the synthetic drugs, including the amphetamines and the barbiturates, were comparable in their pharmacology to the originals was reflected in how rapidly each drug spilled out of the medical context of "treatment" and into the street. Drug prohibitions did not change this. Instead, escalating drug laws were responsible for a radical, negative transformation of all drug use that fell outside the ethical realm. Prohibitionism drove the sharp end of a wedge down the center of America as a drug culture, splitting the drug market into two, one black, the other white. Tobacco and alcohol were kept out of these two markets for the most part, as they were agricultural products indigenous to America. Still, as grey-market drugs, their ethical status remained tenuous, with alcohol experiencing prohibition of various kinds throughout the century and tobacco being increasingly demonized at the century's end.

The creation of black markets, meanwhile, had consequences for society that were immediately negative. The result of a perpetual failure to curb unpopular drug use was that millions, then billions of dollars were spent on what devolved into a drug civil war, a war on a class of drugs and the kind of user that prohibition itself created. For those caught up in the black market, the consequences were also negative, especially when the drug in question was of foreign origin and not a sanctioned synthetic being misused. One million Americans were in jail or prison by the end of the century, a prison epidemic that resulted directly from drug laws, which failed to shut down markets and curb illicit demand, and therefore encouraged even wider markets and in turn even more draconian policies. Huge monies were at stake that capitalized and perpetuated the cycle of the black markets, and those monies only increased as the severity of drug laws increased.

While the notion of drug "war" began as a metaphor, it quickly turned into something more. The brutal consequences that characterized the escalation of military wars also came to be mirrored in America's crusade against a narrow and select group of demonized substances. Drug law after drug law was passed, with each failure to curb illicit use prompting calls for even harsher measures. In the process the "drug abuser" came to be viewed as a stubborn enemy and was vilified as such. The war philosophy of "by-any-means-necessary" that subsequently emerged resulted in an attack not just on drug users but also on American civil liberties. As is true of all great wars, everyone would have to do their bit.

Meanwhile, a "Dutch paradox" had been identified in Europe, based on the observation that lower prices of heroin and higher drug purity were actually translating into less intense and less dangerous forms of drug use (for example, smoking heroin rather than injecting heroin).[2] This was, in essence, the logic of America's drug prohibitions running backwards. If greater legal constraints only made the problem worse, then reversing the influence of the black market should improve the situation. And indeed it did. In stark contrast to this harm-reduction approach was a long-standing American paradox, which continued to loom large as American drug policies persisted, ensuring high prices and low drug purity, as well as higher injection rates and rates of disease, including HIV. The paradox of this failure of policy lay not so much in that drug laws failed to work, for they had never worked to decrease drug use, but rather in how their lasting failure bullet-proofed their logic and fueled their continued escalation.

There was, however, an ever-lurking danger in waging war against these demonized substances, since the "misuse" and "overuse" of prescription drugs had somehow to be kept apart from "abuse" and "addiction" involving illegal drugs, primarily cocaine and heroin, but also marijuana, LSD, and the amphetamines. To facilitate this cultural distinction, drug laws were written and enforced to maintain the double standards of differential prohibition: on the one hand there existed regrettable drug misuse of prescription drugs, which called only for treatment, while on the other hand there was criminal drug abuse, which called first and foremost for punishment. This sharp, culturally constructed distinction also meant that someone arrested for selling a powerful opioid like Oxycontin might receive only a fraction of the punishment received by someone caught selling heroin, or even marijuana. Such a situation is confusing from a pharmacological perspective, but from a historical perspective it makes sense, reflecting as it does the effectiveness of the AMA's efforts to create a separate, ethical realm that safeguarded domestic drug use. With this structure in place, the persecution of illicit drug users and dealers could go forward with wild abandon, and it did.

From the perspective of the AMA's ethical guidelines, the new psychoactive drugs restored "normal" well-being, and the state rightly sanctioned the use of these drugs. Drugs said to destroy, disregard, or expand human wellness, on the other hand, needed to be prohibited and punished. In a kind of Apollonian war on the Dionysian spirit, drug use in America was straight-jacketed by the AMA into a Calvinist doctrine directed toward making a healthier, more moral citizen. In this society, one could not decide on one's own to use drugs (except gray-market drugs), but if one lost the capacity to make good decisions, one could be drugged involuntarily by the state.[3]

The categories of differential prohibition, including "licit versus illicit" and "medical versus recreational," were derivative of this scheme. At the height of the drug war these categories were reinforced and protected via an array of policies and mechanisms spanning numerous institutions and markets. This included drug cartels, the AMA, the private-prison industry, and the White House Office of National Drug Control Policy. Each institution relied on a cult of pharmacology to function, if not prosper, for if drugs could not be classified as having inherent good or evil properties, independent of time, person, or place, such a black-and-white world of pharmacological privilege and punishment could not be sustained.

And thus it was that, by the end of the twentieth century, one could find five mutually reinforcing guilds operating in the service of pharmacological-ism: the pharmaceutical industry, modern biological psychiatry, the bio-medical sciences, drug enforcement agencies (including the DEA, the FBI, and Alcohol, Tobacco, and Firearms), and the American judicial system. Together these institutions formed the two pillars of differential prohibition: the medicopharmaceutical industrial complex (the therapeutic state) and the drug-abuse-prison industrial complex (the prohibitionist state).[4] The principal text that reinforced the first pillar was the *Diagnostic and Statistical Manual* of the American Psychiatric Association; the principal text that reinforced the second was the five-tier classification of drug scheduling, first outlined in the Comprehensive Drug Abuse Prevention and Control Act of 1970 and enforced by the DEA.

What had begun in the 1970s, when illegal drugs were first perceived in the United States as so malignant a threat that President Richard Nixon declared them to be "public enemy number one," had become an all-out war on drugs and drug users. Presidents Ronald Reagan and George H. W. Bush repeated Nixon's call to arms, and a more militant ethos of "zero tolerance" emerged. By the 1990s, when America had amassed the greatest per capita prison population in the world under these policies, the Clinton administration finished out the century clutching nervously to the status quo.[5] William Chambliss, writing on drug policies of the Clinton administration, summarized the bleakness of the situation for American minorities: "It is no exaggeration to say that the lives and futures of young men in the poor Black and Latino communities of the United States are being systematically destroyed and the population of young males permanently alienated by the enforcement of anti-drug laws. Among young Black men between the ages of fifteen and thirty-five, 40 to 50 percent are, at any given moment, either in jail, on probation, on parole or a warrant is out for their arrest."[6]

No doubt the war on drugs will one day rank among the most shameful periods in American history. But this book is not about drug policy. It is, rather, about the basic assumptions concerning "drugs" that underlie such realities. To this end, many particulars of the story of drugs in America have been examined, but a formal consideration of the more general story of what "drugs" are remains to be undertaken. Without such a consideration, one has little hope of appreciating how great was the misadventure that defined drugs in twentieth-century America.

Psychoactive drugs are, after all, not what one thinks they are. The molecular actions of drugs in the body are simply not as all-determining of human experience and behavior as the world has come to believe. Drugs are animated by the ecology of the human settings they enter — psychosocial, cultural, and historical — and it is in these powerful and complex settings that drug discourse and so-called drug effects emerge.

It is also because of these settings that one confronts an immediate problem in understanding drugs, namely, the problem of one's own prejudices about them. Swept up in a cult of pharmacology, psychoactive substances have only rarely been considered outside their politicized and medicalized contexts. What is more, the concept of drugs has been usurped for so long as a tool for executing power and for exerting regulatory control over human behavior that a neutral attitude toward the subject is hard to imagine. Consider the difficulty that those who lived in the seventeenth century had in envisioning themselves as anywhere other than at the center of the universe. People knew what was obvious and thought what was obvious was quite enough to know. The situation is hardly different in the case of drugs. One cannot imagine that the idea that psychoactive drugs exert a special kind of influence on mind and body is hardly more than a myth, just as one cannot imagine that the substances called drugs do not belong to some special molecular universe. Once again, people came to know what was obvious and thought what was obvious was quite enough to know. But another story lies beyond the cult of pharmacology, a story in which drugs have quite a different meaning. And as in Galileo's time, there are those who have, for varying reasons, worked to bring the evidence to light.

Part Three **While at War**

*The truth is addiction is not a voluntary circumstance.
It's not a voluntary behavior. It's more than just a lot of
drug use. It's actually a different state . . . [a] state of
compulsive, uncontrollable drug use.*
—Alan Leshner, interview with Bill Moyers

I n 1954 the *Journal of Comparative and Physiological Psychology* published the article "Positive reinforcement produced by Electrical stimulation of septal area and other regions of rat brain," by James Olds and Peter Milner from McGill University in Montreal.[1] The study went on to become a classic in psychology, behavioral biology, and pharmacology. The reason was simple: Olds and Milner had located what appeared to be the "pleasure center" of the brain. When animals' responses on a switch produced electrical stimulation in the brain's septal area, the animals responded as frequently as several hundred times per hour to keep the stimulation going. Among the many implications of the study was the possibility that certain drugs might be stimulating this "reward" area of the brain, and in doing so, encouraging or even inculcating addictive behavior.

James Olds described the evolution of his seminal discovery a few years later in a piece in *Scientific American*.

In the test experiment we were using, the animal was placed in a large box with corners labeled A, B, C, and D. Whenever the animal went to corner A, its brain was given a mild electric shock by the experimenter. When the test was performed on the animal with the electrode in the rhinencephalic nerve, it kept returning to corner A. After several such returns on the first day, it finally went to a different place and fell asleep. The next day however it seemed even more interested in corner A.

At this point we assumed that the stimulus must provoke curiosity; we did not yet think of it as a reward. Further experimentation on the same animal soon indicated, to our surprise, that its response to the stimulus was more than curiosity. On the second day, after the animal had acquired the habit of returning to corner A to be stimulated, we began trying to draw it away to corner B, giving it an electric shock whenever it took a step in that direction. Within a matter of five minutes the animal was in corner B. After this the animal could be directed to almost any spot in the box at the will of the experimenter. Every step in the right direction was paid with a small shock; on arrival at the appointed place the animal received a longer series of shocks.

After confirming this powerful effect of stimulation of brain areas by experiments with a series of animals, we set out to map the places in the brain where such an effect could be obtained. We wanted to measure the strength of the effect in each place. Here Skinner's technique provided the means. By putting the animal in the "do-it-yourself" situation (i.e., pressing a lever to stimulate its own brain) we could translate the animal's strength of "desire" into response frequency, which can be seen and measured.

The first animal in the Skinner box ended all doubts in our minds that electric stimulation applied to some parts of the brain could indeed provide a reward for behavior. The test displayed the phenomenon in bold relief where anyone who wanted to look could see it. Left to itself in the apparatus, the animal (after about two to five minutes of learning) stimulated its own brain regularly about once very five seconds, taking a stimulus of a second or so every time. After thirty minutes the experimenter turned off the current, so that the animal's pressing of the lever no longer stimulated the brain. Under these conditions the animal pressed it about seven times and went to sleep. We found that the test was repeatable as often as we cared to apply it.[2]

Hundreds of research papers were stimulated by Olds's and Milner's discovery, leading to a variety of findings.[3] Some focused on the generality of the original report, while others provided more insight into the nature of the neurobiological activity of reward. For instance, electrical brain stimulation was replicated in various species, including humans, monkeys, and cats. It was shown even to affect the activity of single brain cells.[4]

Research following the Olds and Milner report also compared brain stimulation with so-called natural rewards, such as food. In one experiment, laboratory rats given the option of pressing a switch that triggered brain stimulation did so almost continuously for twenty days, averaging twenty-nine responses per minute.[5] When such effects were contrasted with those provided by natural rewards, hungry rats and even humans sometimes disregarded food in preference to the electrical brain shock.[6]

Human subjects of brain stimulation sometimes describe the experience as resulting in an odd sense of pleasure or well-being; at other times, however, such subjects describe not so much pleasure as relief from stress, anxiety, or depressed mood. When electrodes were placed in the septum or the thalamus, for example, people described a reduction in their own negative affect — an antidepressant effect.[7] After learning of these findings, psychiatrists saw potential techniques for psychotic patients unresponsive to psychiatric treatment in the institutions, radical new measures that could replace old ones, like frontal lobotomies.[8] Over the next two decades, beginning in the 1960s, patients were taught to push a button to obtain electrical brain stimulation, often responding for hours on end.[9]

In the years following Olds's and Milner's discovery, research also began looking into the neurobiological basis of pleasure, where the focus was less on behavior than on mapping the structures of motivation in the brain. By the end of the century, this research culminated in, among other things, a neurophysiological model of addiction, embraced by many drug scientists as well as various government institutes (including the National Institute of Mental Health and the National Institute on Drug Abuse). Central to this theory was the idea that all habitual drug use could be traced back to a common neural pathway, a pathway that was affected when there was chronic infusion of the drug. The pleasure center of the brain thus became the focus of the search for a unified theory to addiction. Alan Leshner, then the director of NIDA, wrote in 1998, "Although each [abused] drug that has been studied has some idiosyncratic mechanisms of action, virtually all drugs of abuse have common effects, either directly or indirectly, on a single pathway deep within the brain, the mesolimbic reward system."[10]

James Olds followed up his 1954 paper by moving in this direction. In a series of well-received papers published in the early 1960s, he and colleagues found the most robust responding for brain stimulation consistently took place when electrodes were placed in a central area of the brain known as the lateral hypothalamus.[11] This made sense in that that region intersected with a major nerve system — the medial forebrain bundle (MFB) — that interconnected other areas of the brain implicated in pleasure and brain stimulation.

Olds went on to argue in the 1970s that the arrangement in the lateral hypothalamus provided the ideal anatomical structure for the complex interactions known to exist between basic motivations such as hunger and thirst and reward produced via brain stimulation.

There were, however, other theories about the location and structure of the pleasure center in the brain. While it was true that the lateral hypothalamus was important in natural rewards involving hunger and thirst, other areas were also significant, including the ventral tegmental area (VTA), the prefrontal cortex, and the nucleus accumbens.[12] The mesolimbic reward system consisted of neural pathways in the brain linking two of these areas: the VTA in the midbrain and the nucleus accumbens in the limbic system.

As time and research went on, new technologies for brain-mapping research were devised. One of these was autoradiographic labeling, wherein a radioactive glucose solution was entered into the brain in order to track brain metabolism during electrical stimulation. During autoradiographic labeling of the MFB, researchers found a localized, common pattern of neural activation. When put in other areas implicated in brain reward, namely, the prefrontal cortex, common patterns were also observed; however, these common pathways were not the same as those identified by Olds.[13]

As research methods advanced, finding the pleasure center became an even more elusive task. The idea of pleasure center of the brain was a nice metaphor, but was it anything more than a metaphor?[14] Research indicating several anatomically distinct and relatively independent neural circuits involving reward, pleasure, and pain suggested it was not.

Meanwhile, as the debate continued over the anatomical nature of the brain's reward system, neuroscience programs influenced by Olds's and Milner's discovery began to pursue the neurochemical processes involved in reward. One candidate was the neurotransmitter serotonin, a key chemical in the brain that also happens to be the target of the Prozac-class of antidepressants.

Shortly after the 1954 discovery, brain researchers developed a technique to track the neurochemical substrates of reinforcement by staining specific neurochemicals in the brain and observing their subsequent activity. The first two significant neural pathways identified involved not serotonin, but the neurochemicals norepinephrine and dopamine. One prominent researcher in the field at the time was Larry Stein. He promoted an influential "theory of reward" emphasizing norepinephrine over dopamine, a conclusion based on the fact that the latter was not involved in some areas where brain stimulation was reinforcing and that drug studies had shown that blocking the metabolism of dopamine into norepinephrine had a significant impact on the self-administration of brain stimulation.[15]

In the decades that followed, evidence shifted in the other direction, toward a dopamine theory.[16] Researchers exploring the dopamine theory were also employing drugs such as cocaine and amphetamine, for these drugs had direct and immediate effects on dopamine. Several areas of the brain where electrical stimulation had proven effective were also found to be rich in dopamine neurons, including the VTA, the MFB, the nucleus accumbens, and the prefrontal cortex.[17] These areas were especially implicated in the effects of electrical brain stimulation — as well as eating, drinking, sexual behavior, and the use of stimulant drugs — and researchers pushed on in that direction in the 1980s. Eventually a general consensus was reached that dopaminergic pathways play an important role in reward and motivation.

This general conclusion was embraced in part because it was better to lay claim to a discovery while it was fresh and before further news arrived that might ruin everything. But in the four or so decades that had passed since Olds's and Milner's initial discovery, mounting evidence had suggested that the notion of a centralized locus of reward or pleasure was not only elusive but also terribly simplistic. As the physiological psychologist Sebastian Grossman put it, "The notion of a single neural pathway for all types of reinforcement processes seems no longer tenable even if one modifies the original idea."[18]

The entire project was gradually and continuously being overwhelmed by complexity. A harbinger of this complexity was the paper "Escape from self-produced rates of brain stimulation," which appeared in *Science* in 1969.[19] Since the time of Olds's and Milner's initial report, research had reliably shown that animals would work to produce electrical stimulation in certain areas of the brain; that much could be taken for granted. In the 1969 study, however, researchers asked whether brain stimulation would still be pleasurable if it were to occur independent of responding. To test this, researchers first made a temporal recording of each animals' pattern of self-administered brain stimulation, then on another day presented it to each respective animal in exactly the same manner, with no requirement to respond. When electrostimulation was delivered independent of responding in this manner, the animals responded just as reliably, but to turn it off. This indicated a serious hitch in the theory, for if brain stimulation connected to a single neural pleasure switch, why should it matter who throws it?

Even if a pleasure center did exist in the mammalian and bird brain, it seemed pleasure could not be reduced, even in a basic animal model, to a simple matter of stimulating that area. A more interesting but also more complex theory was warranted, suggesting a dynamic interplay between the brain, behavior, and experience. And this made sense: in looking at one's own everyday experience, it is clear that one's sense of pleasure is intricately tied up with an engagement in the activity that produces it.

Such radical findings did not have any great influence on the prevailing pharmacologicalism, however. Studies that raised difficult questions and discouraged reductionist theories about drugs or the brain were all but ignored. Nevertheless, similar findings continued to trickle in, providing further evidence of the ecology of conscious experience, including another paper that appeared in *Science* in 1984. Using more-advanced methods of monitoring the effects of electrical stimulation in the brain, Linda Porrino and colleagues replicated the 1969 study and found that the different behavioral contexts of administered brain stimulation did not just affect the qualitative experience but also led to qualitatively different physiological affects in the brain.[20] That is, whether animals received the stimulation voluntarily or involuntarily changed the manner in which the brain stimulation affected the brain — changes that were also reflected in the finding that the electrical stimulation administered involuntarily produced the opposite behavior effect, that is, avoidance rather than pursuit, another finding replicated by Porrino's study.

Just as the early research on the physiology of reward appeared to have implications for the study of drugs and addiction, so did research revealing the complexity underlying interactions between the brain and behavior. And thus, by the 1980s, when neuroscientists had embraced pharmacologicalism to advance a simple brain-based model of addiction rooted in a dopamine theory, more socially and environmentally oriented researchers, including behavioral pharmacologists, began exploring the interaction between the context of drug use and the impact of drugs on brain and behavior.

A series of studies from the animal laboratory compared the lethal effects of cocaine when it was administered under different environmental conditions.[21] In one of those studies, conducted by Steven Dworkin and colleagues, a group of animals had the opportunity to self-administer intravenous cocaine by responding twice on a switch; animals in another group received intravenous cocaine independent of responding; a third group, the control group, received a drug-free solution consisting of saline, also administered independent of responding. To ensure that the dose and pattern of drug administration was the same for the two groups receiving cocaine, a special methodology was employed: drug administration for each animal in the "involuntary" cocaine group was yoked to the pattern of drug self-administration of their littermate in the first group. That is, animals in the second group received cocaine without responding at a rate identical to the pattern of responding of an animal in the first group. The drug, drug dose, route of administration, and pattern of administration over the several-hour period of drug taking each day were all the same for each pair. If the manner of administration made no difference, as pharmacologicalism predicted, the toxicity should be the same across these two groups and very different from the control group.

The environmental variable of response dependency versus independency "profoundly alter[ed] the lethal effects of cocaine."[22] While none of the animals self-administering cocaine over a several week period died, identical amounts and patterns of cocaine administered independent of responding had lethal effects for five of thirteen animals. While the lethality of the situation was certainly set into motion by the availability of the drug, whether an animal did or did not die in the study was predicted only by the context of cocaine use.[23]

Similar to the approach taken by Porrino and colleagues, Dworkin's group continued their line of research by examining how the basic environmental variable of choice manifested itself in terms of physiological activity in the brain.[24] Their second study was similar in methodology to their first, but the researchers employed morphine rather than cocaine. That is, littermate siblings received either response-dependent intravenous morphine, response-independent morphine (administered in a pattern yoked to the administration of a littermate in the first group), or response-independent saline (also yoked to the pattern of administration of the first animal). In this study, however, radioactive precursors were also employed, which allowed the researchers to measure the neurotransmitter activity in different brain regions following morphine's administration—the same regions probed in the investigations of electrical brain stimulation.

Relative to the saline control condition, the involuntary administration of intravenous morphine increased the animals' dopamine activity an average of 133 percent in the nucleus accumbens and 253 percent in another forebrain structure, the caudate nucleus-putamen (an increase of 100 percent would indicate no difference). These results were straightforward and showed that morphine did have measurable effects on dopamine activity in both regions. However, when these results were compared to those from the animals who responded for morphine voluntarily, very different effects were found. In the nucleus accumbens, the voluntary responders experienced on average less than one-fifth as much activity as the involuntary drug group; in the caudate nucleus-putamen, however, this group experienced a sixfold average increase in activity relative to the involuntary group. Overall, significant differences in the two conditions of morphine administration occurred across various brain regions and neurotransmitter systems. For instance, in nine separate brain regions, self-administered morphine produced more significant effects on GABA activity than did response-independent morphine.[25]

These findings clearly illustrated the dynamics of drug-brain-behavior interactions—dynamics implicated with even greater import in most instances of human drug use. By the 1990s the context of drug administration had been shown to influence the physiological and behavioral effects of cocaine and the opiate morphine, as well as those of electrical brain stimulation. When the "drug taker" was the causal agent responsible for producing the externally derived stimulus (the drug or the shock), the experience and the biobehavioral outcomes changed, including the toxic effects of the drug and the relative experience of pleasure.

From the standpoint of modern pharmacologicalism, such results are upsetting indeed, for they undermine the fundamental notion that a drug's most socially significant effects, such as the mind-altering experience it produces, are derivative only of pharmacology. While modern pharmacologicalism presents a static model of drug determinism that is highly reductionistic—it reduces drug taking and drug effects to the level of molecules tickling a static brain—this research suggests a very different model: drugs do not have a single essence, whether good or bad, addictive or nonaddictive, weak or powerful, that transcends time, person, or place. Because

drugs do not become "drugs" until they enter the ecological mix of environment, behavior, and brain, their status as "drugs" is always contingent and
dynamic, never absolute.

Nevertheless, maintaining its confident absolutism, not to mention its po-
litically correct system of classification of angels and demons, the cult of
pharmacology marched on. In 1994, for example, Alan Leshner, the brain-
oriented psychologist who wrote that "virtually all drugs of abuse have
common effects . . . on a single pathway deep within the brain," took over as
director of National Institute on Drug Abuse.[26]

Leshner replaced C. R. (Bob) Schuster, a psychologist who had headed
the institute since 1986. Prior to directing NIDA, Schuster had had a long
history of scientific research and was one of the founders of behavioral
pharmacology, a field comprising psychologists, pharmacologists, and psychiatrists who studied the interaction between psychoactive drugs and behavior. Schuster had also previously been chair of psychiatry at the University of Chicago, an unusual appointment for a doctor of psychology.

As part of the small group of psychologists and pharmacologists who,
beginning in the 1960s, pioneered the study of biobehavioral processes
underlying drug actions, Schuster and his colleagues had succeeded in demonstrating myriad ways in which environmental and behavioral factors
shape what had previously been defined strictly as pharmacological matters.
Schuster brought his broad understanding of how drugs work to NIDA,
never turning away from its social implications for drugs or drug policy.
This attitude was rare within the U.S. government and was not always
appreciated by his superiors, including Presidents Reagan and Bush. Schuster started NIDA's "behavior therapy development program," for instance,
which emphasized the same social and psychological factors underlying
habitual drug use that had been identified by Alfred Lindesmith. Still, while
Schuster was in a far better position to stem the reductionist tide than
Lindesmith had been decades earlier, he was unable to do so. The field of
neuroscience had grown enormous since the 1970s, and one of the greatest
areas of interest to neuroscientists was drug abuse and its relation to the
brain.

The change from Schuster to Leshner at NIDA marked formally the shift
that had long been taking place in government policy, away from cultural
and psychosocial factors affecting addiction and dependence, and toward a

reductionistic model that would ultimately define addiction as a biological disorder. In a paper entitled "Addiction is a brain disease, and it matters," Leshner, writing as the director of NIDA, opined, "Scientific advances over the past 20 years have shown that drug addiction is a chronic, relapsing disease that results from the prolonged effects of drugs on the brain. . . . Recognizing addiction as a chronic, relapsing brain disorder characterized by compulsive drug seeking and use can impact society's overall health and social policy strategies and help diminish the health and social costs associated with drug abuse and addiction."[27]

A single scientific paper about the brain's reward center in laboratory rats had thus been transformed into official government policy regarding the nature of addiction. Drug dependence and drug addiction involving illegal drugs were effectively encapsulated within a black box of biology that excluded nearly all external factors, whether individual or cultural — the very factors central to acute drug effects and long-term drug outcomes, as demonstrated by numerous sociologists and behavioral pharmacologists, from Lindesmith to Zinberg to Schuster.

According to the disease model, addiction begins before a drug is ever taken. For either genetic or developmental reasons, or both, the brain of an individual fails to produce or release enough dopamine. With the brain in a state of low dopamine activity, and thus pleasure, an individual is prone to seek out drugs that boost his or her dopamine levels.[28] This drug seeking, combined with the negative impact of chronic drug taking on the brain over time, according to the theory, will eventually produce a disease state.[29]

It sounds plausible. The idea that some people might be constitutionally deficient in dopamine seems reasonable, and there is no reason that chronic exposure to a drug might not alter the brain in a manner that promoted dependence. After all, the twentieth century is littered with "medicines," from alprazolam to Zoloft, that are not only habit-forming for the population most likely to use them but also brain-altering such that opting out of chronic use can produce serious withdrawal effects.[30] Some of this withdrawal has been shown to be psychological — a kind of inverse placebo effect — but by no means all of it. In a healthy-volunteer study conducted by GlaxoSmithKline, for instance, company researchers found that, on discontinuation of their drug Paxil, as many as 85 percent of the volunteers suffered agitation, bizarre dreams, insomnia, and other adverse effects.[31]

The shortcomings of the disease model of addiction lie not in the general ideas on which it is premised, but rather in the sheer lack of evidence supporting it. Take, for example, the dopamine changes caused by drug use. Drugs like cocaine and heroin (and nicotine) do have either direct or indirect effects on dopamine systems in the brain. Beyond that, though, many questions remain. For example, since Ritalin produces essentially the same effects on dopamine as does cocaine, should it not, all else being equal, produce the same addiction as cocaine does in those ADHD-diagnosed children who happen to be constitutionally shy of dopamine? The fact that it does not suggests that there is more to addiction and dependence than a drug chronically impacting the brain. There is also the problem that the disease model is directed at the use of illegal drugs, not prescription drugs, even though the drugs that best fit the symptoms of the disease model are not the demon drugs of the twentieth century — cocaine, opium, marijuana, and, to a lesser extent, alcohol — but rather the synthetic angels. Finally, as research in behavioral pharmacology and behavioral neuroscience has demonstrated, changes in dopamine are real, but the nature of these changes is complex and ecological, not simple and pharmacological.[32]

Consider another abused substance that involves dopamine: food. Drugs are not the only substances that affect the mesolimbic system. So are foods. The pleasure one receives from foods depends on various additional factors, including how hungry one is and whether one likes the food that he or she is eating. Physiological research has demonstrated this as well. In one study, when an animal was presented with food, researchers found neurons firing as a function of either the sight or taste of food, but with an important caveat: the neurons fired only when the animal was hungry.[33] If pleasure were as simple as eating foods that triggered the release of dopamine, then one would never stop eating. The same notion applies more or less to drugs. Why should one expect cocaine to be pleasurable at all times or to all individuals when one would never expect this to hold true for even the most beloved foods, such as chocolate, ice cream, or pasta?

The disease model states that chronic use of cocaine or heroin or marijuana or tobacco will lead inevitably to addiction. It also states that, since addiction is a brain disease, the so-called addict inevitably loses his or her power over their drug use. Alan Leshner, interviewed by Bill Moyers on PBS, summarizes this view: "Like most people in this country, I [once] believed that addiction was just a lot of drug use. You use drugs and then you become addicted and you could move back to being just a drug user. And you could just stop any time if you were really serious. A lot of people felt that way, especially about cigarette smoking, but the truth is addiction is not a voluntary circumstance. It's not a voluntary behavior. It's more than just a lot of drug use. It's actually a different state. It's hard for people to understand that, but if you take drugs to the point of addiction, functionally you move into a different state. A state of compulsive, uncontrollable drug use."[34] What Leshner is actually describing here is the disease model of alcoholism adapted to the case of illegal drug abuse. While his description fits the stereotype of addiction and dependence, and soothes the conscience of people like Bill Moyers, who have experienced "drug problems" in their families, the vast literature on careers in drug use flatly contradicts this perspective. In fact, careful work by researchers around the globe has failed to support either of the two core ideas of the disease model: that use leads inevitably to addiction and that addiction, without "treatment," guarantees lifelong use.

The disease model carried on its back a social agenda, which was to ensure that "drug abuse" meant "illegal drugs" in the public imagination and that "use of illegal drugs" translated into "disease." Had the disease model been allowed to stray over to the realm of psychiatric drugs, its raisons d'être would have vanished. Instead, in research, in government, and in the media, the disease model was kept on message: the brains of street addicts were diseased because of dangerous drugs, sold by ruthless criminals amassing huge fortunes.

Bob Schuster, Leshner's predecessor at NIDA, had an influential role in the development of behavioral pharmacology, a role that began in the 1960s and continued during and after his tenure at NIDA. The origins of behavioral pharmacology, however, precede Schuster's arrival on the scene and stem from a series of seminal studies conducted by Peter Dews at Harvard Medical School in the 1950s.[35] Prior to these studies, the field of pharmacology had little interest in behavioral models of drug action, largely because they had little knowledge that there was any need for such models: behavior was an output—an effect—of a drug, not an input on a drug's actions. Since the effects of pharmacological agents unfolded at the physiological level, it was assumed, there was no need to worry about the complexities of behavior. Dews's studies in the psychobiology laboratory at

Harvard turned this view on its head. Pharmacology as it pertained to psychoactive drugs would have to retool, which it did by embracing behavioral pharmacology as a new discipline.[36]

The first in this series of studies, published in the prestigious *Journal of Pharmacology and Experimental Therapeutics*, appeared in print the year after Olds's and Milner's 1954 paper.[37] While Olds and Milner were busy exploring the neurobiological basis of reward, Dews and colleagues were taking an interest in how differences in ongoing behavior altered the direct effects of psychoactive drugs on that behavior. The assumption in pharmacological science at the time was that simple differences in the ongoing rates of behavior — say, high or low — should not alter the nature of the drug outcome. Indeed, what Dews was examining must have seemed like a test of the most straightforward and pointless kind. Yet what he found was anything but straightforward.

Influenced by the radical behaviorist B. F. Skinner — who was also at Harvard, in the Department of Psychology — Dews conducted his original experiment using pigeons trained to peck on a response button to earn food. In technical terms, this is deemed the behavioral baseline: stable rates of responding to obtain a reward (or to avoid an aversive stimulus) are established as a "baseline" prior to a drug's administration; once in place, if responding changes after drug administration, it can be attributed to the drug. Dews's study employed the barbiturate pentobarbital, a depressant. Different schedules of food delivery were used, meanwhile, to organize different rates or baselines of responding. One food schedule, which yielded relatively slow responding, was alternated in the same session with another food schedule, which yielded faster responding; different lights signaled for the animal what schedule was in effect at any given moment. This procedure allowed Dews to ask a simple but adventurous question: would a moderate dose of a barbiturate have a different effect depending on the ongoing rates of responding for food?

Naturally, because the drug employed was a sedative and a central-nervous-system depressant, it was assumed that high enough doses would decrease and eventually eliminate all responding in an animal or person, regardless of the baseline schedule. Dews found, however, that the drug effect at moderate doses did indeed differ in a significant and reliable way depending on the baseline rates of responding for food. These differences were not just quantitative, as one might expect, but also qualitative: a dose of pentobarbital that decreased or eliminated responding on the schedule that yielded slower rates of responding for food actually *increased* response rates on the schedule that produced faster responding, and both effects could be observed within the same experimental session. There was, in other words, a dose or range of doses of the drug that produced behavioral effects in the opposite direction depending on the baseline rates of responding.[38] Every pharmacologist knew that the effect of a drug changed as a function of dose; when plotted on a graph, this is referred to as a drug's dose-response curve. But after a single study by Dews, it appeared as though the effect produced by a drug was not just a function of dose (a pharmacological effect) but also a function of the ongoing rate of behavior (a behavioral effect). In other words, the nature of the drug effect appeared to be both dose-dependent and rate-dependent.

Three years later, Dews published another paper, also in the *Journal of Pharmacology and Experimental Therapeutics*, replicating these same effects.[39] The study was more than just a simple replication, however, for the drug in the study was not a depressant but a stimulant (methamphetamine). Once again, whether the so-called stimulant increased rates of responding to earn food varied as a function of the rate of the behavior prior to drug administration. Rate dependency was not specific to depressant drugs, Dews had shown, but rather was a robust and general finding for all drugs that could directly affect ongoing behavior.

These basic empirical findings by Dews and others were unexpected and profound, and raised fundamental questions about the interactions between drugs and behavior. To wit: how could the same drug — a sedative or a stimulant — decrease rates of one ongoing behavior while increasing rates of another? Dews had not only demonstrated a paradoxical effect that needed explaining but also showed that the behavioral effects of a drug could be examined in a scientific and reproducible fashion in the laboratory. As the behavioral pharmacologist James Barrett wrote years later, "This simple but powerful series of experiments lifted the evaluation and interpretation of drug effects on behavior from that of speculation about ephemeral emotional states to quantitative and observable aspects of behavior that could be manipulated directly and evaluated experimentally."[40]

Sometimes referred to as the "Golden Age of Psychopharmacology," the 1950s were a period of rapid transformation in pharmacology. This was due in part to the discovery of behavioral factors underlying drug effects, but there was another reason as well: the sudden infusion of new, behaviorally active compounds that had immediate significance for psychiatry.[41] As new drugs were introduced for treating problems of "psychosis," as well as for depression and anxiety, there was suddenly a great need for behavioral research that could clarify the nature of these drugs. Key among these compounds was the antipsychotic drug chlorpromazine and the tricyclic antidepressant imipramine.

The study of drugs for psychiatric conditions also focused on a dopamine theory, which posited too much dopamine in the brains of psychiatric patients rather than too little—the hyperdopaminergic theory of schizophrenia.[42] The story of chlorpromazine and the hyperdopaminergic theory had begun in France a decade earlier, when researchers began investigating the treatment of allergic reactions using drugs later determined to be antihistamines. By chance, some researchers had discovered that certain chemical compounds produced a peculiar calming of mental activity in individuals without producing heavy sedation. The first of such compounds to be identified was promethazine, which became the first in a class of drugs called the phenothiazines. Soon thereafter, in the late 1940s, a French drug-company chemist developed chlorpromazine (later branded as Thorazine). The first clinical use of chlorpromazine, however, was in anaesthesiology, administered to patients as a calmative "cocktail" the evening prior to surgery.

Chlorpromazine produces a profile of unique effects on cognition and behavior that is sometimes referred to as the neuroleptic state. Phenothiazines are therefore sometimes referred to as neuroleptics, although they are most commonly known as antipsychotics. The so-called neuroleptic state not only includes a calming effect on the individual but also describes a general blunting of consciousness, such that an individual feels more detached from the world. Naturally, most people do not experience this effect as desirable, and as a class of drugs the antipsychotics are not taken for their acute psychoactive effects and therefore pose no risk for abuse.

Nevertheless, because of these calming effects, drug companies began investigating the usefulness of chlorpromazine and other drugs for the treatment of severe psychological disturbance in the early 1950s.[43] First in France and then in the United States, chlorpromazine and other antipsychotics (such as haloperidol, or Haldol) became widely used in the treatment of institutionalized individuals, often those diagnosed as schizophrenic. Because of their relative success in "managing" the outward symptoms of schizophrenia, the phenothiazines were partly successful in shortening the duration of hospitalization, or preventing it.

A dopamine hypothesis of schizophrenia arose out of these developments, due to the fact that the phenothiazines and other antipsychotics were found to be dopamine antagonists (i.e., they directly block dopamine receptors from receiving dopamine molecules in the brain). If antipsychotics reduced some of the symptoms of schizophrenia, then perhaps the cause of the problem involved the production of excessive activity in dopamine neurons in the brain.[44] The dopamine hypothesis was also rooted in the finding that chronic use of psychostimulants, which increase levels of dopamine in the synapse — the extracellular environment that fills the gap between one neuron and another — can produce psychotic episodes resembling those exhibited by individuals diagnosed as schizophrenic.[45]

As with the dopamine theory of addiction that emerged later, however, research findings either complicated the issue or weighed directly against it. For instance, typical antipsychotics were found to help only in managing the outward, "positive" symptoms of schizophrenia (such as incoherent speech), while the inward, "negative" symptoms went largely unaffected. If dopamine levels formed the basis of the problem, critics charged, changing them should affect both the positive and negative symptoms. Also, like antidepressants, the antipsychotics had direct, immediate effects on dopamine, yet were known to produce many or most of their clinical effects only after repeated administration, which suggested that secondary or "downstream" effects of the drug had to occur for the drug to show any therapeutic effects. Perhaps most important was the fact that researchers were never able to directly demonstrate that those diagnosed with schizophrenia had an excess in dopamine synthesis or release in their brains.[46] Beginning in the early 1980s, symptoms of schizophrenia were traced to dopamine, but also to serotonin, norepinephrine, acetylcholine, GABA, and glutamate.[47]

While the dopamine theory of schizophrenia did not get far, the new drugs on which it was based did, creating a revolution in psychopharmacology and psychiatry. It was in this changing context that Dews published his series of papers on the effects of baseline rates of behavior on drug outcomes. And it was for this reason in particular that the ascent of behavioral pharmacology followed, well suited as it was for the task of studying the suddenly relevant interaction between drugs and behavior.

The implications of Dews's work guided subsequent research in behavioral pharmacology over the next several decades. He had established a new principle for the field, the principle of rate dependency, and had thus taken a crucial first step toward building a new science of drugs and behavior. The principle proved to have another feature also considered important in the philosophy of science: it was parsimonious; it explained more with less. Much of the research that immediately followed the 1950s papers, for instance, showed that drug affects that had previously been attributed to differences in the kind of behavior being studied, such as punished versus reinforced behavior, could be explained by a simpler variable, namely, the different rates of responding associated with those different contexts.[48] Most notable among these reports was a series of investigations by two researchers working with Dews at Harvard, William Morse and Roger Kelleher.

In studies conducted in 1964 Morse and Kelleher looked at the behavioral effects of chlorpromazine and amphetamine, using the method of establishing different baseline rates of responding for food, although they tested the effects in squirrel monkeys rather than birds.[49] They also established an additional baseline in which responding was reinforced not by food but by escape from an aversive stimulus. By establishing nearly identical rates and patterns of responding under these different environmental contexts, Morse and Kelleher could determine whether, as was predicted by the principle of rate dependency, the effect of the drug might be the same regardless of the environmental situation and the kind of behavior it produced, as long as the baseline rates were also the same. Such a study must have seemed quite foreign to most drug researchers at the time, for the behavioral effects of drugs in the 1950s and 1960s were typically explained by reference to interior, emotional states. Nevertheless, rate dependency proved its utility: the studies demonstrated remarkably comparable effects at comparable baseline rates, regardless of the type of environmental contingencies that produced those rates.

These results once again replicated and extended the findings Dews had reported earlier, all of which helped to ease behavioral pharmacology toward the more general theory that psychoactive drugs inevitably entered into a causal stream that included social, environmental, behavioral, and physiological components. From there the impact of Dews's early studies only widened. In demonstrating one kind of basic interaction between psychoactive drugs and behavior, it encouraged behavioral pharmacologists to go looking for others, which were not hard to find.

Researching drug effects in the laboratory using mice, rats, dogs, monkeys, and baboons might seem an odd choice for anyone determined to reveal the complexities involving drugs in human society. And to a degree, the point is valid: no animal model could come close to representing the complex human world in which drugs are taken and experienced. And yet, animal models did ultimately have something to offer, for many drug researchers did not stay content with the idea of creating sterile environments and watching what happened. Instead, they went on to show that the underlying assumptions of America's cult of pharmacology, which by now were being applied in American society on a wholesale basis, were in fact so limited in scope and conservative in implication that even an animal model of drug use was apt to reveal something heretical to the prevailing common sense about drugs.

What Dews had demonstrated in the 1950s was an early example of this, and it was immediately felt within pharmacology and psychiatry. But Dews had studied the effects of drugs on ongoing behavior that was directed toward earning food, and thus was not a model of voluntary human drug use or addiction. Not long after the publication of Dews's findings, however, researchers interested in issues of drug dependence and addiction began to investigate these issues explicitly, which they did by studying drug taking itself.

Prior to his position at the University of Chicago and later at NIDA, Bob Schuster held a joint position in the pharmacology and psychology departments at the University of Michigan. Taking the position was hardly an odd choice, for the chairman of the Department of Pharmacology in the 1960s was M. H. (Mo) Seevers, whom Schuster later described as being the "leading pharmacologist in the world in the area of substance abuse" at the time.[50] Indeed, it was Seevers and colleagues who initiated the study of animal drug taking in the laboratory and who thus laid the groundwork for the emerging behavioral pharmacologists who wanted to explore issues of drug use.

Seevers's first work with animal models of addiction dates back as far as the 1920s and 1930s, and includes a 1936 paper published in the *Journal of Pharmacology and Experimental Therapeutics*, "Opiate addiction in the monkey."[51] As Schuster later remarked, "A little known fact is that in 1929, he [Seevers] had done some studies on cocaine, which are now known as sensitization procedures. He published on the fact that you can give a dog an injection of cocaine once a day at a dose that was not convulsant, but after 8 or 10 administrations became convulsant."[52] Even prior to this, Schuster adds, Seevers had conducted human experimentation into abused drugs, using himself and colleagues as subjects.

> It's also of interest to note that Dr. Seevers and his colleagues had begun some of the earliest work on the behavioral and subjective effects of drugs in humans, when, in the 1930s, they would get together in someone's home and take a drug of the evening. Heroin, cocaine, barbiturates, alcohol . . . sometimes in combination . . . and knowing Dr. Seevers, probably very often in conjunction with gin. He told me one story about, I don't remember specifically who it was, who received an injection of drug, and, as Mo said, turned blue and fell down on the floor. "Scared the shit out of us." The cavalier manner in which drugs were given for experimental purposes to humans during that period of time . . . is remarkable.[53]

Seevers's work and Dews's first came together explicitly in a study that appeared in 1969.[54] In this study Seevers and two other pharmacologists — Gerry Deneau and Tomoji Yanagita — used the same laboratory procedure that Dews had borrowed from the operant psychologist B. F. Skinner, but they reinforced responding not with food but with the intravenous delivery of cocaine. The self-administration paradigm was thereafter widely used as a model of human drug use, largely because a reasonable correlation had been demonstrated between drugs of dependence and drugs self-administered by animals in the laboratory.[55] Among those drugs are not just the opiates and cocaine but most of the artificial angels that were manufactured subsequent to cocaine and the opiates' fall from grace, from amphetamine to Miltown to Seconal to Valium to Ritalin to Oxycontin.

Within pharmacology, the self-administration of drugs was nearly as seminal a discovery as Dews's discovery of rate dependency, and it offered the same promise of parsimony for an area mired in complexity, if not confusion. Prior to the advent of animal models of drug taking in psychopharmacology, the subject of compulsive drug use was still haunted by the ghost in the machine. Notions of mental disease and abnormal personality bogged down theories of addiction, making addiction theory incompatible with scientific study. By contrast, the methodologies of behavioral pharmacology, which produced reliable and robust baselines of drug use, brought the addiction model down to the level of science almost overnight. Not all the implications of this discovery were welcomed, however. The long periods of stable responding for a psychoactive drug that had been demonstrated in much early research looked awfully similar to the patterns of behavior maintained by the delivery of solid and liquid foods. This presented an intellectual if not a professional crisis for some, in that those who studied drug abuse were suddenly faced with a notion that threatened the very raisons d'être of their specialized discipline: everyday drug-taking behavior, including excessive drug use, might be explained in essentially the same terms as those governing eating and drinking.

Whether the rest of society was ready or not, behavioral pharmacologists in the 1970s began making this very point and demonstrating it in the lab.[56] In doing so, they were showing what social scientists were simultaneously reporting from the field, namely, that so-called addictive drugs like cocaine and morphine did not necessarily produce compulsive drug taking. Animals in these studies sometimes administered drugs to excess when the drug was provided in unlimited quantities in an environment devoid of anything else to do. Yet under more limited conditions of drug availability—the same conditions that characterized most human situations involving drug use— patterns of responding were essentially identical to those reinforced by food or water. In one typical example, rhesus monkeys with continuous but not unlimited access to cocaine over long periods "regulated their drug intake to a remarkable degree."[57]

Writing on opiate dependence and addiction in the *Archives of General Psychiatry* in 1976, the Stanford University pharmacologist Avram Goldstein took note of these findings from the lab to suggest that drug seeking and drug use were behaviors that occurred naturally and independently of any underlying pathology. Without the "countervailing influences in human society," Goldstein argued, use of "abused drugs" would become a natural behavior in everyday life, much like it was already in traditional cultures in South America and India.[58] Drug use would not have to be labeled as abnormal behavior, in other words, nor would the realm of domestic drug abuse have to be concealed behind an expanding taxonomy of psychiatric illness.[59]

Dews's basic finding of rate dependency demonstrated that a drug effect is affected by dose as well by the nature of the existing behavior and that the kind of the behavior may be less important in determining the effect of a drug than the rate of behavior. Other behavioral pharmacologists subsequently found that drugs of misuse will maintain stable responding for the drug, a finding with similar implications: the kind of reinforcer — say, candy or alcohol — may be less important in determining the pattern of behavior than the environmental conditions under which the pursuit of the stimulus occurs.

These advances in the behavioral pharmacology of drug abuse, though fundamental, were still relatively basic, and it was not until the 1980s and 1990s that animal drug self-administration was more fully explored as an analog of human drug use. Here, the early findings, however reductionistic, clearly paved the way, for if one can establish stable responding for a drug, then this methodology could also serve as a useful baseline for studying the effects of nonpharmacological — that is, ecological — factors on drug-seeking behavior. A 1986 paper, for instance, replicated research in which animals were provided unlimited access to intravenous cocaine; however, the researchers also examined limited cocaine access by changing half of the animals from unlimited access to access only every other hour. While the unlimited-access group of rats all died within twenty-eight days, none of the rats in the limited-access condition died during the study, which lasted from 90 to 120 days.[60]

Another study of this kind published in 1993 found much the same thing, although in this instance researchers varied both the dose and the degree of access during cocaine self-administration.[61] When the animal could administer up to four doses of cocaine per hour, cyclic rather than compulsive cocaine self-administration was observed. Patterns of self-administration were sometime intense, but the animals did not develop "outward signs of ill health," the researchers noted. In the unlimited-access conditions of that study, problems of toxicity did occur, as in previous studies employing such conditions, but only at the highest of three cocaine doses.

Such studies began to throw a light on the ecology of drug taking: there are instances in which unlimited access to a drug, whether it be alcohol, morphine, or meprobamate (Miltown), have led to compulsive and self-destructive drug taking in people; there are also instances in which unconstrained access does not produce compulsive use or even fails to yield drug use altogether. But human drug problems depend on more than just drug availability. And this, too, was explored in the animal laboratory.

In a 1985 study by Marilyn Carroll at the University of Minnesota, monkeys had access not only to a drug—phencyclidine (PCP), also known as angel dust—but also to a nonpharmacological alternative to drug self-administration.[62] Monkeys could respond to obtain PCP, to obtain a sweet saccharin solution, or to choose some combination of the two. That a meaningful alternative to drug taking might have an effect on drug demand might seem like a case of proving the obvious, but such studies contradicted the growing anti-drug zeal in America, where one could now read in *Rolling Stone*, "Cocaine's power of reinforcement produces its most notorious effects: the desire to keep taking it as long as the drug is available. In one series of experiments . . . scientists let caged monkeys self administer . . . cocaine until they died. . . . The drug made them monomaniacal."[63] What Carroll actually found was that drug use decreased significantly as the sweetness of an alternative, sweet solution increased.[64]

Other researchers, examining other nondrug alternatives with PCP and other drugs, were quick to replicate these findings. A pair of such studies that appeared in 1991 and 1992 presented monkeys with a choice between intravenous cocaine and a sweet food alternative (banana-flavored food pellets). The first of these studies varied the size of the alternative to see if it affected the choices the monkeys made; the second study varied the amount of work required to obtain one or other reinforcer.[65] In each case, the self-administration of cocaine increased as the dose of cocaine increased, all else being equal. More interesting was the sensitivity of cocaine preference to the available of the sweet-food alternative: the demand for cocaine decreased both when the size of the alternative increased and when the work requirement for cocaine increased. In fact, at the largest food size, animals never chose cocaine more than 50 percent of the time, even at the highest cocaine dose.

Drugs that appeared to produce compulsive responding, including morphine and cocaine, were thus shown in the laboratory to be quite responsive to environmental factors, ranging from punishment to nondrug alternatives to the opportunity of social interaction. Researchers even assessed the impact of social dominance on drug abuse, finding that monkeys toward the bottom of a social hierarchy were more prone to cocaine use.[66] In one study, twenty macaque monkeys were placed together for three months to create a dominance hierarchy. While both dominant and subordinate animals self-administered cocaine, only the subordinate monkeys used it heavily. "Enriching the environment can produce large and robust changes" not only in drug use, the principle investigator of the study noted in an interview, but also "in the brain."[67]

Together these studies came to constitute an animal model of human drug use. If this were to be a comprehensive model, however, something still remained to be investigated. Researchers needed to test whether the ecological setting could also influence the *acquisition* of drug use. Most Americans in the twentieth century never experiment with most misused drugs, and thus the question arises as to what factors might influence the onset of drug use. In animal studies that were published in 1989 and 1993, this question was finally investigated. Marilyn Carroll and colleagues took another look at the effects of their sweetened drinking solution, this time employing intravenous cocaine as the drug.[68] Having shown that the sweet alternative decreased drug use, they tested what happened if the alternative was made available prior to making the cocaine available. Across all the conditions of the studies, Carroll found once again that access to the alternative decreased or eliminated drug use: the animals doubled their cocaine use when the sweet solution was removed and significantly reduced their cocaine self-administration when the alternative was presented. More important, however, were the effects of making the alternative available prior to drug availability. Early access to the sweet solution prevented half of the animals from acquiring a habit of cocaine self-administration in the first place and delayed it for many of the others.

As the animal model of human drug use continued to develop, researchers also began looking at psychological factors that influenced the meaning, as it were, of the drug experience. As Alfred Lindesmith and others had demonstrated decades earlier, patterns of drug use are strongly affected by assumptions and attributions about drugs and withdrawal that derive more from the prevailing context of drug use and prevailing placebo texts than from the drug itself. An unlikely factor to explore in the animal laboratory, perhaps, and yet it was explored, and quite successfully.

While behavioral pharmacologists were not going to theorize about the mental states of rats and monkeys, they were interested in an environmental variable that had already demonstrated powerful effects over other human behavior, namely, the conditioned meaning of otherwise meaningless stimuli. In the simplest of terms, this concerned the question of how stimulus elements in the environment acquire meaning or change in meaning because of their association with other, already meaningful stimuli, such as mind-altering drugs[69] Levine's 1974 paper in *Science*, for instance, had demonstrated that, due to repeated pairings, the injection of the hypodermic needle during intravenous drug use came to produce its own positive "drug" experience, independent of the drug.[70]

Behavioral pharmacologists had begun formally to look at such conditioning factors at about the time Levine's paper appeared. These early studies relied on a more complicated procedure.[71] While animals still responded for a drug, the responding resulted in the delivery of multiple stimuli. One stimulus was the drug and the other was a neutral, nondrug stimulus, such as a colored light. Dews and others also used basic environmental stimuli to signal what schedule was in effect during a session; in such instances, the lights would acquire their own significance due to their pairing with the presentation of the drug. In later studies, however, the animals were actually required to respond on a schedule to produce the light stimulus first, and only after the light stimulus was produced some predetermined number of times would the drug stimulus then be presented along with it. This "second-order" schedule is not unlike human drug taking in that considerable amounts of drug-seeking behavior might be carried out, producing a series of stimulus consequences not involving drug administration prior to the use of the drug itself.

When this procedure was first used, in the 1970s, there was a question about whether a neutral stimulus would indeed acquire enough of a positive meaning that its presentation alone would maintain long chains of responding. Thousands of responses might be required to obtain the drug, and without such "conditioned reinforcement," the animals would not complete the overall requirement to earn the drug delivery. In the end, researchers had little difficulty demonstrating such conditioning effects: neutral visual stimuli, paired repeatedly with the delivery of a self-administered drug, acquired a significant "meaning" of their own, such that they, like the drug with which they had first been paired, maintained long periods of responding.[72] As

James Barrett noted, "These procedures seemed to corroborate the view that drug-seeking behavior may be based in part on conditioned reinforcement. . . . These experimental models paralleled the robust drug-seeking behavior shown in drug abusers."[73]

By the 1980s research along these lines was staking an even greater claim of significance. It was one thing to suggest that drug experiences lent meaning to stimuli associated with their use, such that those stimuli gave further encouragement to drug seeking and drug use as drug use continued. But it was quite another thing to suggest that the cycle of repeated drug use itself would become largely the product of such conditioning. Given the finding among people that it was after repeated use of a drug — whether marijuana, opiates, or hallucinogens — that its effects were most appreciated, it was difficult to know to what degree subsequent experiences with drugs involved such a conditioning of meaning. In a report in the *International Journal of the Addictions* in 1973, for example, researchers described a period in the 1960s when heroin's street purity fell to very low levels — as low as one-half of one percent — yet demand for heroin remained largely unaffected. These results led the authors of the study to conclude that most cases of heroin addiction in the United States were at the time a combination of two factors: a pseudo-dependence rooted in the injection of contaminants contained in street drugs (such as quinine), and a psychological addiction rooted in the "ritualism surrounding the acquisition and administration of heroin."[74]

Back in the animal laboratory, investigations of this "ritualism" took a different form, although the results were interpreted much the same. For instance, John Falk at Rutgers University began a series of studies in which he established responding for an oral cocaine solution and then substituted other drugs in its place. Using this procedure he was able to show that ethanol readily substituted for cocaine when the other alternative was water.[75] Caffeine was then substituted successfully for ethanol, after which nicotine was substituted for caffeine. The ease with which Falk was able to accomplish these later substitutions made him "suspicious of [his] good fortune." He worried that the light initially paired with cocaine's self-administration had perhaps become the dominant stimulus reward, biasing the preferences in the favor of any drug substituted for cocaine. In other words, were the animals choosing the presentation of the light that had originally been paired with cocaine more than they were choosing the drug with which the light was now paired? This could be tested easily enough, so Falk returned the animals to a choice of ethanol versus water, then, once the baseline was again stable, substituted a drug that lab animals usually avoided rather than self-administer, namely, lidocaine, an anesthetic. Confirming his suspicion, the animals still self-administered lidocaine as long as the drug was paired with the light.

Further tests by Falk proved more definitively that stimulus conditioning was playing a critical role in drug preference. First, a new group of animals was given the choice between oral cocaine and water, which led to an almost complete preference for the former. When the stimuli paired with cocaine and water were reversed, the animals chose water over oral cocaine. This was an impressive result: with no visual (conditioned) stimulus present, animals clearly preferred cocaine, yet once the visual stimulus was introduced and became a conditioned stimulus, it and water together gained control over cocaine when cocaine was presented alone. The implications were impressive, suggesting as they did that, in at least some instances, the direct physiological consequences of the drug might be less of a sustaining factor in the long run than the larger context that had been associated with drug use in the past.[76] As Falk ultimately concluded, "A drug is not a reinforcer because it has a certain molecular structure capable of exciting specific receptors. The structures and events so described yield, at best, only a potential for reinforcing action that is realized if, and only if, a set of additional conditions are satisfied. Neither is reinforcement a sensory experience that can be experimenter imposed. It is not a thing at all; it is a relational construct."[77]

By the 1990s the modeling of drug use in the animal laboratory had revealed the profound influence nonpharmacological factors can have in the production of drug outcomes. Such demonstrations would not have been of great note had the prevailing cultural models and metaphors of human drug use not become so utterly narrow and reductionistic. The grip of pharmacologicalism had essentially created the need for a radical science of drugs and behavior, a science, that is, that could bridge findings of laboratory research, including neuroscience, with those from naturalistic studies of drug use. However, in taking the next logical step, from controlled animal studies to an experimental analysis of *human* drug use, a host of scientific problems inevitably arose. After all, there are myriad historical and contextual variables that influence drug outcomes, and these factors made interpretations of drug effects inherently difficult. As demonstrated, when recreational or psychiatric drug users were given placebos under blind conditions, they often showed a wide variety of drug effects, even when little or no drug had actually been taken.[78]

One solution to the problem of interpreting drug effects among people was to keep investigations under more controlled conditions. At McMaster University in Canada, Shepard Siegel achieved this by engineering a study that tied together research from the animal lab with research on human drug use in natural settings. Borrowing from animal cocaine studies in which one animal self-administered a drug while another involuntarily received the same pattern of administration, Siegel's 1988 report looked at the effects of identical drug exposure in two groups of drug users, only one of which actually self-administered the drug. That is, he measured drug withdrawal in individuals who either self-administered morphine or had it administered independently.[79] If withdrawal was a simple function of pharmacological exposure to an addictive drug, it should have been the same across all users. And yet Siegel found that withdrawal was notably more severe for the individuals who self-administered the morphine. This finding not only affirmed earlier reports by animal researchers but also provided human experimental evidence for Lindesmith's addiction model, wherein drug withdrawal was said to be not a fixed outcome, but rather one that varies depending on psychological and environmental variables.

Results such as these encouraged psychopharmacologists, including behavioral pharmacologists, to explore the influence of nonpharmacological factors in drug use in human laboratories. Prior to this, in the 1960s and 1970s, most human drug research was not experimental, but instead relied heavily on individual self-reports of drug experiences.[80] Drug addiction and dependence were defined in terms of subjective experiences, with researchers believing that introspections of the drug experience could elucidate how addicts differed from nonaddicts.

Some of the earliest exceptions to this outlook resulted from the creation of the U.S. Public Health Service Hospital in Lexington, Kentucky, an institution that later became the research branch of NIDA. In a move that foreshadowed the incarceration of drug users later in the century, the U.S. Congress authorized the U.S. Public Health Service in 1929 to establish two "narcotic farms . . . for the confinement and treatment of persons addicted to the use of habit-forming narcotic drugs."[81] The first facility opened on 25 May 1935, on a 1,000-acre farm outside Lexington. Although it was a true working farm, it was also essentially a minimum-security prison.[82] A decade or so later its name was changed to the U.S. Public Health Service Hospital, and in 1948 the program became part of the National Institute of Mental Health and was renamed the Addiction Research Center.

Abraham Wikler, one of the founding researchers at the Lexington Hospital, did his residency in psychiatry there and was assigned to a ward dealing with narcotic withdrawal. In 1952 he published an early, influential paper on the subject, in which a single man was given the opportunity to freely self-administer various drugs intravenously. The individual had a history of morphine use and chose morphine almost exclusively over a period of three months. During this time, a stable pattern of drug use emerged, marked by a gradual increase in dosage; in the final, fourth month, his preference for morphine continued and the dosage remained more or less constant. These results, which predated the formal study of animal drug self-administration, were later compared to almost identical patterns of drug use observed in rhesus monkeys. What was important, though, was that Wikler had demonstrated that controlled investigations of human drug taking were possible.[83]

Not until a decade or so later did researchers undertake formal investigations into human drug self-administration. Jack Mendelson and Nancy Mello, at McLean Hospital in Boston, began such work in the 1960s, as did Ira Liebson and colleagues G. Bigelow and R. R. Griffiths at Johns Hopkins University.[84] While early work focused on alcohol use, Mendelson and Mello also examined heroin self-administration in "former heroin addicts." When provided limited access to a button with which they could respond to earn injections of the drug, the subjects earned (i.e., took) all the possible injections over a ten-day period. A similar study by Liebson and colleagues, published in 1979, provided access to drugs at varying dosages in a residential facility, access earned by riding a stationary bicycle.[85] One drug at one particular dose, taken orally, was available over a ten-day period. When a barbiturate (pentobarbital), a benzodiazepine (diazepam), an antipsychotic (chlorpromazine), and placebo were each presented as options under blind conditions, the greatest responding was for the highest dose of the barbiturate. The antipsychotic and the placebo maintained no responding; that is, once those choices had been experienced, they were not chosen again.

Even individuals with a history of drug abuse did not always take these drugs to the fullest extent possible. In another study by Liebson and colleagues, individuals living in a residential facility decreased the number of barbiturate doses earned as the response cost for each dose increased.[86] "Alcoholic" drinkers have also been shown to have greater control over drinking than expected. Henry Fingarette, a drug scholar from the University of California, summarized these studies in his book *Heavy Drinking*: "One research team was able, by offering small payments, to get alcoholics to voluntarily abstain from drink even though drink was available, or to moderate their drinking voluntarily even after an initial 'priming dose' of liquor had been consumed. In another experiment, drinkers were willing to do a limited amount of boring work in order to earn a drink, but when the 'cost' of a drink rose they were unwilling to 'pay' the higher price. Still another experiment allowed alcoholic patients access to up to a fifth of liquor, but subjects were told that if they drank more than five ounces they would be removed from the pleasant social environment they were in. Result: most of the time subjects limited themselves to moderate drinking."[87]

Although laboratory studies of human drug use were never as provocative as animal studies, they were nevertheless successful in bridging the gap between animals' taking of drugs in the laboratory and people's taking of drugs in their everyday lives. Experimental studies of drug use employing animals and humans as subjects revealed that even primitive models were more realistic than the popular views of human drug use and abuse informed by pharmacologicalism.

Chapter Eight **Possessed by the Stimulus**

To return to things themselves is to return to that world
which precedes knowledge, of which knowledge always speaks,
and in relation to which every scientific schematization
is an abstract and derivative sign-language.

—Maurice Merleau-Ponty, *Phenomenology of Perception*

W hen just a boy, Bruce Wayne witnessed an unknown gunman murder his parents in cold blood. According to comic-book legend,
Bruce was the son of Thomas and Martha Wayne: Thomas a well-
respected Gotham physician, and Martha a homemaker. Bruce's parents
were influential in his early life, cultivating in him a deep moral sense. After
seeing his parents shot down by a random thief, Bruce was fundamentally
changed and vowed to spend his life fighting crime. As a young adult, he
worked to this end by traveling the world and becoming a master of martial
arts, acrobatics, science and technology, detective work, even boxing — for,
unlike other comic-book heroes, he had been born with no special human
powers. Having perfected his skills, Bruce Wayne returned home. One
night not long thereafter, he relived the terror of his parents' death and in an
epiphany recognized his destiny: to live out the rest of his life as a bat-man,
bringing justice to crime-riddled Gotham City.

The myth of Batman has nothing whatsoever to do with drugs or pharmacologicalism save one thing: it provides an illustration of the power that
basic stimuli can have on human psychology. The myth describes an immediate and long-lasting transformation of an individual resulting from one
stimulus event: the witnessing of his parent's murder. That an event of this
kind could have such a lasting effect is not hard to imagine; indeed, such
things happen every day in real life. And yet, whether real or imaginary, how
can a brief flutter of auditory and visual stimuli — a puff of air and a splash

of light — have such powerful effects on the workings of a human brain and the subsequent life of a human being?

This question is rarely pondered in part because sights and sounds do not often have such profound effects. Were a boy to witness someone else's parents killed in cold blood or to witness such a thing on television, the traumatizing effect would be quite different. And yet this is exactly the conundrum: how the brief external stimulus events in examples like that of Bruce Wayne — apparently having only the slightest, temporary impact on his eyes, ears, and brain — resulted in such long-lasting effects.

Another reason the question is overlooked is suggested by a comparison to virtual experiences like those on TV. All animals experience more meaning from stimuli than exists in the stimuli themselves; this is sometimes the result of learning, but it is also due to the fact that a process of making meaning is essentially built into the brain. In human beings the capacity to make meaning of naked stimuli according to one's own past history far surpasses that capacity in other animals, and it leads to phenomena like prolonged grief and passion, as well as to the creation of artificial realms of meaning through media like language, art, literature, and film. The mature boy who sees his parents shot dead will interpret that experience according to an evolved system of meaning, in other words, and it is this added meaning that gives basic, stimulus events such potential for influence. What is added is part personal and part cultural, the most important aspect for the boy Bruce Wayne being the immediate and real attack on his and his parents' lives. While the sights and sounds do not cause any physical injury, they leave a profound psychic injury through the very specific and transformative meaning they have for him.

If this digression into the comic realm risks stating the obvious, then one must recognize that the cult of pharmacology has made stating the obvious about drugs a constant and necessary activity. Drugs contain potentialities that lie within the drug's chemical structure, pharmacologicalism posits, and when taken into the body, these potentialities take hold of and transform both brain and behavior. This way of understanding drug outcomes has great efficiency, for it affords society with the opportunity to classify drugs once and for all as angels and demons, independent of time, person, or place. Accordingly, the evil that some drugs pose is determined not by societal conditions or attitudes about drugs — by experience — but by the drug's essence. A century of angels falling from grace did not diminish the popularity of this theory, moreover, since the notion of pharmacological determinism was never judged to be in error; instead, each fallen angel was declared, one after another, to have been inadequately assessed pharmacologically.

In attributing the "cause" of so-called drug effects almost singularly to the drugs themselves, pharmacologicalism differs fundamentally from the stimulus theory just introduced, which asserts that angels fall not because they have fixed properties that are often misidentified, but because their meaning and their effects change over time as their uses and users change. Stated more generally, except at very low or high doses, psychoactive drugs largely function not as so-called drugs — those magical substances deemed to have special powers — but as mere stimuli, with more or less the same, potentially great, powers as other stimuli one experiences and gives meaning to. If the boy Bruce Wayne was greatly affected by simple stimuli, which for him had great significance, so can any drug user, for much the same reason.

Various researchers and scholars, starting with Lindesmith in the 1940s, made it clear that drugs could not be grasped solely as biological or behavioral absolutes. They had to be situated instead in a larger system of understanding involving any number of environmental factors, including the social production of meaning.

To be sure, drugs have effects in the brain that can be generally characterized and classified; for example, cocaine's acute initial effect consists largely of the inhibition of the reuptake of dopamine in the synaptic cleft. But drugs can also acquire effects — effects that mediate and direct these initial physiological effects — simply by virtue of the meanings bestowed on them by reputation (for example, Ritalin is a medicine, and cocaine is a wonderful social excitant). With repeated use, these already complicated effects continue to be influenced by a further accumulation of meanings and expectations. As exemplified by Lindesmith's 1948 book *Opiate Addictions* and Norman Zinberg's 1984 book *Drug, Set, and Setting*, the psychology of meaning and its influence on drug outcomes first came under systematic investigation in the twentieth century. And in the realm of basic science this exploration of meaning began with the appreciation of drugs as stimuli to be carved up with meaning, beginning in the 1960s.

And yet, while there were by the end of the twentieth century hundreds of published reports on the complex ways in which drug outcomes are affected by other stimuli, or on how drugs themselves could function differently as meaningful stimuli, there was essentially no appreciation of these findings outside of pharmacology and substance-abuse research (and to some minor extent, treatment). Conversations regarding what it meant for drugs to function as stimuli and to acquire a powerful meaning for individuals rarely entered the public sphere, in part for reasons that had nothing to do with drugs. The larger theme of stimuli and how they acquire meaning to transform social and physical surroundings into a multidimensional world also never obtained much traction in popular psychology. Mounting a radical challenge against the prevailing cult of pharmacology was thus not only hindered by its unpopular social and political implications, but it was also crippled by the lack of a common language with which to communicate these implications to the public.

Drugs could be treated in such a reductionistic fashion in part because meaning itself had always been similarly understood, that is, as belonging to the thing itself, rather than as a process that emerges out of one's cumulative relationship with objects or events or people. To some extent such *essentialism* of meaning is a natural bias, for meaning seems to flow freely from what one experiences and thus feels as if it's intrinsic to experience. Imagine, for instance, a young girl who spots a shiny new bicycle in a shop window, is overtaken by a sense of wanting the bicycle "more than anything," and then begs her father to "please, please" buy it for her. Not every young girl wants a new bicycle with such intensity, or even at all, but for this girl, at this moment, almost nothing else matters. The meaning of the bicycle exists not in the thing itself but as a historically constructed relationship, with subject and object clashing together. This scenario also illustrates the two fundamental roles that meaning plays in people's lives: the bicycle has meaning for the girl in a *phenomenal* sense, in that it becomes part of the meaning that colors her world (she is attracted to it), and it also has meaning in a *motivational* sense, in that it has the power to evoke certain behaviors (she dwells on it and asks for it). Meaning is thus situated on both sides of human action, a kind of cradle: the stimulus is perceived and experienced as meaningful, behavior is affected accordingly, and, if successful—if the girl eventually gets the bicycle—meaningful consequences of behavior follow.

So, where does the meaning of the bicycle come from in the first place? While the bicycle has clearly acquired a heightened significance for the child, it would be difficult to trace the origins of this and most instances of individual meaning, however strong they might be. Both cultural and personal meanings are involved: the child correctly and unsurprisingly identifies the object as a bicycle, which is part of her general learning of meaning; she also especially likes the object, which is part of her own personal meaning-making. While the origins of culturally based meaning are relatively easy to track down, the personal and idiosyncratic aspects of meaning are of greatest interest, especially in drug studies. After all, it is personal meaning that leads one individual to have no interest in snorting cocaine, another person to have some interest in but experience no great thrill when doing so, and still another person to want to try it, to do so, and then to desire it beyond other things. Each individual knows what "cocaine" is, more or less, but each differs in the meaning cocaine has for him or her, both as a concept and subsequently, if taken, as an experience.

As an individual develops, culture-based meaning and personal meaning co-evolve. The local world is experienced; skills, knowledge and preferences grow; the meaning of the world expands and deepens. But the whole of the world, even of the immediate world, can never be known. One sibling may enjoy swimming while another enjoys bicycling — two different realms of behavior and experience, each with its own surface of meaning and each with its own depth of structure. Depth of structure refers to the hidden world of meaning that awaits someone if he or she is willing and capable of inhabiting that realm over time. The learning of a language, for example, is a deep structure of meaning that applies more or less to everyone: with time and experience, one comes to inhabit a language and language opens up a world of meaning. Playing the violin, landing jumbo jets, and working out theoretical mathematical problems are deep structures that apply to only a few. Whether common or rare, the meaning that defines the experience of knowing a realm more intimately cannot be obtained in an instant: it requires prolonged, firsthand engagement. This is why, for instance, an activity or object can look abstract or boring to most while being totally captivating to a few; the difference lies in meaning, which derives from long-term experience in that particular realm. Writing on "the improvement of discrimination by practice" at the end of the nineteenth century, William James wrote, "One man will distinguish by taste between the upper and the lower half of a bottle of old Madeira. Another will recognize, by feeling the flour in a barrel, whether the wheat was grown in Iowa or

Tennessee. The blind deaf-mute, Laura Bridgman, has so improved her touch as to recognize, after a year's interval, the hand of a person who once has shaken hers; and her sister in misfortune, Julia Brace, is said to have been employed in the Hartford Asylum to sort the linen of its multitudinous inmates, after it came from the wash, by her wonderfully educated sense of smell."[1]

The smoking of marijuana provides a compelling drug example. In his ethnographic research on "becoming a marihuana user," the sociologist Howard Becker conducted dozens of extensive interviews with marijuana users. What he found offered little support for the notion, inherent to pharmacologicalism, that the experience of smoking marijuana was predetermined by its pharmacology. While marijuana created a sensory experience rooted in its pharmacological actions in the brain (later attributed to delta-9-tetrahydrocannabinol), Becker found that the nature of this experience for any individual and at any time was cultivated from a learning process that enhanced and influenced its meaning.[2] Based on his interviews with marijuana users, many of whom were jazz musicians, Becker identified three learned dimensions of efficacious marijuana smoking that positively affected the stimulus effects, or meaning, of the marijuana experience.

Becker showed that novice users must first learn how to take in and hold marijuana smoke in their lungs. When this is achieved, the drug enters the bloodstream and the brain, which then produces unique stimulus effects that may or may not be appreciated. In the second step the individual must learn to identify the stimulus effects and appreciate them for what they are. Summarizing these first two aspects, Becker wrote, "Being high consists of two elements: the presence of symptoms caused by marihuana use and the recognition of these symptoms and their connection by the user with his use of the drug. It is not enough, that is, that the effects have to be present; alone, they do not automatically provide the experience of being high. The user must be able to point them out to himself and consciously connect them with having smoked marihuana before he can have this experience."[3] Research replicating Becker's findings years later reported individuals who might smoke marijuana a dozen, or even thirty to forty, times before ever experiencing a marijuana high.[4]

Once an individual has learned to produce and then discriminate the stimulus effects of marijuana, the signal strength or meaning of these stimuli *as stimuli* seems to increase. At this point, Becker suggests, a third variable comes into play, namely, whether the user, situated in the social milieu of marijuana use, has learned to interpret these effects as desirable. As with step two, the existence of this third factor reveals that experiencing marijuana as a deep structure is not just a matter of pharmacology but also of involvement: by engaging in the practice over time, the psychological processes of perception — processes that govern the influence of all kinds of nondrug stimuli — are mobilized to educate the senses, all of which usually unfolds in a social context. A 1965 British newspaper report on the marijuana scene at Oxford University described a student who believed that "pot" was an acquired taste: "The first half dozen times were disappointing, but Oxford encouraged him in the habit. The University, he thinks, might almost be designed to nourish drug addiction. . . . '[T]he permissive atmosphere about the place means that there's no real form to existence here. Marihuana gives it form. There's this part of the day when you know you'll be happy.'"[5]

The personal and social construction of the drug experience applies to most psychoactive drugs. While the mind-altering effects of one drug, say, LSD, might be more robust than those of another, say, marijuana, each drug presents an ambiguous stimulus array, with a depth of structure that can be probed for years. With more engagement, whether guided by a placebo text that is explicit or not, the meaning of the effects increases and expands. Recall, for instance, Andrew Weil's description of the South American tribe in which all the users of a prepared hallucinogenic substance actually experienced the same hallucinations after ingesting it.[6] Another example derives from an early British investigation into the initial experiential effects of opiates. Two consecutive doses of morphine were given to 150 young males with no previous opiate experience. After finding that only three chose to have the experience repeated and that none believed they would seek out the drug recreationally, the authors concluded, "Opiates are not inherently attractive, euphoric or stimulant" in nature.[7] Clearly, a love of opiates had yet to be cultivated for these individuals.

All of which is not to say that an exploration into the depths of drug experience — turn on, tune in, and drop out — is necessarily something one must aspire to do. Deeper involvements within a stimulus realm can add meaning to one's life, to be sure, but not all meaning will necessarily raise one's life to a higher plane. And, once acquired, meaning is not always easy to push away. Take the problem of chronic pain. As researchers in behavioral medicine have learned, patients can unwittingly stray into a process of selective attention in which they are unwittingly taught by health professionals to detect pain, which makes their chronic pain all the more salient and thus all the more chronic. Much like the skilled marijuana smoker or the cultivated wine drinker, the trained pain patient becomes skillful in discerning what would otherwise be less-detectable sensations; unlike the tasting of fine wines, however, discriminated learning of pain becomes an overwhelming burden that may be hard to tame.

Sociological researchers have provided related examples for drugs. According to Lindesmith's account, addiction is "a learning process extending over a period of time."[8] As in the case of the chronic pain patient, the cultivation of meaning involves the perception of something aversive (namely, drug withdrawal). Encouraged by a fear of withdrawal that is learned from the larger culture—a kind of inverted placebo text—the opiate user becomes trapped in a negative cycle of seeking and using drugs to escape or avoid withdrawal. Fear and the knowledge that there is no drug in the body become the guiding stimuli, conjured up out of a cultural myth about addiction. Lindesmith contrasts this with the less-excitable person who experiences withdrawal but only as a warning sign of possible drug dependence; this user finds a different meaning in the same situation, a meaning that functions to motivate the user to stop using, thus having the opposite effect.

Lindesmith's example can be compared with Becker's in terms of how the drug experience and drug withdrawal differ as deep structures. For Becker the marijuana experience is akin to wine tasting. Discriminating the many aspects of wine—depth, aroma, flavor, texture—requires considerable experience and is part of an acquired appreciation. The same wine does not physically change as one experiences it, yet experience can transform the meaning (or experience) of the wine. In this and in the marijuana example, the stimulus structure is relatively stable: the experienced wine taster experiences and reports on physical attributes of the wine that are also there for the novice but go undetected. Lindesmith's scenario, however, is more involved. Perhaps one could experience withdrawal in much the same way as one appreciates a "fine wine" or "good weed," but it would require an appreciation rather than a dread of the very stimuli one seeks to evaluate. In reality, the stereotypical junky anticipates and experiences withdrawal as a loaded psychological event, pumped with meaning and full of fear. By contrast, those users of opiates (or tobacco or cocaine) who pay less homage to the notion of pharmacological enslavement confront withdrawal in a less-charged form and thus learn from experience that the looming effects are not so great after all. For many or most, however, this learning process is derailed by external factors, where much is added to the experience that need not be there.

Whatever learning takes place during drug use and beyond, the first realms from which a drug's meaning takes form are typically encountered before a drug is ever used: the realms of local and mass culture in which childhood and adolescent development occur. In late-twentieth-century America, for instance, one typically learned that illicit substances like powder and crack cocaine, PCP, methamphetamine, and heroin were inherently addictive and dangerous substances, regardless of who the user was or of the context in which the drug was used. These placebo texts for "hard" drugs thus ensured that most Americans would have little or no actual experience with them, leading their demonization to be constructed in large part independently of any real experience that might contradict it. In this atmosphere any possible exception to the text only seemed to prove the rule.

The lore concerning the use of alcohol, and to a lesser degree marijuana, differed from these teachings. The placebo text that had evolved for alcohol in the latter part of the twentieth century taught the public that the drug was not in fact a drug at all, but belonged to a class of its own; hence the phrase, "drugs and alcohol." The placebo text also taught that men were affected differently by alcohol than were women and that alcohol addiction was unlike addiction involving "dangerous drugs" in that alcoholism stemmed not from exposure to alcohol per se, but rather from exposure combined with a biological predisposition for alcoholism. The lore for alcohol thus maintained all the distinctions necessary for distinguishing alcohol from hard drugs. As the psychiatrist Thomas Szasz wrote in *Ceremonial Chemistry*, Americans in the latter part of the twentieth century also learned that "people who make liquor are businessmen, not the 'members of an international ring of alcohol refiners,'" that "people who sell liquor are retail merchants, not 'pushers,'" and that "people who buy liquor are citizens, not 'dope fiends.'"[9]

For prescribed psychoactive drugs, meanwhile, things were generally different. At least until the 1980s, when tranquilizers and antidepressants began to be marketed directly to the public, most people had little knowledge of what kind of drugs were available via the physician, which was taken to be a sign of the success of the AMA's campaign to have only ethical drugs on the market. It also meant, however, that thousands of Americans were prescribed barbiturates, stimulants, benzodiazepines, and opioids, without having the slightest realization that they were taking drugs that, at least in terms of their pharmacology, were as dangerous as those on the black market.

Meanwhile, although drugs were not being pushed on the public via advertising and mass media, they were nevertheless marketed to physicians along with a variety of pseudo-ailments, from Miltown for the syndromes of being a housewife to Ritalin for the fatigued businessman. Hype for the new ethical medicines appeared as advertisements in medical journals and as literature that was handed out to physicians. All of this proved highly effective. Typically physicians would embrace a new drug as a breakthrough, use would increase, and the lore surrounding the latest panacea would spread person-to-person, entering the public imagination. To the extent that such sanctioned drug use followed the script of the pharmaceutical establishment and did not overflow into the hands of recreational drug users and "addicts" who had their own ideas, each of these drugs was swallowed along with its own well-crafted placebo text. Dependence might ensue for some users, but the medical context would usually conceal this until it existed on a vast scale.

The creation of the antidepressant-drug market exemplified that process. As soon as drug makers had a new pill on their hands, they began to envision new drug markets that might be expanded or created to serve it. For the compounds sold as antidepressants, the industry held seminars, had books published, and underwrote public-health campaigns to "educate" the public about the signs and symptoms of anxiety, depression, panic, and social anxiety. In the early 1960s, for instance, Merck, the largest pharmaceutical company at the time, wanted to boost demand for their new antidepressant. But general practitioners rarely diagnosed depression. To overcome this rather considerable obstacle, Merck bought 50,000 copies of a new book entitled *Recognizing the Depressed Patient* and sent copies to general practitioners and psychiatrists.[10] The intention was to transform the meaning of these mood states such that they would be interpreted not as vague, background sensations hailing from the mind but as vivid, foreground symptoms stemming from a defective brain.

In Japan, decades later, antidepressants again followed this course. By the 1990s Japan was the last holdout among industrial nations in terms of the prescribing of SSRIs and other antidepressant drugs. Antidepressants had simply never been very popular in Japan, in part because benzodiazepines like Valium and Xanax were used there long after they had been discontinued in the West. Since Big Pharma acquired its fortunes by pushing high-priced, patented new drugs, creating an antidepressant market in Japan promised to be a highly profitable venture. But how to crack the cultural code? Once again, the drug industry began not by pushing drugs directly on the public, but by first cultivating a new cultural meaning of what it meant to be depressed in the first place. In an insightful piece in the *New York Times* magazine, Kathryn Schulz explained, "If you had lived in Japan for the last five years, you would know by now that your kokoro is at risk of coming down with a cold. Your kokoro is not part of your respiratory system. . . . Your kokoro is your soul, and the notion that it can catch cold (kokoro no kaze) was introduced to Japan by the pharmaceutical industry to explain mild depression to a country that almost never discussed it."[11]

"Kokoro no kaze" was not exactly the idea that one had a mild form of depression: it was a whole new cultural meme. The meaning of the word for depression in Japanese, *utsubyo*, had always been used exclusively for serious depressive disorders. Thus, rather than attempting to mainstream this traditional and rather grave notion, the drug industry hijacked a milder notion—the common cold. And it worked. Within a few short years, kokoro no kaze transformed the Japanese's thinking about the ebbs and flows of mood as a medical disorder. In the five years subsequent to the construction of kokoro no kaze, for instance, 177 books on "depression" were published, compared with only twenty-seven titles in the preceding five years.[12] But this was only half the plan. Drug makers did not just medicalize the meaning of an age-old attitude that had ancient roots in Buddhism; they also provided its cure. In 1999 the Japanese company Meiji Seika Kaisha began selling the SSRI Depromel and was among the first companies to employ the notion of kokoro no kaze. GlaxoSmithKline followed a year later with their SSRI Paxil.

The effect of such campaigns, whether in the United States, Japan, or elsewhere, was to raise awareness about an inner experience and then alter its meaning. To have thus artificially altered perceptions is a remarkable phenomenon, representing nothing less than the transformation of the interior psychological world of an entire society. As this transformation took hold in Japan with regard to the SSRIs, admitting to having less than a perfect sense of mood from day to day went from having a negative connotation, to be ignored and never to be discussed in public, to having a positive social status. "Mild depression is not contagious," Schulz continued in the *Times*, "but it can be considered, in the root sense of the word, communicable — and for the last five years, the pharmaceutical industry and the media have communicated one consistent message: your suffering might be a sickness. Your leaky vital energy, like your runny nose, might respond to drugs."[13]

While the people in Japan, like those back home in America, had little grasp of how the meaning of their private experiences was being heightened and then socially reconstructed by the drug industry, Big Pharma knew exactly what was under way. By heightening and redefining the meaning of a person's inner experience, transforming it from a psychological to a medical landscape, new drug markets could be made, billions of pills could be sold, and billions of dollars could be reaped.

A drug sold is a drug taken. Once a drug is administered into the body, the meaning of the drug prior to taking it joins with and influences the meaning of the drug experience as it unfolds. Sometimes this experience is nothing like expected, and either the person's "mind is blown" or he or she is disappointed. At other times there are no surprises, and the person is more or less satisfied by the results, whether religious, recreational, or therapeutic in nature. And at other times those experiences, like the ones described by Becker, may not at first match one's expectation, but change toward them over time.

No surprise then that the origins of the drug experience are not always clear. Consider, for example, the nineteen-year-old college student who developed "disturbing and self-destructive thoughts" two weeks after starting on Prozac.[14] What was the meaning of those thoughts? Were they a sign of the problem getting worse, such that more of the drug or a different drug would be justified? Or were they an unwanted side effect of the drug? It is not that the stimuli presenting themselves subsequent to Prozac's use are subtle; it is just that they lack a clear and coherent meaning about their origins. Instead, the stimuli hover there, momentarily naked, waiting for an attribution to clothe them. In this case, the young woman was not very fortunate. Because her physicians interpreted her thoughts as due to the "disease" — there was no record of what her own attributions were — they increased her dosage of Prozac from 20 mg to 40 mg to 60 mg and then to 80mg. With each increase, the physicians assured the woman (and themselves) that her disturbed thoughts had nothing to do with the drug. By the time the dosage reached 80 mg, however, the woman was violently banging her head and mutilating herself. When this finally convinced her doctors to discontinue Prozac, the troubling side effects vanished.

MacAndrew's and Edgerton's *Drunken Comportment* also showed how background assumptions and attitudes regarding the meaning of a drug effect join with and alter those very effects. The intoxicating effects of alcohol were shown to have different meanings for different Native American tribes, and these meanings appeared to have been inherited not from the spirits contained in alcohol, as believed, but from the examples of others.[15] According to the cult of magical spirits, both ancient and modern, a drug's effects on one's comportment are a direct function of its essence (and dosage). But MacAndrew's and Edgerton's findings suggested something different: as in the Becker example, the drug does have a stimulus effect, but it is often the meaning that is attached to those stimulus effects that ultimately determines the drug experience.

How the stimulus effects of drugs acquire meaning from sources other than the drug was also revealed in studies in which users were blind or mislead about the drug they are using, for example, the studies conducted at the University of Chicago, Yale University, and Johns Hopkins University, in which cocaine users mistook lidocaine, amphetamine, or caffeine for cocaine when they were "blind" to what exactly they were given. The effects of the other substance, along with the uncertainty about the drug, the drug setting, and the subjects' expectations, all provided enough of a stimulus set to encourage the belief, at least for many subjects, that they were experiencing cocaine.

In America's cult of pharmacology, psychoactive drugs were believed to have a unique capacity to produce stimulus effects; that is, the stimuli that derive from drugs were said to have unique powers. And yet research in behavioral pharmacology and elsewhere seemed to indicate that there was nothing psychologically, physiologically, or behaviorally unique to the stimuli that derive from drugs, that they were in fact comparable to stimuli experienced via the senses that came from other realms of experience.

In the 1990s gambling addiction's parallels to drug addiction were extolled at length. The analogy was apt, but it was drug addiction that was clarified by gambling addiction, not vice-versa. To be sure, gambling and drug use can both become self-destructive activities for some individuals, and compulsive gambling has been linked to effects on dopamine in much the same way as have various drugs (including cocaine and Ritalin). But other important similarities were rarely noted. The vast majority of people involved in gambling are not compulsive players, for instance, just as most users of so-called addictive drugs, including cocaine, heroin, and alcohol, are not compulsive users. Gambling also made it clear, or should have, that one does not have to ingest something into their bloodstream for it to exert a profound influence over their experiences, their choices, and their habits — something that both drugs and gambling do when they acquire a heightened, all-consuming meaning for an individual. Given that gambling involves only external, or "exteroceptive," stimuli (like the murder of Bruce Wayne's parents), the "interoceptive" nature of drug stimuli appears to be only a superficial difference.

According to pharmacologicalism, a drug's ability to enter into the bloodstream, cross the blood-brain barrier, and directly impact the brain renders it capable of exerting special powers. But were psychoactive drugs really ever shown to be potent molecules that have special access to the brain? While drugs are ingested into the body and from there unleash a cascade of physiological and chemical effects, sometimes even deadly ones, evidence accumulated by the 1990s had demonstrated not only that drug actions in the brain were mediated by ongoing biobehavioral processes but also that drug stimuli impact the body, the brain, and behavior in much the same manner as do other, exteroceptive stimuli. As Thomas Szasz argued in his book *Ceremonial Chemistry*, the notion that psychoactive drugs belong under a special discipline of pharmacology, roped off from the study of all other human activities, was a highly dubious one: "If . . . textbooks of pharmacology legitimately contain a chapter on drug abuse and drug addiction, then, by the same token, textbooks of gynecology and urology should contain a chapter on prostitution; textbooks of physiology, a chapter on perversion; . . . textbooks of mathematics, a chapter on gambling syndicates; and, of course, textbooks of astronomy, a chapter on sun worship."[16]

Because of the twentieth-century emphasis on addiction and dependence on "dangerous drugs," drugs were easily segregated from other kinds of experience, even though the latter, including gambling, also involved obsessions and compulsions. If drugs were attributed special powers, in other words, it was due to the belief that drugs had a unique capacity to affect the brain and behavior. It was also due to the fact that some drugs were deemed acutely dangerous because of their risk of overdose. But is this really a unique attribute of drugs? Indeed, this assumption was rarely compared with the obvious, perhaps too obvious, fact that stimuli that derive from the exteroceptive realm posed similar risks. The same kind of stimuli that makes someone aware that a person is behind him or her, such as a hit on the back, could also injure or even kill if delivered with great enough force. The natural light that allows someone to see his or her surroundings can also blind that person if he or she stares at the sun for too long. One can also overdose on auditory stimuli, as when artillery fire or playing in a rock band causes hearing loss. These "overdoses" have long been examined with scientific precision, moreover, via the science of psychophysics. But what of it? Psychophysics no more explains Nietzsche's love of music than pharmacology explains Freud's love of cocaine.

Another difference assumed to distinguish drugs from other sensorial experiences is the fact that psychoactive substances can impact the brain with great speed and force, as does, say, crack cocaine. As with the notion of overdose, this assumption has rarely, if ever, been evaluated. Neuroscience demonstrated long ago that exteroceptive stimuli travel to the brain with a speed and force that exceeds that of drugs. Light, for example, is electromagnetic energy that is transformed by the visual system into electrochemical impulses, which then travel to the brain. Known as sensory transduction — the translation of energy entering the body into electrochemical activity that travels within it — this process occurs for all the senses and can lead to quick and dramatic changes in the brain. Consider a first kiss, or sexual intercourse. By contrast, does the nicotine contained in smoke, which enters the lungs, then the blood and the brain, really act so directly and so powerfully on the brain?

The suggestion of a link between drug outcomes and the psychological process of making meaning first emerged in sociological and anthropological research, including that of Weil, MacAndrew and Edgerton, Becker, and Lindesmith. In the second half of the twentieth century these areas of study rejected the reductionism common to other disciplines investigating drugs.

They were not "hard sciences," however, and when it came to influencing American policy for either illicit or medically sanctioned drug use, their findings were easily ignored. The findings coming out of the behavioral-pharmacology laboratory, on the other hand, were very much the product of basic science. Much of this research was federally funded and thus had a greater impact on American drug policy and drug treatment. And yet the effect was still quite small.

But behavioral pharmacology also had another influence. In engineering a science of drugs and behavior, it had the potential for acting as a powerful empirical and theoretical bridge connecting the drug theories of the social sciences with the physiological findings of neuroscience and psychopharmacology. Unfortunately, such connections were rarely made. The social sciences distrusted the reductionism of the laboratory — even the behavioral-pharmacology laboratory — and the psychopharmacologists and neuroscientists distrusted the constructionist views of the social scientists. By the end of the century, enough pieces were in place for building an alternative, interdisciplinary account of voluntary drug use that effectively tore down modern pharmacologicalism, but the builders remained holed up in their respective disciplines and never gathered to build it.

In the meantime, research continued. As evidence of the social production of meaning in drug use and drug effects surfaced in the social sciences, research in the behavioral-pharmacology laboratory explored the stimulus functions of drugs. While an animal model of the social production of drugs was not a realistic goal, researchers found it possible to study basic learning processes involving drugs as stimuli. In fact, so dynamic were these processes in animals that they begged the greater question of how deep the ecology of drug outcomes might run in humans. After all, was meaning-making not believed to be a quintessentially human affair?

In addition to the research involving the self-administration of drugs maintained by the conditioned stimuli associated with drug administration, a second, parallel area of research had its roots in research by Peter Dews and others, who explored the effects of drugs on behavior generally. At its most radical moments, this animal research brought into question the entire distinction between drug and nondrug stimuli.

One rather curious but illustrative study explored whether environmental stimuli could substitute for interoceptive, drug stimuli, producing the same behavioral effect.[17] Rats were first trained to discriminate between a drug that typically made them anxious and saline solution (a placebo). When a drug injection was administered before an experimental session, responses on one button would be reinforced with food; when the saline was administered before a session, responding on a different button led to food. Animals had only the interoceptive stimuli produced (or not produced) by the injection to determine which button to press.

After the rats were trained to discriminate reliably between a particular dose of the drug and the saline, the researchers then tested whether the presentation of an exteroceptive stimulus that produced anxiety—a cat dowsed in catnip—would substitute for the anxiogenic drug. That is, would the presentation of the cat as a "stimulus" result in responding on the "I'm anxious" button for food, as though the rat had been administered the anxiety-producing drug? Such an effect might seem bizarre: why would an animal respond according to an external stimulus when it had never learned to do so? However, if the drug and the cat were functionally equivalent in their ability to produce certain interoceptive stimuli (namely, anxiety), and the interoceptive stimuli were the deciding factors, regardless of their origin, then the animal should do just this. And indeed, the latter result prevailed: when the composite visual-olfactory stimulus was presented to the animal, all the animals reliably pressed the button that was associated with the anxiogenic drug. The question thus arose: drug stimuli may affect behavior, but was this a unique effect to be explained by pharmacological principles, or was this a general effect that could be explained largely by psychological principles?

Overall, studies have suggested the latter. In a simple but elegant study by Chia-Shong Chen, published in 1968, rats were injected with alcohol to test its effects on performance in running a maze to earn food.[18] The animals were sorted into two groups: one received alcohol prior to running the maze for each of the three sessions, whereas the second group received alcohol after completion of the maze. Thus, animals in both groups were exposed to exactly the same amount of alcohol across the three trials, but only one group completed the maze while "under the influence" of alcohol. On the fourth trial, alcohol was administered to both groups prior to the session. With alcohol exposure having been the same for both groups, and with both having had the same amount of practice running the maze, one might predict that each group would, on average, do equally well. The group of rats who received alcohol prior to the first three test sessions might, on the other hand, do more poorly on the fourth trial, since their learning of the maze could have been hindered by the depressant effects of alcohol, especially given that the animals in this group had learned the maze with more difficulty during the initial trials than had those in the other group.

But there was also another prediction, one that emphasized alcohol's general effects as a stimulus and more or less ignored alcohol's effects as a so-called depressant drug: with the drug's stimulus effects being part of the context of learning a task, they might be incorporated into that learning such that the later removal of these stimuli could actually disrupt the performance. At the same time, if alcohol was not part of the context of learning, as for the second group, its administration prior to the fourth trial might prove to be disruptive, since unfamiliar (drug) stimuli were being introduced to the behavioral context.

In general, as learning occurs, stimuli become part of what guides the behavior, from running down a staircase to remembering a person's name; remove any of the stimuli and the performance naturally degrades. For example, one becomes accustomed to one's own car—the location and resistance of the brake, the gas, the shifter, the wheel, the turning radius—and thus one can drive it with little conscious attention paid to the mechanics of getting in, starting, stopping, shifting, or turning. However, in an unfamiliar car, such fluidity disappears; one must focus on the task and learning must begin again. At this point, stimuli and relations between stimuli in the new environment once again become embedded within the learning in order to guide behavior better.

Learning of this kind turned out to be quite evident in Chen's study. On average, the animals who had run the maze under the influence of alcohol on the first three trials were considerably more successful than the other group in running the maze on the fourth trial. The former animals not only completed more correct trials during the test trial than they had in any previous trials, they also completed more correct trials than the other group for that trial; in fact, the second group performed terribly, completing only 10 percent as many trials as they had averaged in the previous sessions. Given that both groups had exactly the same alcohol exposure up to that point, the effect of the injection of alcohol before the final trial cannot be explained as a drug effect per se. This is true by definition, since the same drug administration had different effects on the same task. These effects can be explained, however, by reference to alcohol as a stimulus. Because of the training procedure, the stimuli had come to function for one group as meaningful stimuli, and it was this difference in learning—not a difference in drug exposure—that accounted for the differences in the performance of two groups in the final trial.

Chen did not, however, complete the other half of the test. On the one hand, Chen's study showed that the *administration* of the drug to the second group just prior to the trial disrupted performance because it produced a change in the (nondrug) stimulus conditions under which the task had originally been learned. What was not tested was whether the *removal* of the alcohol stimuli for the other group would have disrupted their performance in the same way and for the same reason. From the standpoint of pharmacologicalism, this idea is heretical, since it suggests that, depending on the animal's learning history with a psychoactive drug, its removal for one individual might actually have the same effect as its presentation for another. While Chen did not test for this outcome, other researchers did.

A 1973 paper examined the "disruptive" effects not of alcohol (a depressant), but of amphetamine (a stimulant).[19] Robert Carey trained laboratory rats to earn food by responding on a button in a particular temporal pattern: if no responses occurred for a fixed amount of time, the first response after that time led to the presentation of food; by contrast, any premature response caused the clock to reset back to zero, with no food delivered. Naturally, this schedule of reinforcement resulted in efficient, occasional responding, as rats and other animals are quite good at learning temporal discriminations. Once the so-called reinforcement schedule was learned, with the animals reliably responding at a slow rate and receiving most or all of the food possible in a session, they were injected with amphetamine prior to subsequent sessions. Having had no experience with the stimulant drug, rates of responding initially shifted in an upward direction. As a result, the drug disrupted performance: responding was more often premature, causing less food to be earned.

From this point on, animals continued to do the task with amphetamine administered prior to each session; those animals that performed "under the influence" showed tolerance to amphetamine's initial disruptive effects, with their levels of performance eventually returning to their previous, optimal levels. The drug stimuli were now part of the learned context for responding for food and thus were no longer disruptive. Now Carey had the opportunity to conduct a test equivalent to the missing test in Chen's rat-maze study: the drug was no longer injected prior to each session. If amphetamine was functioning as part of the stimulus environment governing slow but effective responding, amphetamine's removal should lead to the same disruption in responding as had the initial presentation of amphetamine — and it did. When saline was administered in place of amphetamine, the animals showed a relative *increase* in responding; with a shift from 5.1 to 6.2 responses per minute, this also resulted in a loss of food.

As with alcohol in the rat-maze study, amphetamine in the Carey study appeared to have both direct pharmacological effects and learned, stimulus-controlling effects. What was more, over time the nature of the drug effect changed. When first administered, amphetamine increased rates of responding; this was partly because it was a stimulant but also because the behavior of responding slowly for food had never been learned in the context of a drug. With the disruption of food, however, the animals quickly learned to respond at optimal rates while under the influence of amphetamine; in fact, this learning was so well established that the removal of amphetamine now disrupted responding in the same manner as its initial presentation had. While a drug can be classified as a stimulant or depressant, such effects on behavior are not predetermined by the molecules contained within. Processes of learning can alter their effects, and perhaps even reverse them.

These kinds of learned effects came to be defined by behavioral pharmacologists as *behavioral tolerance*, distinguishable from traditional kinds of tolerance because it results from a learning process rather than a physiological one.[20] In the rat-maze study, for instance, all rats were exposed to the same amount of alcohol and therefore should have shown the same level of drug tolerance, at least as traditionally defined. Instead, in the test session, only those animals with the experience of completing the task after alcohol injections showed (behavioral) tolerance.

The original conceptualization of behavioral tolerance dates back to 1966, when Bob Schuster and his colleagues employed a clever procedure to demonstrate in a single animal and within the same sessions, what Chen and then Carey demonstrated using groups of animals across multiple sessions.[21] Schuster and his group did this by training laboratory rats on two concurrent schedules of food reinforcement, one signaled by a constant light and the other signaled by a flashing light. As in the Carey study, one of the schedules required the animals to wait a fixed duration before responding, with premature responses resetting the clock and resulting in a loss of reward. Food reinforcement during the other schedule also required a response after a fixed amount of time, but premature responses did not reset the clock, having no effect. The result was two distinct patterns of responding prior to the drug administration.

Once the animals had mastered these two schedules, which were presented in sequence, one after the other, within each session, amphetamine was administered prior to the session. As in the Carey study, this typically led to an increase in responding under both schedules. Because this increase in responding had a negative consequence in only one of the two schedule conditions, which it did by disrupting the acquisition of food in the schedule wherein premature responses reset the clock, behavioral tolerance was predicted to develop only in that condition. After repeated sessions with the administration of amphetamine, tolerance appeared in just that manner, evident only for the schedule that required longer periods without responding. Viewed traditionally, behavior was essentially tolerant and not tolerant to the drug at the same time, depending on the prevailing stimulus conditions (i.e., the constant versus flashing light). As a result, each time the experimenters administered amphetamine, they observed a rate-increasing "drug effect" when one light stimulus was present and no rate-increasing effect when the other light stimulus was present. As Schuster and colleagues concluded,

> Clearly the common physiological mechanisms responsible for drug tolerance cannot be appealed to as an explanation. If the tolerance observed were attributable to changes in absorption or metabolism, there would be no explanation for the differential development of tolerance in the different behaviors. . . . Behavioral tolerance will develop in those aspects of the organism's behavioral repertoire [only] where the action of the drug is such that it disrupts the organism's behavior in meeting the environmental requirement for reinforcements. Conversely, where the actions of the drug enhance, or do not affect the organism's behavior in meeting reinforcement requirements we do not expect the development of behavioral tolerance.[22]

With the demonstration of behavioral tolerance, behavioral pharmacologists had delivered another blow to pharmacologicalism. For centuries it had been known that with repeated exposure to a drug, some of the effects might diminish, and that by increasing the dose, some or all of these effects could be recovered, at least for a time. This pattern came to be known as drug tolerance. But with the discovery of behavioral tolerance in the 1960s and 1970s, drug tolerance was shown to involve more than basic physiological or metabolic processes. Whereas some forms of tolerance did result from drug exposure, other forms of tolerance were in fact a kind of learning — learning that was contingent on the drug acting not as a drug per se, but simply as one of any kind of stimulus, interoceptive or exteroceptive in origin. Learning processes were beginning to appear as at least as powerful in psychopharmacology as the drugs themselves. What made this finding all the more impressive was that these learned effects were not restricted to the behavioral effects of a drug. Behavioral tolerance could be demonstrated for other drug effects as well.

One study along these lines began by injecting two groups of animals with equal doses of morphine.[23] Morphine was employed in part because it produces hyperthermia (that is, it raises body temperature). Thus, after a series of morphine injections, tolerance could be measured in terms of the hyperthermic reaction. To assess whether tolerance was merely the result of physiological adaptation, however, the researchers also tested the two groups in different environments. One group was kept in the same environment in which they had always received morphine, whereas the other group received the drug in a new environment.

What the study found was that the animals exposed to morphine in the novel setting did in fact show more hyperthermia (i.e., less tolerance) than did the animals kept in the familiar one. As with previous studies, tolerance to the drug's effect — in this case, a standard physiological effect of hyperthermia — was clearly mediated by processes of learning and adaptation that was specific to the environment in which the drug was administered: when the environment in which the learning occurred was removed, significantly less tolerance was observed.

While such findings continued to raise fundamental questions about the extent to which drug effects could be explained strictly in pharmacological terms, they also had immediate, real-world implications. Shepard Siegel, the author of the morphine-hyperthermia study, was aware of anecdotal reports of overdose when habitual drug users were displaced from their usual injection sites.[24] Such cases were considered a mystery, for why would an addict overdose and perhaps die from a dose that he or she had tolerated just the day before? From his own research Siegel knew it was because tolerance was learned in a specific context, so when addicts experienced a change of setting, they also experienced an unexpected and dangerous loss of tolerance. Siegel then set out to document this phenomenon, reporting his findings in "Heroin 'overdose' death: Contribution of drug-associated environmental cues," a 1982 paper published in *Science*.

Meanwhile, anti-drug crusaders and a cadre of obliging researchers were making a concerted effort to show that cocaine produced a withdrawal syndrome, defined as "craving," and that this problem was a pure product of the drug. The reason was simple. The classic metaphor of addiction in the twentieth century derived from opiate addiction, and the ability of a drug to induce withdrawal thus became a defining feature of an addictive drug. In the 1960s, for instance, the WHO's Expert Committee on Addiction-Producing Drugs upheld a sharp distinction between "physical dependence" and "psychic dependence."[25] Peter Laurie described the outlook at the time, writing, "In many people's minds, the most important and dangerous quality of a drug is its addictiveness . . . [a term] applied to drugs that cause physical changes in the body, perpetuating their use. That is, 'tolerance' is established in the 'addict,' and he needs more of the drug to hold off withdrawal symptoms or to reach the same intensity of effect."[26]

Where cocaine was concerned, this definition of a dangerous drug posed a problem. It was already understood, at least among psychopharmacologists and some international organizations of health, that cocaine does not produce either tolerance or withdrawal. Therefore, it could not be classified as a typically addictive substance. And yet, by the 1980s cocaine had been defined in the public imagination as the most dangerous and rapidly addicting drug, having pushed opiates aside as the model of drug addiction. "Cocaine-driven humans will relegate all other drives and pleasures to a minor role in their lives. . . . If we were to design deliberately a chemical that would lock people into perpetual usage, it would probably resemble . . . cocaine."[27]

A concerted effort was made to overcome this contradiction, with millions of federal dollars spent on "proving" that the craving caused by cocaine was in fact comparable to the withdrawal experienced from opiates. The effort succeeded. Via a convoluted chain of logic about cocaine's addiction-like properties, cocaine was redefined as a classically addictive drug, and the key to addiction was now the craving that resulted after its continuous use. "Cocaine produces no gross physiological withdrawal symptoms," wrote one researcher, "demonstrat[ing] that subjective experiences or symptoms other than physiological discomfort are crucial in addiction to cocaine and to other substances of abuse. . . . Investigators are now exploring how psychological symptoms in drug withdrawal, particularly unpleasant mood states and craving for drug euphoria, maintain chronic drug addiction."[28]

The hype concerning cocaine's addictive cravings was ironic, for while cocaine never really met the standard profile of withdrawal and dependence, many prescription medicines at the time did, including the barbiturates. Although these problems of dependence were easily ignored, since "ethical medicines" by definition had nothing to do with "drug abuse" and "addictive drugs," one other problem remained: the government's own data showed cocaine's power to induce addiction was a myth. The 1990 National Household Survey of Drug Abuse found, for instance, that for those who had used the drug in the last year, only one in three had used the drug twelve or more times, and only one in ten took cocaine more than once per week.[29] A Canadian survey found a similar pattern, with only one in twenty active users taking cocaine once per month or more.[30] More in-depth studies also showed this. One researcher tracked fifty regular cocaine users for over a decade and found that only five of them became compulsive users.[31] Erickson and her colleagues at the University of Toronto tracked inner-city crack users and found a similar pattern, with heavy or continuous use occurring in only about a third of the seventy users.[32]

The science of craving fared no better. Researchers and so-called policy experts could tie cocaine to the opiate addiction wagon, but this did not eliminate the fact that, as had been demonstrated well before the 1980s, even the link between opiate withdrawal and addiction was tenuous. And thus it was that, with the proclamation that cocaine was one of the most addictive drugs, a few researchers began publishing research that suggested otherwise. Much of this research focused on the role of stimuli in drug use and threw considerable doubt on the importance of craving as an inevitable cause of compulsive drug abuse.

Among these researchers was, once again, Bob Schuster. No longer the director of NIDA, Schuster was free to question the government-sponsored focus on craving and did so in a study that appeared in 1995.[33] Along with his colleagues, he examined opiate withdrawal and measured the cravings individuals reported during their withdrawal, where withdrawal was induced in habitual opiate users via an opiate antagonist. The study had its origins in earlier research showing that craving for opiates, as well as for cigarettes, fluctuated according to the immediate availability of the drug. Craving was a dynamic psychological variable, it had been shown, that hinged on the knowledge that drugs were present.[34] What Schuster and colleagues found was consistent with this. Drug users were asked to rate their craving in terms of whether they felt "like shooting up," and these reports were measured relative to the intensity of their physical withdrawal. There was no reliable correlation. Increases in withdrawal, whether measured physiologically or as self-reports of mood, were not strongly associated with reports of craving. What was more, craving did not predict increased drug taking during the experiment. As Schuster and colleagues concluded, "Craving is not causally related to increased drug taking."[35]

What was bad news for opiates was even worse news for cocaine. In a series of studies done in the 1990s, the researchers Marian Fishman and Richard Foltin at Columbia University found little if any relationship between cravings, rated on an "I want cocaine" scale, and the self-administration of cocaine by habitués residing in a clinical research ward. In one study a therapeutic drug was administered to reduce craving, and it did, but self-administration of cocaine did not change.[36] In another study a different therapeutic drug was administered. While not lowering self-reports of craving, it still led to decreases in cocaine self-administration.[37]

All this was consistent with what was being demonstrated at the time for nicotine and cigarette smoking. As was now claimed with regard to cocaine, nicotine withdrawal was also said to control the user by overwhelming him or her with a craving for the drug, creating a cycle of addictive behavior. Nicotine substitutes like the transdermal patch were then marketed as a method to break this cycle. However, studies looking for such a link found instead that while a nicotine substitute might reduce smoking to some minor degree, it did so without having any effect on craving. Even a study by Jack Henningfield, a leading government scientist behind the effort to link the smoking habit to nicotine, found a strong dissociation between the desire to smoke and the likelihood of smoking.[38]

Has a contradiction surfaced here? If stimuli and their meaning are involved in drug seeking, drug use, and drug outcomes, including stimuli produced by the drugs themselves, why then would craving—a potentially strong stimulus—not reliably affect drug use? Craving is certainly a real and measurable phenomena that has a relationship to drug desire and drug use. Yet as an experience, it does not appear to necessarily cause drug seeking or drug use. After craving was redefined in the 1980s in an attempt to cast cocaine as an inherently addictive drug, the burden on the concept simply became too great. Withdrawal and craving may be greater after repeated drug use, but the meaning and thus the impact of these experiences have been shown to stem from a variety of nondrug factors, including personality, placebo texts, situations, and personal beliefs. And for this reason, whether across cultures or among different individuals or groups, drug effects are necessarily diverse. As Peter Laurie noted, "Cannabis was, and is, used in the Far East to assist meditation and religious out-of-self-ness; the assassins or Haschischiens took it to make them ferocious; in Cairo in the thirties it was the centre of a nationalist, anti-British movement; American jazz musicians use it socially, and feel it improves their musical sensitivity; students here [in the UK] take it as an emblem of rebellion."[39]

However strong the stimuli produced by a drug or its absence might be, reports in the twentieth century showing that they yield uniform effects were rare. By contrast, considerable ethnographic, correlational, and empirical research showed seemingly wild unpredictability in drug outcomes across context, cultures, and placebo texts. Perhaps the most powerful demonstration of the ambiguous nature of drug stimuli was provided in a study that did not even employ a drug.

In what became a classic study, Stanley Schachter and Jerome Singer reported in 1962 that giving human subjects an injection of epinephrine (adrenaline) did not produce any consistent psychological effects.[40] Subjects were told that they were in a study examining the effects of a vitamin, and when they were administered the stimulant, no consistent experience or emotion emerged. Intrigued by this, Schachter and Singer asked the following question: might the injected substance serve as a kind of physiological primer—a chemical canvas on which they could paint different experiences by concurrently exposing subjects to different emotions? To encourage such emotions, they exposed subjects to social contexts designed to make them either cheerful or angry. The researchers found, as they had hoped, that it was indeed possible to place varying emotional states on the top of the stimulus's effects merely by suggestion. The epinephrine was not irrelevant, however, since the social contexts were far less effective in creating emotions when there was no epinephrine in the injection. "Given a state of physiological arousal for which an individual has no immediate explanation," Schachter and Singer explained, echoing the words of MacAndrew and Edgerton, "he will label this state and describe his feelings in terms of the cognitions available to him."[41] That is, if the drug is a vessel with which to sail on an experiential sea, the placebo text becomes the compass that guides its course.[42]

As researchers continue to demonstrate, withdrawal *from* drugs and cravings *for* drugs are not parts of a hard-wired circuit leading inevitably to abuse and dependence. Instead, another kind of circuit, one that is ecological in nature, is revealed: a circuit that runs between environment, behavior, experience, and the brain. The metaphor of an ecological circuit has the advantage of acknowledging not only that drug outcomes are dynamic but also that the connection between drugs and drug dependence can be short-circuited. While stimuli associated with drug use and drug abstinence are undeniably real and potentially important, their causal role in drug use has in fact never been shown to be strong, let alone absolute.

But of course none of this mattered at the end of the twentieth century. With or without empirical support, cocaine remained at the top of the dangerous-drug charts through the 1980s and 1990s. One reason was crack cocaine.

With fears of a crack epidemic dominating the public imagination in the mid- to late 1980s, the criminal sentencing for possession of crack increased steadily until it was several times more severe than for powder cocaine. Like the decline of alcohol, opiates, and cocaine in the first half of the century, crack's immediate fall from grace focused not just on a drug but also on its users. Crack in the 1980s was an inner-city drug used by poverty-stricken minorities. Powder cocaine, meanwhile, remained a more fashionable, upper-class drug used primarily by whites. The diverging criminal realities for these two forms of cocaine stemmed not from any significant pharmacological differences, for smoking cocaine differs from snorted or injected cocaine to no greater degree than smoking of opiates differs from injecting heroin. What mattered were public perceptions, perceptions cultivated by hysterical media reports about crack.

In the months leading up to the 1986 presidential election, NBC News ran more than 400 separate stories on crack and powder cocaine.[43] In May of that year, the nightly news anchor Tom Brokaw reported that crack was not only becoming "America's drug of choice," it was also "flooding" across America. *USA Today* reported, "Addicts spend thousands of dollars on binges, smoking the contents of vial after vial in crack or 'base' houses—modern-day opium dens—for days at a time without food or sleep. They will do anything to repeat the high, including robbing their families and friends, selling their possessions and bodies." When these media claims were investigated following allegations of racial bias, crack was not found to be a uniquely harmful or dangerous drug. As a report the U.S. Sentencing Commission sent to Congress in 1995 concluded, "The media and public fears of a direct causal relation between crack and other crimes do not seem to be confirmed by empirical data. . . . [S]tudies report that neither powder nor crack cocaine excite or agitate users to commit criminal acts and that the stereotype of a drug-crazed addict committing heinous crimes is not true for either form of cocaine."[44]

It was an apt note on which to close the twentieth century. When the hysteria surrounding crack collided with the conclusions of the sentencing commission—a body created by and almost always respected by Congress—again nothing happened. That the conclusion of a conservative body like the sentencing commission could not influence the media or government, even when buttressed by volumes of evidence in its favor, all but forces the conclusion that an ideology of angels and demons underlies America's troubled policies regarding prescription drugs, street drugs, and store drugs. The science of drugs that was in the news was not erecting any pillars of wisdom. Instead it was serving as a front organization for the institutions of differential prohibition and safeguarding their central tenet: whether angels or demons, drugs have magical powers that can transform both mind and behavior.

Chapter Nine **Ideology**

*The concept of progress acts as a protective mechanism to
shield us from the terrors of the future.*

—Frank Herbert, Dune

As the twentieth century ended, much had been learned about the complex, ecological nature of drug outcomes. It was a dramatic chapter in the long history of human interactions with drug substances, even if the most radical discoveries remained buried under an almost universally accepted reductionism of drugs, the brain, and human agency. Those aspects of drugs that created societal spectacle—from intoxication and other altered states of consciousness to psychiatric utility to addiction and dependence—were shown to vary dramatically across users and contexts. Researchers made true breakthroughs in understanding how drugs worked, as pharmacological effects were decoupled from potent psychological and social variables that interacted with and shaped them. This awakening unfolded under the long shadow of the cult of pharmacology, however, which left American society ill-situated to benefit from new insights. Instead, a differential prohibition of drugs was built on a foundation of pharmacologicalism, erected in the midst of scandal, intrigue, violent crime, corporate crime, and congressional hearings, all of which resulted from American policies and attitudes toward drugs as often as from the drugs themselves.

The story of drugs in twentieth-century America is thus a story of angels and demons, of how psychoactive substances and their users were segregated into two general categories, the ethical and the immoral. It is a dark story in American history, if not a terribly unique one. The cult of pharmacology had its origins in an ancient magicalism surrounding drugs, the notion that certain substances contain powerful spirits that give them special capabilities. But it also had its origins in a common ideological process that unfolded steadily throughout the century, a process that involved the relentless social production of the meaning of drugs, an ideology of otherness that was hardly specific to drugs.

Throughout history societies have deemed drugs a special other, assigning them to a realm all their own. In America this made two things possible. First, the study of psychoactive drugs was absorbed into a scientific discipline, pharmacology, which was not equipped to grapple with the powerful dialectic that existed between drugs, their users, and the historical and immediate contexts of use. Indeed, pharmacology was a rather unwitting parent to psychoactive drugs, ignoring most of those aspects that distinguished them from drugs that were not active in the brain. Second, and perhaps more important, with drug effects roped off as a source of unique powers, drugs retained the status of other, as they had for millennia. Drugs remained in the hands of specialized disciplines — psychiatry, pharmacology, psychopharmacology, behavioral neuroscience — where they continued to be treated as an exceptional mode of influence on mind and body, qualitatively distinct from experiences mediated by the senses.

The empirical disciplines neither reigned in drugs nor took them out of the realm of the magical to bring them within the earthly constraints of the natural sciences. In fact, the opposite happened, with those disciplines actually ensuring that drugs remained in the realm of the alien and exotic. Substances believed to have special healing powers were deemed good drugs, or "medicines," while demonized substances, or "drugs," were imbued with destructive and enslaving powers. This is why, in 1936, one could read in *Scientific American* that "marihuana produces a wide variety of symptoms in the user, including hilarity, swooning, and sexual excitement."[1] And why a half-century later one could read that a medicine called PCP, a drug created by Parke Davis and Company in 1956, promoted violence while endowing its users with superhuman strength.

Still defined as a special "other," drugs remained within the long tradition wherein influential groups and bodies, both in the public or private sphere, wielded control over the social production of meaning and thereby acquired or maintained influence over the thoughts and actions of the public.

This is not an active conspiracy, but rather the simple play of the mechanisms of power oriented toward persuading and influencing others, perhaps even with the goal of doing good.

There are numerous other examples. Nazism is a nondrug example of the invention of a special other for purposes of persuasion. Germany in the 1930s believed in the possibility of reviving a pure and noble race, a possibility that according to Nazi ideology was racially and culturally compromised by impure and inferior others, including the Jew. Like the angel drug and the demon drug, the Aryan and the Jew were constructed as distinct and distinguishable categories that gave meaning to and thereby excused extraordinary political, social, and scientific measures. According to the logic of Nazism, the Germanic race deserved the servitude of the entire world, while the Semitic race required total eradication. What these extremes really represented was a powerful racist ideology by which, via the construction of meaning and the shaping of people's perceptual attributions, the German public was persuaded to see what was never there, while becoming blind to what was. To give the whole affair a look of modern legitimacy, meanwhile, a science of race was introduced as propaganda. This science was said to establish a hierarchy of racial purity among true Germans based on family history (i.e., racial mixing). The result was that a diverse ethnic reality rooted in culture and history was eliminated, replaced by a pseudoclassification of ideal types. Purported to be based on genetics, this biological reductionism reigned supreme as a kind of scientific fundamentalism in much the same way as pharmacological reductionism was employed to determine whether certain drugs and drug users were good or evil.

Nazism also paralleled pharmacologicalism in its attempts to hold a tenuous middle ground that lay between the extremes. Nazi ideology treated the British as racially acceptable, for instance, just as American pharmacologicalism permitted the existence of grey-market substances like alcohol and tobacco. While the angel drug and the demon drug are only limited metaphors for the Aryan and Jew, for drugs are not people, this hardly matters. For as the differential prohibition of drugs emerged, the positive and negative attributions bestowed on different drugs were also bestowed on their users. Use of drugs like barbiturates and SSRIs defined one kind of drug user—the patient—while use of drugs like heroin and cocaine defined another—the drug abuser.

The storyline of drugs in the twentieth century, therefore, was not without precedent or comparison. Indeed, Nazism is only one of several notable examples of how a powerful ideology of the other could be used to turn irrational, even insane, views and policies into "commonsense" notions of progress.

Orientalism, as outlined by Edward Said in his book by the same name, also compares to modern pharmacologicalism.[2] Said defined and critiqued orientalism as a self-serving Western ideology for shaping the West's understanding of the Orient and its people. He who defines a thing controls a thing, Said believed, and by mystifying the East as an alien other, the West was able to define it to its own advantage. If Arabs were characterized as a people forever mired in religion and myth, for instance, they could be dismissed wholesale as a crude people of a backwards culture, as the enemies of science, democracy, and material progress. A similar mystification of the other was also clear in the history of drugs: those who had the opportunity to construct the meanings of drugs used their power to reconfigure which drugs could properly be used, how, and by whom. The decades-long history of Harry J. Anslinger and his Federal Bureau of Narcotics and Dangerous Drugs was one notable example. The modern pharmaceutical industry, which by the end of the century had overtaken the FDA to reinstitute the patent-medicine industry, is another.

In Said's historical analysis, which appeared in 1979, the division drawn was between the Orient as a singular Eastern other, painted in broad strokes, and the Occident, defined as the diverse but familiar reality of the West. Said's framework proves useful for clarifying the ideology of drugs in the twentieth century in that it points to orientalism, like pharmacologicalism, as a "Western style for dominating, restructuring, and having authority over" all that which was deemed part of the other.[3] Applied to pharmacologicalism, this framework can be understood as a system for rendering something so alien, exotic, or special that even the most bizarre notions about it become believable. Thus, just as "orientalism approaches a heterogeneous, dynamic, and complex human reality from an uncritically essentialist standpoint," according to Said, so does pharmacologicalism reduce the complexities of drug phenomena down to static drug essences, rendering them as an almost exclusively pharmacological and biochemical concern.[4]

The analogy to Said's East versus West does not apply to angels versus demons, however, but to the exotic realm of drugs (including both angels and demons) versus the traditional realm of everyday sense experience. After all, the core myth underlying the cult of pharmacology is that drugs are unique from other, traditional modes of experience. Whether it is a different realm of experience (the Orient) or a different modality of experience (the pharmacological) does not matter. For both orientalism and pharmacologicalism, the underlying realities are repressed and denied, replaced by a harsh pseudoreality that conforms to carefully guarded and historically evolved social, moral, and political imperatives. Thus it is that psychoactive substances are deemed exotic and granted special powers that translate into essential moral properties. Once established, these moral objects must be appropriately classified and managed by the state, affirming a differential prohibition of drugs that, like orientalism and Nazism, knows no bounds.

From alcohol's prohibition to the tobacco wars to marijuana hysteria to the media's crack overdose, America's cult of pharmacology offered a unique story. However, the social forces by which pharmacologicalism gave rise to a differential prohibition of angels and demons — the process of creating meaning around a special other called drugs — was also part of a more general history of power, of how power flows and functions in society, and of how it is used to exert control over the social production of meaning.

Looking back at a century or so of failed prohibitionist policies in America, asking how it could be that the rise of differential prohibition in the twentieth century correlated with such a vast proliferation of all kinds of drugs, from the street, the store, and the pharmacy, one might wonder whether the prohibition of demons and the medicalization of angels really had anything to do with improving or safeguarding people's health. If the goal had been to decrease people's use of unregulated drugs of abuse, or to minimize the toll that black markets have on individuals and society, or even just to decrease the domestic demand for dependence-producing synthetic medications, "other, more effective policies would have been embraced long before the twentieth century's end.[5]

The cult of pharmacology must therefore have served a different purpose than the elimination of dangerous drugs and the sanctioning of psychiatric medications. With regard to pharmaceuticals: during the twentieth century, the competitiveness of the drug market and the fact that one or two successfully approved and marketed compounds could raise a company from rags to riches almost overnight made for an increasingly aggressive and reckless industry. The medicopharmaceutical industrial complex that subsequently emerged benefited directly from differential prohibition, moreover, in that the demonization of certain natural substances — marijuana, cocaine, and opiates — helped set them apart from "ethical" pharmaceutical compounds, even if the latter had equal or greater toxicity.

Drug prohibition followed a somewhat different path. While it also involved (black) market forces that acted on society and individuals, it represented the evolving problem of managing the growing availability of synthetic drugs. Along these lines, the present historical period, considered by most as an era of drug prohibition, compares to the Victorian era, widely held to be a time of sexual repression. In *The History of Sexuality* Michel Foucault argued that the popular understanding of sexual repression in the classical period was inadequate because it could not account for the explosion of sexual content in bourgeois, Victorian society.[6] Sexuality was not so much repressed, Foucault argued, as it was reproduced to fit new standards of the human body, standards that concerned the supervision and disciplining of the body, not necessarily the extinguishing of it as a source of pleasure. Foucault wrote, "We are dealing not nearly so much with a negative mechanism of exclusion as with the operation of a subtle network of discourses, special knowledge, pleasures, and powers."[7] Repression of the body was secondary to establishing control over it and thereby exerting a differential regulation over the uses of the body, as well as the uses of pleasure.

Foucault's analysis of Victorian sexuality may not be a perfect mirror for the history of drugs in twentieth-century America, but one aspect of his analysis does stand out: just as Foucault saw sexual practices being reconstructed and strengthened at the very time when they were thought to be repressed, one also sees in the twentieth century a vast reconstruction and proliferation of psychoactive drugs emerging alongside a centralized regime of control erected alongside a myth of prohibition. Like Victorian puritanism, drug prohibitions were really more about the management and control of the body and the behavior of the masses than about total negation. The purpose of drug policies was therefore mistaken to be quantitative in nature — aimed at decreasing drug use generally — when in fact it was qualitative — aimed at defining and constraining, from a moral American standpoint, proper and acceptable forms of drug use.

The story of drugs in twentieth-century America is in the end really two stories that emerged side by side. One of these stories is specific to the twentieth century and involves the elaborate construction of a bifurcated world of medicinal angels and all-possessing demons. The other is more general and marginal, and concerns the genuine pursuit of knowledge regarding how drugs work in society. Both stories draw from the same source — the American drug scene — but they do so in very different ways. Pharmacologicalism appeared as a great influence on both the illicit and domestic drug scene as the century progressed, while the radical critique of *what drugs are* was little more than a footnote to that relentless progression.

The social production of drugs thus remained in the twentieth century much what it had been since ancient times — a powerful human enterprise for endowing certain molecules with potency and meaning. The gradual awareness and characterization of the powerful but distorting process of pharmacologicalism, and how it encouraged drugs to be seen and experienced as a unique other in twentieth-century America, was not an exception or even a threat to this long affair. It was simply another example of the diversity of drug-related phenomena that the social production of drug outcomes had yielded for millennia.

ESCALATION OF AMERICAN DRUG LAWS
IN THE TWENTIETH CENTURY

1909 *Opium Exclusion Act.* Essentially an import act, it prohibited the importation of opium and its derivatives, except for medical use. At this time,
it was still legal to use and manufacture opium in the United States,
although opium-poppy growing in the United States had to be licensed.

1914 *Harrison Act.* Essentially a drug-distribution act, it specified lawful dis-
tributors for the sale of poppy and coca derivatives, including physicians, dentists, and veterinary surgeons, if registered. All other dealing
and dispensing of these drugs became illegal.

1918 *Eighteenth Amendment to the U.S. Constitution.* Prohibited the manufacture, sale, and transportation of alcohol. (It was repealed in 1933 by the
Twenty-First Amendment.)

1922 *Jones-Miller Act.* Established the Federal Narcotics Control Board, raised
penalties for the illegal dealing of poppy and coca derivatives, and restricted importation to crude (versus refined) forms of the drugs.

1924 The manufacture of heroin became illegal in the United States.

1930 Congress passed legislative changes that led the Federal Narcotics Control Board to be replaced by the Bureau of Narcotics of the Treasury
Department.

1937 *The Marijuana Tax Act.* Established regulation by taxation of all levels of
marijuana production, sale, and use. (It was ruled unconstitutional in
1969.)

1951 *Boggs Amendment* (to the Harrison Act). Established minimum mandatory sentences for all offenses involving derivatives of opium, coca, and
cannabis.

1956 *The Narcotic Drug Control Act.* Raised minimum mandatory sentences and
included a provision that made selling heroin to a minor a capital offense.

1968 The Bureau of Narcotics of the Treasury Department became the Bureau of Narcotics and Dangerous Drugs of the Justice Department.

1970 *Comprehensive Drug Abuse Prevention and Control Act.* Replaced the Harrison Act of 1914 and federalized all drug laws, regardless of state laws
concerning interstate commerce. Overall, it represented a shift from
regulation by taxation to the direct criminalization of drug practices.
The law also established a five-tier scheduling of drugs (that excluded
alcohol) and a Commission on Marijuana and Drug Abuse, which led
to a 1973 report recommending the legalization of marijuana.

1970s *Racketeer-Influenced and Corruption Organizations (RICO) and Continuing Criminal Enterprises (CCE) Statutes.* Allowed the forfeiture of

personal assets for individuals and organizations charged with drug trafficking.

1982   *Department of Defense Authorization Act.* Diverted select parts of the armed forces and NASA to the task of drug enforcement.

1984   *Comprehensive Crime Control Act.* Initiated the trend toward a federal "zero-tolerance" stance with regard to drugs by increasing the length of sentences for drug offenses, including drug cultivation, trafficking, possession, and use.

1986   *Anti-Drug Abuse Act.* Enlarged on the 1984 act.

1988   *Anti-Drug Abuse Amendment Act* and *Zero Tolerance.* A White House drug policy initiative that further focused drug prohibitions against users, it stated that both supply and demand were crucial to illegal drug markets, that drug abusers began as willful agents, not as powerless victims, and that self-destruction was not an individual freedom. This initiative spawned a number of states to enact "three strike" laws that significantly raised minimum mandatory sentences for repeat drug offenders.

U.S. REGULATIONS ALLOWING A WHITE MARKET
FOR DRUGS IN THE TWENTIETH CENTURY

1906   *Pure Food and Drugs Act.* Essentially a labeling act, it established the federal government's role in the regulation of drugs. It focused in part on the "misbranding" of patent medicines, which had the intended effect of forcing manufacturers to reveal the true active ingredients contained in the product.

1912   *Shirley Amendment.* Further clarified the issue of misbranding, forbidding any therapeutic claims that were "false and fraudulent."

1938   *Food, Drug, and Cosmetic Act.* Essentially a product-safety act, it required that drug manufacturers demonstrate product safety when used as directed. Manufacturers had to submit to the FDA a "new drug application" that reported testing for toxicity. This and other provisions created a more active role for the FDA and encouraged a partnership between the agency and the pharmaceutical industry. It also led to an increase in prescription (versus over-the-counter) drugs.

1951   *Humphrey-Durham Amendment.* Created three classes of prescription drugs: those that must be labeled with a warning of "habit forming"; those the FDA said posed too great a risk for toxicity unless administered by a physician; and those deemed to be "new" drugs.

1962   *Kefauver-Harris Amendment.* Essentially a drug-efficacy act, it established that any drug "applied for" since 1938 had to show both clinical efficacy and safety when used as directed. It also stipulated that advertisements must include a summary of possible adverse reactions. In the years that followed, the FDA commissioned research councils and review panels to further establish and clarify regulations for both prescription and over-the-counter drugs.

1 H. C. Shelley, *Inns and taverns of old London* (London: Pitman, 1908).
2 For a history along these lines, see D. B. Heath, U.S. drug control policy: A cultural perspective, *Daedalus* 121.3 (1992): 269–91.
3 P. Laurie, *Drugs: Medical, psychological and social facts* (Baltimore: Penguin, 1967); A. Lindesmith, *Addiction and opiates* (Chicago: Aldine, 1968); S. Peele, *The meaning of addiction: Compulsive experience and its interpretation* (Lexington, Mass.; Lexington Books, 1985); O. Ray, *Drugs, society, and human behavior* (St. Louis: Mosby, 1983); E. Schlosser, Reefer madness, *Atlantic Monthly*, August 1994, 45–63; E. Schlosser, Marijuana and the law, *Atlantic Monthly*, September 1994, 84–94; T. S. Szasz, *Ceremonial chemistry* (Garden City, N.Y.: Anchor Press, 1974); A. Weil, *The natural mind* (Boston: Houghton Mifflin, 1972); N. E. Zinberg, *Drug, set, and setting* (New Haven, Conn.: Yale University Press, 1984).
4 Weil, *The natural mind*.
5 A. Weil and W. Rosen, *From chocolate to morphine: Everything you need to know about mind-altering drugs* (Boston: Houghton Mifflin, 1983), 27.

Chapter One Mama Coca

In *Margaret, the Last Real Princess*, Noel Botham details how Princess Margaret snorted cocaine in the dressing room of the Rolling Stones in 1967 London. She kissed Mick Jagger on the cheek and said, "I'm going to enjoy your concert even more after that."

1 N. D. Volkow et al., Is methylphenidate like cocaine? Studies on their pharmacokinetics and distribution in the human brain, *Archives of General Psychiatry* 52 (1995): 350.
2 R. J. DeGrandpre, *Ritalin nation: Rapid-fire culture and the transformation of human consciousness* (New York: Norton, 1999).
3 J. Rayburn, Educator jailed, *Deseret News*, 1 April 2000.
4 K. Thomas, Stealing, dealing and Ritalin: Adults and students are involved in abuse of drug, *USA Today*, 27 November 2000.
5 DeGrandpre, *Ritalin nation*.
6 Thomas, Stealing, dealing and Ritalin.
7 Ibid.
8 DeGrandpre, *Ritalin nation*.
9 Ibid.
10 See Drug Enforcement Administration, Office of Diversion Control, Conference report: Stimulant use in the treatment of ADHD (Washington: Drug

Enforcement Administration, 1996); G. Feussner, Diversion, trafficking, and the abuse of methylphenidate: A report from the DEA (presentation, NIH Consensus Conference on ADHD, Bethesda, Md., November 1998).

11 Feussner, Diversion, trafficking, 11.

12 R. J. DeGrandpre, ADHD: Serious psychiatric problem or all-American cop-out? *Cerebrum*, summer 2000.

13 Feussner, Diversion, trafficking, 201. Field agent Feussner also provided the following sample of findings for Indiana, South Carolina, and Wisconsin.

A. Indiana

— a 14 year old sold his girlfriend's MPH medication to an undercover agent
— a 16 year old crushed his MPH tablets and brought the powder to school
— an 18 year old female student was encountered with crushed MPH powder at school and admitted to abusing it for longer than a year
— a school nurse reported missing/stolen MPH from supplies held at school
— 12 high school students were trafficking MPH at school
— a student was stealing MPH medication from another student's medication bottle. Although prescribed MPH, he said he needed more.

B. South Carolina

— a father brought a MPH tablet to the police for identification: son later admitted he was snorting Ritalin
— a 16 year old was arrested for marijuana possession and was found to be carrying 65 MPH tablets. He admitted to crushing the tablets and snorting the powder
— school officials reported MPH theft from the nurse's office
— several students were suspended from school for distributing MPH on the school bus
— four male Citadel students were expelled for non-medical use of MPH.

C. Wisconsin

— 12 students were suspended or expelled for selling MPH on the school bus
— a 13 year old boy was selling his brother's medication at school
— a 16 year old male was found to be trading his MPH medication for marijuana
— A female student distributed her MPH medication on the school bus. She had left home with 60 tablets and arrived at school with 4
— three schools were broken into and MPH medication was taken.

14 Drug Enforcement Administration, Conference report; Feussner, Diversion, trafficking.

15 K. Goldberg Goff, Parents, schools need to control Ritalin access, *Washington Times*, 6 May 2001.

16 Drug Enforcement Administration, Conference report.

17 Cited in Goff, Parents, schools need to control Ritalin access.

18 See C. Tennant, The Ritalin racket, online article, 1997, copy in author's files.

19 Three factors, when taken in concert, in all likelihood made the epidemic of Ritalin misuse inevitable: the quantity of the drug infused into schools in the 1980s and 1990s, the quality of the drug relative to the cost and unavailability of

street amphetamines and cocaine, and the growing recreational use of psychoactive substances generally by American adolescents, which more than doubled during the 1990s. Trends toward recreational use of Ritalin have continued into the twenty-first century, even attracting the attention of Washington. In September 2000 the U.S. House Judiciary Committee, chaired by Henry Hyde III, wrote to the General Accounting Office, "Virtually every data source available confirms what the US Drug Enforcement Administration, state and local law enforcement, and various media outlets have documented: widespread theft, diversion and abuse of Ritalin and drugs like it, within public schools throughout the country" (quoted in Thomas, Stealing, dealing and Ritalin). The United Nations' International Narcotics Control Board also expressed concern, asking why the world's power gave so many stimulants to its children and noting that North Americans generally seem attracted to "uppers" while western Europeans seem more attracted to "downers" (Report of the International Narcotics Control Board [New York: United Nations, 2000]).

20 N. Volkow et al., Decreased striatal dopaminergic responsiveness in detoxified cocaine-dependent subjects, *Nature* 386 (24 April 1997): 830.

21 C. E. Johanson and C. R. Schuster, A choice procedure for drug reinforcers: Cocaine and methylphenidate in the rhesus monkey, *Journal of Pharmacology and Experimental Therapeutics* 193 (1975).

22 For example, see J. Bergman et al., Effects of cocaine and related drugs in nonhuman primates: III. Self-administration by squirrel monkeys. *Journal of Pharmacology and Experimental Therapeutics* 251 (1989): 150–55.

23 See Feussner, Diversion, trafficking, table 2.

24 See ibid., table 1.

25 H. May, Principal arrested in theft of medication: Ritalin tablets disappear from Orem grade school, *Salt Lake Tribune*, 1 April 2000, D2.

26 J. Rayburn, Principal arrested in Ritalin theft, *Deseret News*, 1 April 2000.

27 Quoted in L. H. Diller, Does attention deficit disorder really exist? (letter), *New York Times*, 7 September 1997.

28 See R. M. Julien, *A Primer of Drug Action*, 5th ed. (New York: Freeman, 1988), table 5.2.

29 M. M. Schweri et al., [^{3}H]Threo-(+/-)-methylphenidate binding to 3,4-dihydroxyphenyl ethylamine uptake sites in corpus striatum: Correlation with the stimulant properties of ritalinic acid esters, *Journal of Neurochemistry* 45 (1985): 1062–70; A. S. Unis et al., Autoradiographic localization of [3h]-methylphenidate binding sites in rat brain, *European Journal of Pharmacology* 113 (1985): 155–57. See also N. D. Volkow et al., Is methylphenidate like cocaine? Studies on their pharmacokinetics and distribution in the human brain, *Archives of General Psychiatry* 52 (1995): 350–53.

30 Volkow et al., Is methylphenidate like cocaine?, 457.

31 N. D. Volkow et al. (1999). Dopamine transporter occupancies in the human brain induced by therapeutic doses of oral methylphenidate, *American Journal of Psychiatry* 155 (1999): 1325–31.

32 Ibid., 1329.

33 Ibid., 1330.

34 J. Talan, Ritalin as pill not addictive, *Newsday*, 30 September 1998, A21.

35 He was preceded as drug czar by William Bennett (1989–1991), Robert Martinez (1991–1993), and Lee Brown (1993–1996).

36 Despite McCaffrey's many military honors, he has also been accused of committing war crimes during his command in Desert Storm (see S. Hersh, Overwhelming force, *New Yorker*, 22 May 2000, 49–82).

37 The colonel's wife loves cocaine, CNN, 27 August 2000.

38 From "The evolving drug threat in Colombia and other South American source zone Nations," a talk given to the Senate Committee on Foreign Relations on 6 October 1999.

39 The colonel's wife loves cocaine, CNN, 27 August 2000.

40 William Bastone first reported on these events in an article that appeared on the *Village Voice* website (http://www.villagevoice.com) on 5 August 1999. The article by Bastone (Colombian coke caper) then appeared in the 11–17 August 1999 issue.

41 What follows comes in part from research and reporting by Gabriella Gamini, Latin American correspondent to the *London Times*; for example, see "The colonel, his wife, the chauffeur and cocaine," *London Times*, 1 November 1999.

42 Note that, in March 2005, five U.S Army soldiers came under investigation for allegedly smuggling thirty-two pounds of cocaine out of Colombia aboard a U.S. military aircraft.

43 M. Gladwell, Java man, *New Yorker*, 30 July 2001, 76.

44 L. Kipnis, *Against love: A polemic* (New York: Pantheon, 2003), 185–86.

45 C. Van Dyke and R. Byck, Cocaine, *Scientific American,* March 1982, 128.

46 Ibid.

47 M. W. Friedman et al., Cardiovascular and subjective effects of intravenous cocaine administration in humans, *Archives of General Psychiatry* 33 (1976): 983–89.

48 C. R. Rush et al., Intravenous caffeine in stimulant drug abusers: Subjective reports and physiological effects, *Journal of Pharmacology and Experimental Therapeutics* 273 (1995): 351–58.

49 In still other studies, recreational cocaine users have reported comparable effects from using amphetamine, except that the effects of the latter have a longer duration. Also, beliefs about the effects of stimulants have been shown to significantly alter the "effects" of a placebo administered in its place (see M. Fillmore and M. Vogel-Sprott, Expected effect of caffeine on motor performance predicts the type of response to placebo, *Psychopharmacology* 115 [1992]: 383–88).

50 Van Dyke and Byck, Cocaine, 128.

51 A. Weil, The new politics of coca, *New Yorker*, 15 May 1995, 70.

52 Ibid.

53 W. Schivelbusch, *Tastes of Paradise* (New York: Pantheon, 1992).

54 Ibid., 153, 156.

55 J. Durlacher, *Cocaine: Its history and lore* (London: Carlton, 2000).
56 World Health Organization, Publication of the largest global study on cocaine use ever undertaken, WHO/20, 14 March 1995, press release.
57 Ibid.
58 Even this is an exaggeration of the risks, however, since the report does not offer a representative sample of the general population, because most of the general population have no interest in taking cocaine or other illicit substances.
59 See P. G. Erickson et al., *The steel drug: Cocaine in perspective* (Lexington, Mass.: Lexington Books, 1987); P. G. Erickson and B. K. Alexander, Cocaine and addictive liability, *Social Pharmacology* 3 (1989): 249–70.
60 In an interview the drug-policy analyst Ethan Nadelman said, "The US Government put extensive pressure on WHO to keep [the] report from being released" (B. Weinberg, Changing the prohibition regime, *High Times*, October 1995, 60).
61 WHO forty-eighth world health assembly, Geneva, 1–12 May 1995; see S. T. Martin, U.S. policy not limited to border, *St. Petersburg Times*, 29 July 2001.
62 Quoted in Martin, U.S. policy not limited to border.
63 WHO forty-eighth world health assembly, Geneva, 1–12 May 1995.
64 R. J. DeGrandpre, Constructing the pharmacological: A century in review, *Capitalism, Nature, Socialism* 30 (2000): 75–104.
65 See, for example, T. K. McKenna, *Food of the gods: The search for the original tree of knowledge* (New York: Basic Books, 1992); B. Inglis, *The forbidden game: A social history of drugs* (New York: Scribner, 1975).
66 Gutiérrez-Noriega's work had ties to a plan for the reduction of coca cultivation, which was first made in 1929 by Dr. Carlos A. Ricketts (see L. Grinspoon and J. B. Bakalar, *Cocaine: A drug and its social evolution* [New York: Basic Books, 1985]).
67 Weil, The new politics of coca.
68 T. G. Aigner and R. L. Balster, Choice behavior in Rhesus monkeys: Cocaine versus food, *Science* 201 (1978): 534–35; M. A. Bozarth and R. A. Wise, Toxicity associated with long-term intravenous heroin and cocaine self-administration in the rat, *JAMA* 254 (1985): 81–83; G. Deneau, T. Yanagita, and M. H. Seevers, Self-administration of psychoactive drugs by the monkey: A measure of psychological dependence, *Psychopharmacologia* 16 (1969): 30–48; C. E. Johanson, R. L. Balster, and K. Bonese, Self-administration of psychomotor stimulant drugs: The effects of unlimited access, *Pharmacology, Biochemistry, and Behavior* 4 (1976): 45–51; T. Yanagita et al., Evaluation of pharmacological agents in the monkey by long term intravenous self or programmed administration, *Excerpta Medica International Congress Series* 87 (1965): 453–57.
69 Specifically, the studies showed that animals prefer cocaine to food (Aigner and Balster, Choice behavior), will more often die from cocaine than heroin (Bozarth and Wise, Toxicity), and will self-administer cocaine until death or near-death (Aigner and Balster, Choice Behavior; Bozarth and Wise, Toxicity; Deneau, Yanagita, and Seevers, Self-administration of psychoactive drugs; Johanson, Balster, and Bonese, Self-administration of psychomotor stimulant drugs).

70 See S. Peele and R. J. DeGrandpre, Cocaine and the concept of addiction, *Addiction Research* 6 (1998): 235–63.

71 Cited in J. P. Morgan and L. Zimmer, Animal studies of self-administration of cocaine: Misinterpretation, misrepresentation and invalid extrapolation to human cocaine use, *Rolling Stone*, February 1989, 72; reprinted in P. Erickson et al., eds., *Harm reduction: A new direction for drug policies and programs* (Toronto: University of Toronto, 1997).

72 D. G. McNeil Jr., Why there's no methadone for crack, *New York Times*, 14 June 1992, sec. 4, p. 7.

73 C. Holden, Flipping the main switch in the central reward system? *Science*, 15 December 1989, 1378–79.

74 See R. J. DeGrandpre and W. K. Bickel, Drug dependence in consumer demand, in *Advances in behavioral economics*, edited by L. Green and J. Kagel (Norwood, N.J.: Ablex, 1996), 3:1–36; W. L. Woolverton, Determinants of cocaine self-administration by laboratory animals, in *Cocaine: Scientific and social dimensions*, edited by G. R. Bock and J. Whelan (West Sussex, U.K.: Wiley, 1992), 149–64.

75 See B. K. Alexander et al., Adult, infant, and animal addiction, in *The meaning of addiction: Compulsive experience and its interpretation*, edited by S. Peele (Lexington, Mass.: Lexington Books, 1985), 73–96.

76 See M. A. Nader and W. L. Woolverton, Effects of increasing the magnitude of an alternative reinforcer on drug choice in a discrete-trial choice procedure, *Psychopharmacology* 105 (1991): 169–74; M. A. Nader and W. L. Woolverton, Effects of increasing response requirement on choice between cocaine and food in Rhesus monkeys, *Psychopharmacology* 108 (1992): 295–300.

77 See S. Dworkin et al., The effects of 12-hour limited access to cocaine: Reduction in drug intake and mortality, in *Problems of drug dependence*, edited by L. S. Harris (Washington: U.S. Government Printing Office, 1986), 221–25.

78 Johanson, Balster, and Bonese, Self-administration of psychomotor stimulant drugs.

79 See N. Heather et al., eds., *Psychoactive drugs and harm reduction* (London: Whurr, 1993); E. Nadelman, Position paper on harm reduction, in *The harm reduction approach to drug control: International progress* (New York: Lindesmith Center, 1994). See also Going Dutch, *Economist*, 15 January 2000, 55–56; P. D. Cohen and A. Sas, Cocaine use in Amsterdam in nondeviant subcultures, *Addiction Research* 2 (1994): 71–94.

80 Cited in T. S. Szasz, *Ceremonial chemistry: The ritual persecution of drugs, addicts, and pushers* (Garden City, N.Y.: Anchor, 1974).

81 G. Stix, Lollipop, lollipop: A candied sedative with a kick arouses opposition from doctors, *Scientific American*, May 1994, 113.

82 R. Mathias, NIDA initiative tackles methamphetamine use, *NIDA Notes* 13 (1998): 10–11. *NIDA Notes* is a periodical published by the National Institute on Drug Abuse.

83 E. Nieves, Drug labs in Valley hideouts feed nation's habit, *New York Times*, 3 May 2001.

84 Desoxyn review taken from http://remedyfind.com.

85 S. Stokley, Rubidoux woman sentenced to prison, *Press Enterprise*, 11 January 2000.

86 D. E. Beeman, Boy's meth abuse may haunt his life: Rubidoux woman gave drug to son, 9, *Press Enterprise*, 17 January 2000.

87 S. Stokley, Rubidoux woman sentenced to prison.

Chapter Two **Cult of the SSRI**

1 Jury rules out drug as factor in killings, *New York Times*, 13 December 1994 (online).

2 Ibid.

3 S. Boseley, They said it was safe, *Guardian*, 30 October 1999, A1; as health editor at the U.K.'s *Guardian* newspaper, Sarah Boseley covered the SSRI saga unflinchingly and more thoroughly than any other reporter in the world. Her reporting also had considerable influence on an award-winning BBC television report (Panorama) that was highly critical of the SSRIS.

4 Cited in ibid.

5 For a more detailed discussion, see C. Medawar, The antidepressant web, 1997, www.socialaudit.org.uk; P. R. Breggin, *Talking back to Prozac* (New York: St. Martin's Press, 1994).

6 See, for example, W. C. Wirshing et al., Fluoxetine, akathisia, and suicidality: Is there a causal connection? *Archives of General Psychiatry* 49 (1992): 580–81.

7 Boseley, They said it was safe, A1.

8 From D. Healy, Zoloft suicide: Causal mechanisms, *The Healy Report*, www.justiceseekers.com.

9 Ibid.

10 M. H. Teicher et al., Emergence of intense suicidal preoccupation during fluoxetine treatment, *American Journal of Psychiatry* 147 (1990): 207–10. A total of six cases were reported.

> Case 1 was a 62-year-old woman who began experiencing suicidal thoughts and other adverse side effects eleven days after starting Prozac, but then experienced a complete reversal of these effects three days after stopping the drug. She described the experience as "uniquely bad," stating that "death would be a welcomed result."
>
> Case 2 was a 39-year-old man who developed a serious preoccupation with suicide and fantasies of self-destruction one month after starting Prozac. The sudden change in his manner led his elderly mother and former wife both to make "emergency calls" to his medical-care providers. Several weeks after the drug was discontinued there were no signs of any Prozac-related problems.
>
> Case 3 was a 19-year-old female college student who developed "disturbing and self-destructive thoughts" two weeks after starting Prozac. When the dose was in-

creased from 20–40mg, the problems became worse, and then worse again after the dose was increased from 40–60mg. Inexplicably, she then had her dose increased from 60–80mg, which led her to banging her head and mutilating herself. She did not show marked improvement until three months after the drug was discontinued.

Case 4 was a 39-year-old woman who experienced a worsening of depression and the emergence of suicidal thoughts two weeks after starting Prozac. For the first time she began to have thoughts of buying a gun and killing herself. She improved markedly after Prozac was discontinued.

Case 5 was a 39-year-old woman who, after going on Prozac, experienced the return of suicidal thoughts for the first time in years. However, "in contrast to her past experience with suicidal feelings, she now embraced these impulses and hid them from the clinicians." Suicidal thoughts diminished about 11 days after Prozac was discontinued.

Case 6 was very similar to Case 4.

11 Ibid., 207.
12 From David Healy's declaration to the court in U.S. District Court, *Susan Forsyth v. Eli Lilly and Company*, Civil No. 95–00185.
13 Wirshing et al., Fluoxetine, akathisia, and suicidality, 580–81.
14 A. J. Rothschild and C. A. Locke, Reexposure to fluoxetine after serious suicide attempts by three patients: The role of akathisia, *Journal of Clinical Psychiatry* 52 (1991): 491–93.
15 S. Boseley, They said it was safe, A1.
16 Ibid.
17 Ibid. This remark was from an internal memo by Leigh Thompson, a chief scientist at Eli Lilly.
18 C. M. Beasley et al., Fluoxetine and suicide: A meta-analysis of controlled trials of treatment for depression, *British Medical Journal* 303 (1991): 685–92.
19 This critique comes from D. Healy, From the psychopharmacology file, in *The Psychopharmacologists III* (London: Altman, 2000), xii–xxiii. In 1995 a report was published in the *British Medical Journal* that offered a more credible comparison of suicide rates for Prozac than the 1991 Beasley report. Looking at ten antidepressants used by a total of 170,000 patients in primary-care settings in the United Kingdom, the researchers found that Prozac, the only SSRI included in the study, was associated with a suicide rate at least twice that of other antidepressants. The reported rate of suicide for Prozac in the so-called Jicks' study was about 189 suicides per 100,000 years of patient use of the drug. (Patient years are calculated because individuals taking older drugs will have often taken them for longer periods.) Lilly claims that this rate is lower than the overall suicide rate among depressed patients, which is about 600 suicides per 100,000 years. This higher rate, however, derives from data for severely depressed patients only, whereas the vast majority of people listening to Prozac experience only mild to moderate depression. As Lilly's own packaging stated in 1996, Prozac's efficacy "was established in 5- and 6-week trials with depressed outpa-

tients. . . . [T]he antidepressant action of Prozac in hospitalized depressed patients has not been adequately studied." See S. Jick et al., Antidepressants and suicide, *British Medical Journal* 310 (1995): 215–18.

20 From a timeline presented to the jury in *Forsyth v. Eli Lilly* during closing arguments by the plaintiffs (http://www.bhagd.com/media/timeline.html).

21 Ibid.

22 Eli Lilly documents; see www.baumhedlundlaw.com.

23 R. Bourguignon, Dangers of fluoxetine, *Lancet* 349 (1997): 214.

24 From David Healy's declaration to the court in U.S. District Court, *Susan Forsyth v. Eli Lilly and Company*, Civil No. 95–00185. Another study put the rate as high as 25 percent (see J. F. Lipinski et al., Fluoxetine induced akathisia: Clinical and theoretical implications, *Journal of Clinical Psychiatry* 50 [1989]: 339–42).

25 Ibid.

26 Steven Paul, a psychiatrist and vice president of Lilly Research Laboratories, quoted in R. Raphael, A dark side to Prozac, 21 June 2000, ABCNews.com.

27 The statistic "years of patient use" controls for the fact that older antidepressants have been used for longer periods by individuals taking them than new ones (see D. Healy, *The creation of psychopharmacology* [Cambridge, Mass.: Harvard University Press, 2002]; O. Hagnell et al., Suicide rates in the Lundby study: Mental illness as a risk factor for suicide, *Neuropsychobiology* 7 [1981]: 248–53).

28 D. Healy, *Let them eat Prozac: The unhealthy relationship between the pharmaceutical industry and depression* (New York: New York University Press, 2004).

29 D. Healy, Antidepressant induced suicidality, *Primary Care Psychiatry* 6 (2000): 23–28.

30 The two-week period was shortened if the drug was not well tolerated.

31 Healy, Antidepressant induced suicidality.

32 S. Boseley, Prozac class drug blamed for killing, *Guardian*, 26 May 2001.

33 S. Boseley, Murder, suicide: A bitter aftertaste for the 'wonder' depression drug, *Guardian*, 11 June 2001 (online).

34 Boseley, Murder, suicide.

35 By the 1970s, researchers had learned that, when someone goes off their anti-anxiety drug and feels overwhelmed with anxiety, they not only kept taking the drug, they also became convinced that the drug was effective. People failed to realize that, to great benefit of the pharmaceutical industry, the drug produces its own withdrawal syndrome, characterized largely by anxiety. Not only does the drug not cure the problem, it actually has the capacity, even in non-anxious people taking benzodiazepines for other reasons, to create it. That the same story of dependence would emerge for users of SSRIs (and the infants of mothers taking SSRIs) had become clear by the end of the century; see M. J. Spencer, Fluoxetine hydrochloride (Prozac) toxicity in a neonate. *Pediatrics* 92 (1993): 721–22.

36 From papers filed in a legal action by Baum Hedlund (http://www.baumhedlundlaw.com).

37 Medawar, The antidepressant web.
38 See, for example, J. G. Modell et al., Comparative sexual side effects of bupro-
   pion, fluoxetine, paroxetine, and sertraline, *Clinical Pharmacology and Therapeutics* 61 (1997): 476–87.
39 Healy, *The creation of psychopharmacology*, 372.
40 As one critic of psychiatric drugs put it, "Anxiety is now on the back-burner and
   depression has become the dominant 'disease.' Then we were anxious, now we
   are depressed. Valium out, Prozac in" (Medawar, The antidepressant web).
41 P. Tyrer and R. Owen, Gradual withdrawal of diazepam after long-term therapy,
   Lancet 1, no. 8339 (1983): 1402–6.
42 D. Healy, *The antidepressant era* (Cambridge, Mass.: Harvard University Press,
   1997).
43 D. T. Wong et al., Prozac (fluoxetine, Lilly 110140), the first selective serotonin
   reuptake inhibitor and an antidepressant drug: Twenty years since its first publication, *Life Sciences* 57 (1995): 411–41.
44 Healy, *The antidepressant era.*
45 Ibid.
46 See Healy, *Let them eat Prozac.*
47 D. Healy, The marketing of SHT: Anxiety or depression, *British Journal of
   Psychiatry* 158 (1991): 737.
48 Healy, *The creation of psychopharmacology*, 373.
49 Healy, *The antidepressant era.*
50 Healy, The marketing of SHT, 737.
51 The advertisement appeared in the *New York Times* magazine, October 2001.
52 A. Khan, How do psychotropic medications really work? *Psychiatric Times*,
   October 1999, 11.
53 S. I. Dworkin et al., Response-dependent versus response-independent presentation of cocaine: Differences in the lethal effects of the drug, *Psychopharmacology*
   117 (1995): 262–66.
54 See S. I. Dworkin and J. E. Smith, Behavioral contingencies involved in drug-
   induced neurotransmitter turnover changes, *Research monographs of the National
   Institute of Drug Abuse* 74 (1986): 90–106; J. E. Smith et al., Brain neurotransmitter turnover correlated with morphine-seeking behavior in rats, *Pharmacology, Biochemistry and Behavior* 16 (1982): 509–19; J. E. Smith et al., Limbic
   acetylcholine turnover rates correlated with rat morphine-seeking behaviors,
   Pharmacology, Biochemistry and Behavior 20 (1984): 443–50.
55 This appears to have been the case, for instance, with the woman from Randolph, Vermont, who, almost three months after doubling her dose of Prozac,
   took a .22-caliber pistol and killed her eight-year-old son, four-year-old daughter, and herself.
56 Peter Kramer, *Listening to Prozac* (New York: Viking, 1993).
57 The popular media reacted to Prozac's release with the same zeal it offers any
   other scientific breakthrough, a zeal in which "mere change is mistaken for

progress and innovation for improvement" (G. Dukes, editorial, *International Journal of Risk and Safety in Medicine* 10 [1997]: 67).

58 "Beyond Prozac," *Newsweek*, 7 February 1994, 36–40.

59 Ibid.

60 "The Mood Molecule," *Time*, 29 September 1997, 55–62.

61 Ibid.

62 Ibid. The contradiction was possible because the article never explicitly stated that norepinephrine was the "dirty" neurochemical affected by the tricyclics.

63 "Beyond Prozac."

64 See R. J. DeGrandpre, Antidepressants: Progress or promotion? *Cerebrum*, Winter 2004, 67–82.

65 Ibid. See also R. J. DeGrandpre, Trouble in Prozac nation, *Nation*, 5 January 2005, 6.

66 Straight talk, *Eli Lilly 2000 annual report*, 9.

67 D. Wong et al., Duloxetine- and veulafaxine-induced increases in extracellular levels of serotonin and norepinephrine in the cat brain, New Clinical Drug Evaluation Unit poster session III-38 (2001).

68 L. Kowalczyk, Lilly pins hopes on new antidepressant drug, *Boston Globe*, 16 December 2001.

69 Horgan's op-ed piece appeared on 28 March 1999, A17.

70 As a review of antidepressant effectiveness in the *Journal of the American Medical Association* concluded in 1964, "Depression is, on the whole, one of the psychiatric conditions with the best prognosis for eventual recovery with or without treatment. Most depressions are self-limited and the spontaneous or placebo-induced improvement rate is often high. For example, in a series of nine controlled studies on hospitalized patients, 57% of the patients given placebo therapy showed improvement in two to six weeks" (J. O. Cole, Therapeutic efficacy of antidepressant drugs: A review, *JAMA* 190 [1964]: 124–31).

71 Praise for the SSRIs is from an on-line chat session (cited in Medawar, The antidepressant web).

72 M. Enserink, Can the placebo be the cure? *Science*, 9 April 1999, 238–40.

73 Ibid., 239.

74 Lee Park and Lino Covi, Nonblind placebo trial, *Archives of General Psychiatry* (1965), 336–45.

75 Ibid.

76 Ibid.

77 S. Blakeslee, "Placebos prove so powerful that even experts were surprised," *New York Times*, 13 October 1998.

78 See I. Kirsch and G. Sapirstein, Listening to Prozac and hearing placebo, *Prevention and Treatment*, June 1998, www.journals.apa.org/prevention/volume 5/. Kirsch and Sapirstein reported that nearly all the variation in the efficacy of antidepressants across studies could be accounted for by variation in the magnitude of the placebo effect. They also found that active placebos—drugs that

should have no pharmacological or clinical efficacy in the treatment of depression — were just as effective as the antidepressants. See also S. Fisher and R. P. Greenberg, *The limits of biological treatments for psychological distress* (Hillsdale, N.J.: Erlbaum, 1989). For an overview of these ideas see S. Fisher and R. Greenberg, Prescriptions for happiness, *Psychology Today* (September–October 1995): 32–37. See also J. Horgan, *The undiscovered mind* (New York: Free Press, 1999).

79 This estimate is from Kirsch and Sapirstein, Listening to Prozac and hearing placebo.

80 One arrives at this same conclusion when looking at three studies Lilly submitted to the FDA for drug licensing. The dangerous adverse effects of Prozac might have been moot if the FDA had just upheld rigorous scientific standards; that is, had they relied only on data from patients receiving Prozac alone, Lilly's drug might have gone the way of Merck's MK-869. When the results of the 135 patients taking benzodiazepines are removed from the data set that Lilly submitted, the statistical advantage of Prozac over placebo vanishes. That a benzodiazepine might make Prozac look like an effective antidepressant comes as no surprise, moreover, since anxiety has long been known to play a role in depressive syndromes. The fourth study Lilly submitted to the FDA, which did not allow the concurrent use of anti-anxiety drugs, never showed any effect at all; that is, there was never any statistically significant difference between Prozac and placebo (for a more detailed discussion, see Medawar, The antidepressant web).

Chapter Three The Emperor's New Smokes

1 D. Kessler, *A question of intent: A great American battle with a deadly industry* (New York: Public Affairs, 2001), 26.
2 Ibid.
3 As related in ibid., 24.
4 Ibid., 63.
5 Ibid.
6 Ibid., 64.
7 C. E. Koop, *Nicotine addiction: The health consequences of smoking: A report of the surgeon general* (Washington: Office of the Surgeon General, 1988).
8 D. Kessler, *A question of intent*, 156.
9 Ibid., 75.
10 Ibid., 76.
11 Ibid., 81.
12 See O. Ray, *Drugs, society, and human behavior* (St. Louis: Mosby, 1983).
13 Kessler, *A question of intent*, 86.
14 Ibid., 93.
15 Ibid., 101, 102.
16 Ibid., 104.

17 O. Ray, *Drugs, society, and human behavior*, 190.

18 Kessler, *A question of intent*, 122.

19 Ibid., 123.

20 Ibid., 172, 173.

21 Ibid., 153. Whether this testimony was actually given is not clear; the statement comes from an advanced copy that Kessler received.

22 Ibid., 168.

23 Ibid., 246. See also House Committee on Energy and Commerce, Subcommittee on Health and the Environment, *Regulation of tobacco products*, 103rd Cong., 2nd sess., 21 June 1994, pt. 3.

24 Kessler, *A question of intent*, 246.

25 Ibid., 227.

26 Ibid., 228.

27 Ibid., 252; P. Hilts, Tobacco company was silent on hazards, *New York Times*, 7 May 1994.

28 Kessler, *A question of intent*, 255.

29 The hearings before the Subcommittee on Health and the Environment took place in 1994 on 25 March, 14 April, 28 April, and 21 June.

30 Kessler, *A question of intent*, 160–61.

31 Koop, *Nicotine addiction*, 5.

32 J. Foulds et al., Effect of transdermal nicotine patches on cigarette smoking: A double blind crossover, *Psychopharmacology* 106 (1992): 426. Another study that appeared in *Psychopharmacology* found that the combined use of nicotine patch and nicotine gum was more effective. However, this improvement is not likely to be due to nicotine, which is absorbed in good quantity via the patch, but rather due to the addition of the nonpharmacological activity of gum chewing (K. O. Fagerstrom, Effectiveness of nicotine patch and nicotine gum as individual versus combined treatments for nicotine withdrawal symptoms, *Psychopharmacology* 111 [1993]: 271–77).

33 G. Sutherland et al., Randomised controlled trial of nasal nicotine spray in smoking cessation, *Lancet* 340 (1992): 324–29.

34 *Clinical practice guideline: Treating tobacco use and dependence* (Washington: Office of the Surgeon General, 2000).

35 With regard to the patch, see T. Abelin et al., Effectiveness of a transdermal nicotine system in smoking cessation studies: Methods and findings, *Experimental and Clinical Pharmacology* 11 (1989): 205–14; T. Abelin et al., Controlled trial of transdermal nicotine patch in tobacco withdrawal, *Lancet* 1, no. 8628 (1989): 7–10; R. D. Hurt et al., Nicotine patch therapy for smoking cessation combined with physician advice and nurse follow-up: One-year outcome and percentage of nicotine replacement, *JAMA* 271 (1994): 595–600. With regard to the inhaler, see A. Hjalmarson et al., The nicotine inhaler in smoking cessation, *Archives of Internal Medicine* 157 (1997): 1721–28; N. G. Schneider et al., Efficacy of a nicotine inhaler in smoking cessation: A double-blind, placebo-controlled trial, *Addiction* 91 (1996): 1293–1306; P. Tonnesen et

al., A double-blind trial of a nicotine inhaler for smoking cessation, *JAMA* 269 (1993): 1268–71. With regard to the gum, see S. M. Hall et al., Nicotine gum and behavioral treatment: A placebo controlled trial, *Journal of Consulting and Clinical Psychology* 55 (1987): 603–5; M. J. Jarvis et al., Randomised controlled trial of nicotine chewing-gum, *British Medical Journal* 285 (1982): 537–40. With regard to the nasal spray, see G. Sutherland et al., Randomised controlled trial of nasal nicotine spray in smoking cessation, *Lancet* 340 (1992): 324–29.

36 Similar results were found during a study of smokers conducted at the University of Michigan Medical School in 1967. In that fifteen-day study a catheter was placed in the arm of each subject so that either saline solution or nicotine could be administered. The participants were told nothing about the nicotine, nor were they informed that the study concerned smoking. They also could not detect when nicotine was administered. They simply sat in an isolated room for six hours, with reading and other activities available and permission to smoke. On days when no outside nicotine was administered, the smokers averaged 10.1 cigarettes per session. When nicotine was delivered, they smoked an average of 7.3 cigarettes and smoked the cigarettes less completely. As did later studies, this study suggested that nicotine reduced but did not eliminate the desire to smoke. (B. R. Lucchesi et al., The role of nicotine as a determinant of cigarette smoking frequency in man with observations of certain cardiovascular effects associated with the tobacco alkaloid, *Clinical Pharmacology and Therapeutics* 8 [1967]: 791.)

37 J. K. Finnegan et al., The role of nicotine in the cigarette habit, *Science* 102 (1945): 94–96.

38 A. Dunhill, *The gentle art of smoking* (New York: Putnam, 1954), quote from the jacket; see also his introduction, xi–xiii.

39 W. Schivelbusch, *Tastes of paradise* (New York: Pantheon, 1992), 111, 115.

40 Ray, *Drugs, society, and human behavior*, 188.

41 R. Klein, *Cigarettes are sublime* (Durham, N.C.: Duke University Press, 1993), 20–21.

42 D. Shapiro, Smoking tobacco: Irrationality, addiction, and paternalism, *Public Affairs Quarterly* 8 (1994): 197.

43 B. Mausner et al., *Smoking: A behavioral analysis* (Elmsford, N.Y.: Pergamon, 1971).

44 All quotes in this paragraph are from Mausner, *Smoking*, chap. 13, p. 354.

45 "Behavioral aspects," in J. B. Richmond, *The health consequences of smoking* (Washington: Office of the Surgeon General, 1981), 9.

46 Kessler, *A question of intent*, 162.

47 Ibid., 151.

48 Ibid., 162.

49 Among the earliest reports was S. R. Goldberg et al., Persistent behavior at high rates maintained by intravenous self-administration of nicotine, *Science* 214 (1981): 573–75. Goldberg et al.'s conclusions must be tempered, however, because they used a methodology that, through operant conditioning, can pro-

mote the administration of drugs that are not misused by humans (on this, see J. L. Falk, The discriminative stimulus and its repetition: Role in the instigation of drug abuse, *Experimental and Clinical Psychopharmacology* 2 [1994]: 43–52; W. A. McKim, *Drugs and behavior* [Upper Saddle River, N.J.: Prentice Hall, 2000]).

50 M. E. Jarvik, Further observations on nicotine as the reinforcing agent in smoking, in *Smoking behavior: Motives and incentives*, edited by W. L. Dunn (Washington: Winston, 1973), 33–49; cited in W. A. McKim, *Drugs and behavior* (Upper Saddle River, N.J.: Prentice Hall, 2000).

51 G. A. Deneau and R. Inoki, Nicotine self-administration in monkeys, *Annals of the New York Academy of Sciences* 142 (1967): 277–79.

52 U.S. Department of Health and Human Services, The surgeon general's call to action to prevent and decrease overweight and obesity (Rockville, Md.: U.S. Department of Health and Human Services, Public Health Service, Office of the Surgeon General, 2001).

53 John Leo, Thank you for not smoking, *U.S. News and World Report*, 15 July 1996.

54 Quoted in Banks, A case study of tobacco regulation by the Food and Drug Administration, 2002, www.law.syr.edu/faculty/banks/public law/syl1 _ 02 .pdf.

55 From Jacob Sullum's op-ed essay, "Give Dole a break," *New York Times*, 12 July 1996.

56 J. Klein, The tobacco election, *Mother Jones*, May–June 1996.

57 See R. J. DeGrandpre, Just cause, *Sciences*, March–April 1999, 14–18; G. A. Marlatt and W. H. George, Relapse prevention: Introduction and overview of the model, *British Journal of the Addictions* 79 (1984): 261–73; G. A. Marlatt and J. R. Gordon, *Relapse prevention: Maintenance strategies in addictive behavior change* (New York: Guilford, 1984). See also Shapiro, Smoking tobacco, 197.

58 D. Shapiro, Smoking tobacco, 197.

59 S. Peele and R. J. DeGrandpre, Cocaine and the concept of addiction, *Addiction Research* 6 (1998): 235–63.

60 Ibid.

61 *Diagnostic and statistical manual of mental disorders*, 4th ed. (Washington: American Psychiatric Association, 1994).

62 S. E. Hyman, Shaking out the cause of addiction, *Science*, 2 August 1996, 611.

63 Jaffe's conceptualization is outlined in Goodman and Gilman's authoritative pharmacology text, *The pharmacological basis of experimental therapeutics* (J. J. Jaffe, Drug addiction and drug abuse, in *Goodman and Gilman's the pharmacological basis of therapeutics*, 6th ed., edited by A. G. Gilman et al. [New York: Macmillan, 1980]). B. K. Alexander, *Peaceful measures: Canada's way out of the "war on drugs"* (Toronto: University of Toronto Press, 1990); it is Alexander's common-sense system that, with a few noted exceptions, is employed herein.

64 J. Shedler and J. Block, Adolescent drug use and psychological health, *American Psychologist* 45 (1990): 612–30.

65 Cited L. D. Harrison, Cocaine using careers in perspective, *Addiction Research* 2

(1994): 1–20. See also Peele and DeGrandpre, Cocaine and the concept of addiction.

66 D. B. Kandel, D. Murphy, and D. Karus, Cocaine use in young adulthood: Patterns of use and psychosocial correlates, in *Cocaine use in America: Epidemiologic and clinical perspectives*, edited by N. J. Kozel and E. H. Adams (Washington: U.S. Government Printing Office, 1985), 76–110.

67 As a veteran psychopharmacologist makes clear, physical dependence and tolerance "are two manifestations of the same phenomenon, a biologically adaptive phenomenon which occurs in all living organisms and [for] many types of stimuli, not just drug stimuli" (H. Kalant, Drug research is muddied by sundry dependence concepts [paper presented at the annual meeting of the Canadian Psychological Association, Montreal, June 1982]).

68 A. T. McLellan and C. Weisner, Achieving public health and safety potential of substance abuse treatments, in *Drug policy and human nature*, edited by W. K. Bickel and R. J. DeGrandpre (New York: Plenum, 1996), 61–80.

69 R. Brown and R. Middlefell, Fifty-five years of cocaine dependence, *British Journal of Addiction* 84, no. 8 (1989): 946.

70 See, for a review, P. Cohen and S. Arjan, *Ten years of cocaine: A follow-up study of 64 cocaine users in Amsterdam* (Amsterdam: Department of Human Geography, University of Amsterdam, 1993).

71 Quoted in Mausner, *Smoking*, chap. 13, p. 354.

72 *Nicotine addiction* (Washington: National Institute on Drug Abuse, 1998), NIH Pub. no. 01–4342.

73 Shapiro, Smoking tobacco.

74 R. Nemeth-Coslett and J. E. Henningfield, Effects of nicotine chewing gum on cigarette smoking and subject and physiological effects, *Clinical Pharmacology and Experimental Therapeutics* 39 (1986): 625–30.

75 The following studies all examined the long-term effects of nicotine exposure on the brain, and not one of them correlated these effects to any meaningful outcome: Y.-S. Ding et al., Mapping nicotinic acetylcholine receptors with PET, *Synapse* 24 (1996): 403–7; J. S. Fowler et al., Inhibition of MAO B in the brains of smokers, *Nature* 379 (1996): 733–38; J. S. Fowler et al., Brain monoamine oxidase A inhibition in cigarette smokers, *Proceedings of the National Academy Sciences* 93 (1996): 14065–69; J. M. Stapleton et al., Nicotine reduces cerebral glucose utilization in humans, *NIDA Research Monograph* 132 (1993): 106; N. D. Volkow et al., Imaging the living human brain: Magnetic resonance imaging and positron emission tomography, *Proceedings of the National Academy Sciences* 94 (1997): 2787–88.

76 Shapiro, Smoking tobacco.

77 R. Kluger, *Ashes to ashes: America's hundred year cigarette war, the public health, and the unabashed triumph of Phillip Morris* (New York: Knopf, 1996), xiv–xv.

1 Quoted in D. F. Musto, America's first cocaine epidemic, *Wilson Quarterly* 13 (1989): 59–64.

2 See O. Ray, *Drugs, society, and human behavior* (St. Louis: Mosby, 1983); D. Healy, *The antidepressant era* (Cambridge, Mass.: Harvard University Press, 1997).

3 Quoted from an 1821 article in *North American Review* in H. Fingarette, *Heavy drinking* (Berkeley: University of California Press, 1989).

4 Ray, *Drugs, society, and human behavior*, 308.

5 For a general discussion of these issues, see D. Healy, *The creation of psychopharmacology* (Cambridge, Mass.: Harvard University Press, 2002).

6 B. Hodgson, *Opium: A Portrait of the Heavenly Demon* (San Francisco: Chronicle Books, 1999), 3, 5.

7 From the Johns Hopkins University website, http://www.med.jhu.edu.

8 E. M. Brecher et al., *Licit and illicit drugs* (Boston: Little Brown, 1972).

9 W. Penfield, Halsted of Johns Hopkins, *JAMA* 210 (1969): 2214–18.

10 Ibid.

11 Ibid., 2215.

12 E. M. Brecher et al. (1972). *Licit and illicit drugs*. Boston: Little Brown.

13 Osler, quoted in Penfield, Halsted of Johns Hopkins, 2216.

14 Ibid.

15 Brecher et al., *Licit and illicit drugs*, 35.

16 Whatever conclusions are drawn for morphine also apply to heroin, which, although more potent than morphine, is derived from morphine and has essentially identical effects when taken at comparable doses (see C. A. Bassett and R. J. Pawluk, Blood-brain barrier: Penetration of morphine, codeine, heroin and methadone after carotid injections, *Science* 178 [1972]: 984–86; R. B. Haemmig and W. Tschacher, Effects of high-dose heroin versus morphine in intravenous drug users: A randomized double-blind crossover study, *Journal of Psychoactive Drugs* 33 [2001]: 105–10.

17 W. C. Cutting, Morphine addiction for 62 years: A case report, *Stanford Medical Bulletin* 1 (1942): 39.

18 Ibid.

19 Ibid.

20 Ibid., 41.

21 M. Booth, *Opium: A history* (London: Simon and Schuster, 1996), 29.

22 Ibid., 39–40, 48.

23 Brecher et al., *Licit and illicit drugs*, 36. The Anslinger material comes from H. J. Anslinger and W. Oursler, *The murderers* (New York: Farrar, Straus, and Cudahy, 1961).

24 Brecher et al., *Licit and illicit drugs*, 36.

25 Ibid., 37.

26 Ibid.

27 E. J. Morhous, Drug addiction in upper economic levels: A study of 142 cases, *West Virginia Medical Journal* 49 (1953): 189 (cited in Brecher et al., *Licit and illicit drugs*).

28 Morhous quoted in Brecher et al., *Licit and illicit drugs*, 38.

29 T. S. Szasz, *Ceremonial chemistry* (Garden City, N.Y.: Doubleday Anchor, 1974), 85.

30 R. Davenport-Hines, *The pursuit of oblivion* (London: Weidenfeld and Nicolson, 2001), 139.

31 One version of the report is: L. Singh and T. Brassey. *First report of the Royal Commission on Opium with minutes of evidence and appendices* (London: H. M. Stationery Office, 1894–95). The commission was "To report on the effects of prohibition of the growth and sale of opium, except for medical purposes, in British India and whether this could be extended to the Native States."

32 Davenport-Hines, *The pursuit of oblivion*.

33 Ibid., 140.

34 Ibid., 141.

35 Ibid.

36 Ibid., 141.

37 Ibid., 139.

38 N. E. Zinberg and R. C. Jacobson, The natural history of "chipping," *American Journal of Psychiatry* 133 (1976): 37–40.

39 Ibid., 37.

40 Ibid.

41 Ibid., 38.

42 Ibid., 39.

43 W. S. Burroughs, Kicking drugs: A very personal story, *Harper's*, July 1967, 39–42.

44 Brecher et al., *Licit and illicit drugs*, 33.

45 L. N. Robins and G. E. Murphy, Drug use in a normal population of young negro men, *American Journal of Public Health* 57 (1967): 1580–96.

46 I. Chein et al., *The road to H: Narcotics, delinquency, and social policy* (New York: Basic Books, 1964), 159.

47 J. A. O'Donnell, A follow-up of narcotic addicts: Mortality, relapse, and abstinence, *American Journal of Orthopsychiatry* 34 (1964): 948–54; L. Robins, *Deviant children grown up: A sociological and psychiatric study of sociopathic personality* (Baltimore: Williams and Wilkins, 1966); C. Winick, Maturing out of narcotic addiction, *U.S. Bulletin on Narcotics* 14 (1962): 1–7; C. Winick, The life cycle of the narcotic addict and of addiction, *U.S. Bulletin on Narcotics* 16 (1964): 1–11.

48 Winick, The life cycle of the narcotic addict.

49 For a review of these findings, see D. Waldorf, Natural remission from opiate addiction: Some social-psychological processes of untreated recovery, *Journal of Drug Issues* 13 (1983): 237–80.

50 L. N. Robins et al., Narcotic use in Southeast Asia and afterward, *Archives of General Psychiatry* 32 (1980): 955–61.

51 L. N. Robins et al., Drug use by U.S. Army enlisted men in Vietnam: A follow-up on their return home, *American Journal of Epidemiology* 99 (1974): 235–49; Robins et al., Narcotic use in Southeast Asia. See also N. E. Zinberg, Heroin use in Vietnam and the United States: A contrast and critique, *Archives of General Psychiatry* 26 (1972): 486–88.

52 Robins et al., Drug use by U.S. Army enlisted men.

53 D. Waldorf and P. Biernacki, Natural recovery from heroin addiction: A review of the incidence literature, *Journal of Drug Issues* 9 (1979): 281–89.

54 D. N. Nurco, Addict careers: II. The first ten years, *International Journal of the Addictions* 16 (1981): 1327–56.

55 Ibid.

56 Waldorf and Biernacki, Natural recovery from heroin addiction; D. Waldorf and P. Biernacki, The natural remission from opiate addiction: Some preliminary findings. *Journal of Drug Issues* 11 (1981): 61–74; Waldorf, Natural remission from opiate addiction.

57 Waldorf and Biernacki, The natural remission from opiate addiction, 71.

58 S. Peele and R. J. DeGrandpre, Cocaine and the concept of addiction, *Addiction Research* 6 (1998): 235–63.

59 A. R. Lindesmith, A sociological theory of drug addiction, *American Journal of Sociology* 43 (1938): 593–613.

60 A. Lindesmith, *Addiction and opiates* (Chicago: Aldine, 1968), 8.

61 Both scenarios are portrayed in the film *The People vs. Larry Flynt*, the latter of which applies to Larry Flynt and the former to his wife.

62 See Waldorf and Biernacki, The natural remission from opiate addiction.

63 "The critical experience in the fixation process is not the positive euphoria produced by the drug but rather the relief of the pain that invariably appears when a physically dependent person stops using the drug. This experience becomes critical, however, only when an additional indispensable element in the situation is taken into account, namely, a cognitive one. The individual not only must experience relief of withdrawal distress but must understand or conceptualize this experience in a particular way. He must realize that his distress is produced by the interruption of prior regular use of the drug" (Lindesmith, *Addiction and opiates*, 8).

64 For a general discussion of this idea, see R. J. DeGrandpre, A science of meaning, *American Psychologist* 55 (2001): 721–39.

65 P. Laurie, *Drugs: Medical, psychological and social facts* (Baltimore: Penguin, 1967), 13.

66 C. MacAndrew and R. B. Edgerton, *Drunken comportment: A social explanation* (Chicago: Aldine Publishing, 1969).

67 Ibid., 4.

68 A. Weil, *The natural mind* (Boston: Houghton Mifflin, 1972).

69 Report of the Mayor's Committee on Drug Addiction to the Honorable R. C. Patterson, Jr., commissioner of correction, New York City, *American Journal of Psychiatry* 10 (1930–1931): 509.

70 Lindesmith, *Addiction and opiates*, ch. 2.

71 Ibid.

72 Report of the Mayor's Committee on Drug Addiction, 518.

73 Ibid.

74 Lindesmith, *Addiction and opiates*, 37.

75 Ibid. A similar situation took place in India while it was still under British colonial rule, wherein the blind administration of opiates was used to distinguish true pain patients from habitués seeking opiates, and thus demonstrated that the placebo text regarding opiate addiction was not restricted to the West (Psychological aspects of opium addiction, *Indian Medical Gazette*, 1931, 663).

76 D. G. Levine, "Needle freaks": Compulsive self-injection by drug users, *American Journal of Psychiatry* 131 (1974): 297–300.

77 Lindesmith, *Addiction and opiates*, 39.

78 B. J. Primm and P. E. Bath, Pseudoheroinism, *International Journal of the Addictions* 8 (1973): 231–42.

79 J. F. Richards, Indian empire and peasant production of opium in the nineteenth century, *Modern Asia Studies* 15 (1981): 59–82.

80 Ibid.

81 J. F. Richards, Opium and the British Indian empire, *Modern Asia Studies* 36 (2002): 375–420.

82 The idea of opium eating had its origin in de Quincey's *Confessions of an English Opium-eater* and, with the exception of opium smoking (via the opium pipe), came to refer to consumption of the opiates generally, including morphine.

83 Ray, *Drugs, society, and human behavior*.

84 B. A. Hartwell, The sale and use of opium in Massachusetts, *Annual Report of the Massachusetts Board of Health* 22 (1889): 137–58.

85 O. Marshall, The opium habit in Michigan, *Annual Report of the Michigan State Board of Health* 6 (1878): 61–73; L. P. Brown, Enforcement of the Tennessee anti-narcotic law, *American Journal of Public Health* 5 (1914): 323–33.

86 D. F. Musto, *The American disease: Origins of narcotic control* (New York: Oxford University Press, 1987), 5.

87 Quoted in W. F. Crafts et al., *Intoxicating drinks and drugs in all lands and times* (Washington: International Reform Bureau, 1911), 14.

88 Quoted in Ray, *Drugs, society, and human behavior*, 308.

89 Lindesmith, *Addiction and opiates*.

90 D. T. Courtwright, *Dark paradise: Opiate addiction in America before 1940* (Cambridge, Mass.: Harvard University Press, 1982).

91 C. W. Earle, The opium habit: A statistical and clinical lecture, *Chicago Medical Review* 2 (1980): 442–46 (cited in Courtwright, *Dark paradise*).

92 R. L. Swarns, Mayor wants to abolish use of methadone, *New York Times*, 21 July 1998, B1.

93 Musto, *The American disease*.

94 Peele, *The meaning of addiction*, 7.

95 Ray, *Drugs, society, and human behavior*, 151.

96 G. Milner, quoted in ibid., 132.

97 Lindesmith, *Addiction and opiates*, 211.

98 Brecher, *Licit and illicit drugs*, 36.

99 C. J. Acker, *Creating the American junkie: Addiction research in the classic era of narcotic control* (Baltimore: Johns Hopkins University Press, 2002).

100 Courtwright, *Dark paradise*, 3.

101 Ibid., 215.

102 Musto, America's first cocaine epidemic.

103 J. L. Corning, The growing menace of the use of cocaine, *New York Times*, 2 August 1908. See also Negro cocaine fiends, new southern menace, *New York Times*, 11 February 1914.

104 Quoted in Musto, America's first cocaine epidemic.

105 R. Ashley, *Cocaine: Its history, uses and effects* (New York: Warner Books, 1976), 89.

106 J. A. Inciardi, *The war on drugs II* (Mountain View, Calif.: Mayfield, 1992).

107 Quoted in Lindesmith, *Addiction and opiates*, 219.

108 Ibid., 221.

109 L. Sloman, *Reefer madness: The history of marijuana* (New York: St. Martin's, 1979).

110 J. L. Himmelstein, *The strange career of marijuana: Politics and ideology of drug control in America* (Westport, Conn.: Greenwood Press, 1983).

111 Reported from Mexico City, 6 July 1927; quoted in J. A. Inciardi and K. McElrath, *The American drug scene* (Los Angeles: Roxbury Publishing, 1998), 62.

112 Marijuana menaces youth, *Scientific American*, March 1936, 150–51.

113 J. Johnston, *Chemistry of common life* (Edinburgh, U.K.: Blackwood, 1855).

114 Again, Courtwright and others typically cloud the significance of the massive nonaddicted use of opiates in the nineteenth century by claiming local observers were unaware of the genuine nature of addiction and thus missed the large numbers who manifested withdrawal and other addictive symptoms. Courtwright struggles to explain how the commonplace administration of opiates to babies "was unlikely to develop into a full-blown addiction, for the infant would not have comprehended the nature of its withdrawal distress, nor could it have done anything about it" (*Dark paradise*, 58; see also V. Berridge and G. Edward, *Opium and the people: Opiate use in nineteenth-century England* [New York: St. Martin's Press, 1981]).

Chapter Five America's Domestic Drug Affair

1 In another trend the FDA and other government bodies have embraced nicotine as a treatment drug for cigarette smokers, exemplifying what might be called "medical conversions," where, in the name of treatment, white-market drugs are substituted for black-market drugs. By this route NIDA came to work alongside the pharmaceutical industry in developing such "treatment" compounds.

See, for example, P. Zickler, Clinical trials network will speed testing and delivery of new drug abuse therapies, *NIDA Notes* 14 (1999): 1, 4.

2 O. Ray, *Drugs, society, and human behavior* (St. Louis: Mosby, 1983).

3 Cited in C. G. Murdock, *Domesticating drink: Women, men, and alcohol in America, 1870–1940* (Baltimore: Johns Hopkins University Press, 1998).

4 Ray, *Drugs, society, and human behavior*.

5 Read P. Starr, *The social transformation of American medicine* (New York: Basic, 1982).

6 Ibid.

7 T. R. Pegram, *Battling demon rum* (Chicago: Ivan R. Dee, 1998).

8 Ibid.

9 Cited in Murdock, *Domesticating drink*, 82.

10 A. Sinclair, *Era of excess: A social history of the prohibition movement* (New York: Harper-Colophon, 1964).

11 R. A. Campbell, *Demon rum or easy money* (Ottawa: Carleton University Press, 1991).

12 Quoted in Campbell, *Demon rum or easy money*, 24–25.

13 C. E. Terry and M. Pellens, *The opium problem* (New York: Bureau of Social Hygiene, 1928), 962–63.

14 From S. H. Snyder, *Drugs and the brain* (New York: Scientific American, 1996).

15 K. K. Chen et al., A comparative study of synthetic and natural ephedrines, *Journal of Pharmacology and Experimental Therapeutics* 33 (1928): 237–58.

16 M. Joseph, *Speed* (London: Carlton Books, 2000).

17 Ibid.

18 Ibid.

19 Ibid.

20 On a bender with Benzedrine, *Everybody's Digest* 5 (1946): 50.

21 Joseph, *Speed*, 24.

22 Although amphetamine was first brought to market as a nasal decongestant, the amphetamines became such popular angels for the same reason as cocaine had half a century earlier. Amphetamines and cocaine are identical neither in their chemical structures nor in their mechanisms of action in the dopamine centers of the brain, but the immediate psychoactive effects of these drugs can rarely be differentiated even by experienced users under blind conditions.

23 Joseph, *Speed*.

24 Quoted in Ray, *Drugs, society, and human behavior*, 304.

25 Methamphetamine fact sheet; see www.chestnut.org.

26 For one of the earliest examinations of this issue, see H. Isbeel, The newer analgesic drugs: Their use and abuse, *Annals of Internal Medicine* 29 (1948): 1003–12.

27 D. Blair, *Modern drugs for the treatment of mental illness* (London: Staples Press, 1963), 105.

28 J. Parker, *Tranx: Minor Tranquilizers, Major Problems* (Tempe, Ariz.: Do It Now Foundation, 2000), 5.

29 For a review and related findings, see F. M. Berger, Anxiety and the discovery of the tranquilizers, in *Discoveries in biological psychiatry*, edited by F. J. Ayd and B. Blackwell (Philadelphia: Lippincott, 1970), 142–54.

30 Ibid.

31 D. Healy, *The creation of psychopharmacology* (Cambridge, Mass.: Harvard University Press, 2001).

32 Ibid., 99.

33 From Wallace Laboratories, Physical reference manual, in *Miltown: The tranquilizer with muscle relaxant action*, 4th ed. (New Brunswick, N.J.: Wallace Laboratories, 1960), 6.

34 Ibid., 51.

35 E. J. Morhous, Drug addiction in upper economic levels: A study of 142 cases, *West Virginia Medical Journal* 49 (1953): 189.

36 J. A. Ewing and T. M. Haizlip, A controlled study of the habit forming propensities of meprobamate, *American Journal of Psychiatry* 114 (1958): 835.

37 O. Ray (1983). *Drugs, society, and human behavior*. St. Louis: Mosby.

38 B. Jackson, "White-collar pill party," *Atlantic*, August 1966, 36–37.

39 See Ray, *Drugs, society, and human behavior*, chap. 14.

40 Blair, *Modern drugs for the treatment of mental illness*, 105.

41 Ray, *Drugs, society, and human behavior*, 288.

42 In January 1880 the *Quarterly Journal of Inebriety* noted:

> The persons who become habituated to chloral hydrate are of two or three classes, as a rule. Some have originally taken the narcotic to relieve pain, using it in the earliest application of it for a true medicinal and legitimate object, probably under medical direction. Finding that it gave relief and repose, they have continued the use of it, and at last have got so abnormally under its influence that they cannot get to sleep if they fail to resort to it.
>
> A second class of persons who take to chloral are alcoholic inebriates who have arrived at that stage of alcoholism when sleep is always disturbed, and often near impossible. These persons at first wake many times in the night with coldness of the lower limbs, cold sweatings, startings, and restless dreamings. In a little time they become nervous about submitting themselves to sleep, and before long habituate themselves to watchfulness and restlessness, until a confirmed insomnia is the result. Worn out with sleeplessness, and failing to find any relief that is satisfactory or safe in their false friend alcohol, they turn to chloral, and in it find for a season the oblivion which they desire and which they call rest. It is a kind of rest, and is no doubt better than no rest at all , but it leads to the unhealthy states that we are now conversant with, and it rather promotes than destroys the craving for alcohol. In short, the man who takes to chloral after alcohol enlists two cravings for a single craving, and is double-shotted in the worst sense.
>
> A third class of men who became habituated to the use of chloral are men of extremely nervous and excitable temperament, who by nature, and often by the labors in which they are occupied, become bad sleepers. A little thing in the course of their

daily routine oppresses them. What to other men is passing annoyance, thrown off with the next step, is to these men a worry and anxiety of hours. They are over-susceptible of what is said of them, and of their work, however good their work may be. They are too elated when praised, and too depressed when not praised or dispraised. They fail to play character-parts on the stage of this world, and as they lie down to rest they take all their cares and anxieties into bed with them, in the liveliest state of perturbation. Unable in this condition to sleep, and not knowing a more natural remedy, they resort to the use of such an instrument as chloral hydrate. They begin with a moderate dose, increase the dose as occasion seems to demand, and at last, in what they consider a safe and moderate system of employing it, they depend on the narcotic for their falsified repose. (Abuse of chloral hydrate, *Quarterly Journal of Inebriety* 4 [1880]: 53–54)

43 Ibid.
44 E. M. Brecher et al., *Licit and illicit drugs* (Boston: Little, Brown, 1972), 249.
45 H. Isbell, Chronic barbiturate intoxication, AMA *Archives of Neurology and Psychiatry* 64 (1950): 8.
46 The subjects were in fact volunteers, although they volunteered within a prison-type setting.
47 Brecher et al., *Licit and illicit drugs*.
48 A. Tatum, *Physiological Reviews* 19 (1939): 472–502.
49 D. R. Wesson and D. E. Smith, *Barbiturates: Their use, misuse, and abuse* (New York: Human Sciences Press, 1977), 15.
50 From R. King, *The drug hang-up: America's fifty year folly* (Springfield, Ill.: Charles C. Thomas, 1972).
51 Ibid.; quoted in T. S. Szasz, *Ceremonial chemistry* (Garden City, N.Y.: Anchor Books, 1974).
52 Federal study links sleeping pills to 5,000 deaths yearly in the US, *New York Times*, 28 November 1977.
53 M. Nyswander, *The drug addict as a patient* (New York: Grune and Stratton, 1956), 34; the quote given by Nyswander is from A. Wikler, *Drug addiction* (Hagerstown, W.V.: W. F. Prior, 1953).
54 W. S. Burroughs, *Naked lunch* (1959; London: Harper, 2005), 225.
55 From a summary of barbiturates at http://www.drugscope.org.uk.
56 Wesson and Smith, *Barbiturates*, 15.
57 See Brecher et al., *Licit and illicit drugs*, chap. 30.
58 From King, *The drug hang-up*.
59 E. Brecher et al., *Licit and illicit drugs*, 254.
60 S. Cohen, statement before the Subcommittee to Investigate Juvenile Delinquency, U.S. Senate Committee on the Judiciary on Drug Abuse, 15 December 1971.
61 See, for example, M. C. Cumberlidge, The abuse of barbiturates by heroin addicts, *Canadian Medical Association Journal* 98 (1968): 1045–49; E. Hamburger, Barbiturate use in narcotic addicts, *JAMA* 189 (1964): 366–68.

62 This claim is made by the FDA on its website, http://www.fda.gov.

63 Ray, *Drugs, society, and human behavior*, 313.

64 D. Zwerdling, Methaqualone: The "safe" drug that isn't very, *Washington Post*, 12 November 1972, B3.

65 The Quaalude scam, *Newsweek*, 28 September 1981, 93.

66 From the FDA website, http://www.fda.gov.

67 In 1973, with officials becoming aware of its similarities to barbiturates, methaqualone was reclassified as a Schedule II drug, that is, as having medical use but also a high potential for abuse.

68 Jackson, "White-collar pill party," 37.

69 L. Sternbach, The benzodiazepine story, *Journal of Medicinal Chemistry* 22 (1979).

70 On the latter possibility, see M. C. Smith, *Small comfort: A history of the minor tranquilizers* (New York: Praeger, 1985).

71 D. Ramchandani, *The librium story*, 2002, http://www.benzo.org.uk.

72 See, for example, L. Randell et al., The psychosedative properties of methaminodiazepoxide, *Journal of Pharmacology and Experimental Therapeutics* 129 (1960): 163–71; L. Randell (1961). Pharmacology of chlordiazepoxide (Librium), *Diseases of the Nervous System* 22 (1961): 7–15.

73 Dallek, *An unfinished life*.

74 D. Healy, *The antidepressant era* (Cambridge: Harvard University Press, 1997), 226.

Chapter Six **War**

1 E. Nieves, Drug labs in Valley hideouts feed nation's habit, *New York Times*, 3 May 2001.

2 See D. Gardner, When the damage is done, *Ottawa Citizen*, 27 July 2003, C3.

3 An exception has been made for gray-market drugs like alcohol; another exception to the hegemony of pharmacologicalism is the limited medical use of certain demon drugs, which consists mainly of acknowledging that some substances believed to have nefarious qualities may have limited use under very circumscribed conditions (e.g., morphine, meperidine, and methylphenidate). In terms of the formal DEA drug scheduling, such drugs are identified as Schedule II drugs.

4 The last words written on behalf of the therapeutic state in the twentieth century were penned by U.S. Surgeon General David Satcher in a report issued on mental health in America, *Mental health: A report of the Surgeon General* (Rockville, Md.: U.S. Department of Health and Human Services, 1999). For criticism of the report, see R. J. DeGrandpre, Surgeon General report laudable but misleading, *Los Angeles Times*, 20 December 1999; T. Szasz, Mental disorders are not diseases, *USA Today*, 20 January 2000. Regarding the rise of the prohibitionist state, the annual costs at the end of the century were estimated to be $18 billion, with the cost of "drug abuse" in society estimated at approximately $100 billion in 1992 (see J. W. Shenk, America's altered states: When does legal relief

of pain become illegal pursuit of pleasure? *Harper's*, May 1999, 38–52; G. Boyd and J. Hitt, This is your Bill of Rights on drugs, *Harper's*, December 1999, 57–61; N. Swan, Drug abuse costs to society set at $97.7 billion, continuing steady increase since 1975, *NIDA Notes* 13 [1998]: 1, 12). Remarking on the growing costs of the war on drugs in 1973, Michael R. Sonnenrich, executive director of the *National Commission on Marijuana and Drug Abuse*, noted, "The budget estimates that have been submitted indicate that we will exceed the $1 billion mark. When we do so, we become, for want of a better term, a drug abuse industrial complex" (quoted in T. S. Szasz, *Ceremonial chemistry* [New York: Anchor, 1974]).

5 On this, see E. Schlosser, Marijuana and the law, *Atlantic Monthly*, September 1994, 84–94; L. Wacquant, L'emprisonement des "classes dangereuses" aux États-Unis, *Le Monde Diplomatique*, July 1998, 20–21. See also D. S. Bell, The irrelevance of research to government policies on drugs, *Drug and Alcohol Dependence* 25 (1990): 221–24.

6 W. Chambliss, Clinton just says "no": Don't confuse me with the facts, *New Left Review* 204 (May 1994). See also E. Currie, *Reckoning: Drugs, the cities, and the American future* (New York: Hill and Wang, 1993).

Chapter Seven **The Drug Reward**

1 J. Olds and P. Milner, Positive reinforcement produced by electrical stimulation of septal area and other regions of rat brain, *Journal of Comparative and Physiological Psychology* 47 (1954): 419–27.

2 J. Olds, Pleasure centers in the brain, *Scientific American* (October 1956): 107–8.

3 A. Wauquier and E. T. Rolls, eds., *Brain-stimulation reward* (Amsterdam: Elsevier, 1976).

4 See, for example, J. Olds and T. Hirano, Conditioned responses of hippocampal and other neurons, *Electroencephalography and Clinical Neurophysiology* 2 (1969): 159–66J; Olds et al., Single unit patterns during anticipatory behavior, *Electroencephalography and Clinical Neurophysiology* 26 (1969): 144–58.

5 E. S. Valenstein and B. Beer, Continuous opportunity for reinforcing brain stimulation, *Journal of the Experimental Analysis of Behavior* 7 (1964): 183–84.

6 For example, see A. Routtenberg and J. Lindy, Effects of the availability of rewarding septal and hypothalamic stimulation on bar pressing for food under conditions of deprivation, *Journal of Comparative and Physiological Psychology* 60 (1965): 158–61.

7 For example, see R. G. Heath, Pleasure response of human subjects to direct stimulation of the brain: Physiologic and psychodynamic considerations, in *The role of pleasure in human behavior*, edited by R. G. Heath (New York: Hoeber, 1964), 219–43. See also Wauquier and Rolls, *Brain-stimulation reward*.

8 Writing on the subject by the physiological psychologist Sebastian Grossman can be found at http://www.wireheading.com.

9 C. W. Sem-Jacobsen, Electrical stimulation and self-stimulation in man with chronic implanted electrodes: Interpretation and pitfalls of results, in *Brain-stimulation reward*, edited by A. Wauquier and E. T. Rolls (Amsterdam: Elsevier, 1976), 505–26. See also J. Delgado, *Physical control of the mind: Toward a psychocivilized society* (New York: Harper and Row, 1969); C. W. Sem-Jacobsen, *Depth electrographic studies of the human brain and behavior* (Springfield, Mo.: Thomas Publishers, 1968).

10 A. I. Leshner, Addiction is a brain disease, *National Institute of Justice Journal* (1998): 4. See also A. I. Leshner, Addiction is a brain disease, and it matters, *Science* 278 (1997): 45–47. A similar view was also taken by Steven Hyman when he was serving as director of the National Institute of Mental Health: "Repeated doses of addictive drugs—opiates, cocaine, and amphetamine—cause drug dependence and, afterward, withdrawal" (Shaking out the cause of addiction, *Science* 273 [1996]: 611–12).

11 See J. Olds, Hypothalamic substrates of reward, *Physiological Review* 42 (1962): 554–604; M. E. Olds and J. Olds, Approach avoidance analysis of rat diencephalons, *Journal of Comparative Neurology* 120 (1963): 259–95; R. H. Wurtz and J. Olds, Amygdaloid stimulation and operant reinforcement in the rat, *Journal of Comparative Physiological Psychology* 56 (1963): 941–49; R. H. Ursin and J. Olds, Self-stimulation of hippocampus in rats, *Journal of Comparative Physiological Psychology* 61 (1966): 353–59.

12 For example, see M. Wolske, Activation of single neurons in the rat nucleus accumbens during self-stimulation of the ventral tegmental area, *Journal of Neuroscience* 13 (1993): 1–12.

13 C. R. Gallistel et al., A portrait of the substrate for self-stimulation, *Psychological Review* 108 (1981): 228–73; L. J. Porrino et al., The distribution of changes in local cerebral energy metabolism associated with brain stimulation reward to the medial forebrain bundle of the rat, *Brain Research* 511 (1990): 1–6; E. Yadin et al., Unilaterally activated systems in rats self-stimulating at sites in the medial forebrain bundle, medial prefrontal cortex, or locus coeruleus, *Brain Research* 266 (1983): 39–50.

14 See E. S. Valenstein, The anatomical locus of reinforcement, in *Progress in physiological psychology*, edited by E. Stellar and J. Sprague (New York: Academic Press, 1966), 1:149–90.

15 L. Stein, Secondary reinforcement established with subcortical stimulation, *Science* 127 (1958): 466–67; L. Stein, Norepinephrine reward pathways: Role in self-stimulation, memory consolidation and schizophrenia, in *Nebraska symposium on motivation*, vol. 22, edited by J. K. Cole and T. B. Sonderegger (Lincoln: University of Nebraska Press, 1974); L. Stein, Reward transmitters: Catecholamines and opioid peptides, in *Psychopharmacology: A generation of progress*, edited by A. Lipton et al. (New York: Raven Press, 1978), 569–81.

16 R. A. Wise and P-P. Rompré, Brain dopamine and reward, *Annual Review of Psychology* 40 (1989): 191–225.

17 R. A. Frank, Cocaine euphoria, dysphoria, and tolerance assessed using drug-

induced changes in brain-stimulation reward, *Pharmacology, Biochemistry, and Behavior* 42 (1992): 771–79; R. A. Wise, Action of drugs of abuse on brain reward systems, *Pharmacology, Biochemistry, and Behavior* 13 (1980): 213–23.

18 See http://www.wireheading.com.

19 S. S. Steiner et al., Escape from self-produced rates of brain stimulation, *Science* 163 (1969): 90–91.

20 L. J. Porrino et al., Metabolic mapping of the brain during rewarding self-stimulation, *Science* 224 (1984): 306–9.

21 S. I. Dworkin et al., Response-dependent versus response-independent presentation of cocaine: Differences in the lethal effects of the drug, *Psychopharmacology* 117 (1995): 262–66.

22 Ibid., 262.

23 A similar study investigated a sedative-hypnotic drug (midazolam, a benzodiazepine), although rather than testing the toxicity of the drug, the researchers tested the ability of the animals to detect the stimulus effects of the drug after they had experienced it earlier, either voluntarily or involuntarily. (Just as an experienced barbiturate user might be able to detect the effects of a dose of a barbiturate from placebo, so animals can discriminate the stimulus effects of one drug from another; in fact, laboratory mammals are generally better than humans at drug discrimination.) The study showed that animals with a history of self-administering the drug were significantly better discriminators than were animals given the history of involuntary drug administration. Again, such differences did not correlate with differences in drug exposure, since the animals in the two groups were given the same exposure. However, they did correlate with a nonpharmacological variable, namely, whether drug administration was contingent or noncontingent on responding (N. A. Ator and R. R. Griffiths, Differential sensitivity to midazolam discriminative-stimulus effects following self-administration versus responses-independent midazolam, *Psychopharmacology* 110 [1992]: 1–4).

24 J. E. Smith and S. I. Dworkin, Behavioral contingencies determine changes in drug-induced neurotransmitter turnover, *Drug Development Research* 20 (1990): 337–48.

25 GABA is an amino acid that acts as a neurotransmitter in the brain.

26 Leshner, Addiction is a brain disease, 4.

27 Leshner, Addiction is a brain disease, and it matters, 45.

28 See K. Blue et al., Reward deficiency syndrome, *American Scientist* 84 (March–April 1996): 132–45.

29 Hyman, Shaking out the cause of addiction.

30 For a similar discussion regarding antipsychotic drugs, often administered involuntarily (and thus outside the purview of this book), see R. Bentall, *Madness explained: Psychosis and human nature* (Allen Lane: London, 2003).

31 S. Boseley, Murder, suicide: A bitter aftertaste for the "wonder" depression drug, *Guardian*, 11 June 2001.

32 Other complexities also bedevil the dopamine hypothesis of addiction. First, dopamine antagonists (neuroleptics) have been shown to antagonize the self-

administration of cocaine in animals, suggesting that the reinforcing effects of cocaine may in fact be mediated by dopamine activity; however, drugs that antagonize acetylcholine also have been shown to antagonize the self-administration of both cocaine and morphine (see M. C. Wilson et al., Cholinergic influence on intravenous cocaine self-administration by rhesus monkeys, *Pharmacology, Biochemistry, and Behavior* 1 [1972]: 643–49; W. M. Davis and S. G. Smith, Central cholinergic influence on self-administration of morphine and amphetamine, *Life Sciences* 16 [1975]: 237–46). Similarly, drugs that block receptors activated by norepinephrine have been shown to affect animal self-administration of both cocaine and morphine (see W. M. Davis et al., Noradrenergic role in the self-administration of morphine and amphetamine, *Pharmacology, Biochemistry, and Behavior* 3 [1975]: 477–84; S. R. Goldberg and F. A. Gonzalez, The effects of propranolol on behavior maintained under fixed-ratio schedules of cocaine injection or food presentation in squirrel monkeys, *Journal of Pharmacology and Experimental Therapeutics* 198 [1976]: 626–34). Once again, from the view of behavioral neuroscience, the involvement of biochemistry in psychological problems is more complex than typically assumed.

33 M. J. Burton et al., Effects of hunger on the responses of neurons in the lateral hypothalamus to the sight and taste of food, *Experimental Neurology* 51 (1976): 668–77.

34 Bill Moyers interview with Alan Leshner on PBS, Close to home, 1998, www.pbs.org.

35 P. B. Dews, Studies on behavior: I. Differential sensitivity to pentobarbital of pecking performance in pigeons depending on the schedule of reward, *Journal of Pharmacology and Experimental Therapeutics* 138 (1955): 393–401.

36 J. E. Barrett, Reflections: The emergence of behavioral pharmacology, *Molecular Interventions* 2 (2002): 470–75; see http://molinterv.aspetjournals.org/.

37 Dews, Studies on behavior; P. B. Dews, Stimulant actions of methamphetamine, *Journal of Pharmacology and Experimental Therapeutics* 122 (1958): 137–47.

38 See also W. H. Morse, An analysis of responding in the presence of a stimulus correlated with periods of non-reinforcement, Ph.D. diss., Harvard University, 1955.

39 P. B. Dews, Stimulant actions of methamphetamine, *Journal of Pharmacology and Experimental Therapeutics* 122 (1958): 137–47.

40 Barrett, Reflections: The emergence of behavioral pharmacology, http://molinterv.aspetjournals.org/.

41 Ibid.

42 G. Sedvall, Monoamines and schizophrenia, supplement to *Acta Psychiatrica Scandinavica* 82 (1990): 7–13.

43 The original report is J. Delay and P. Deniker, Le traitement des psychoses par une methode neurolytique derivée d'hibernothéraphie: Le 4560 RP utilisée seul une cure prolongée et continuée, *Comptes Rendus Congès des Médecins Aliénistes et Neurologistes de France et des Pays de Langue Française* 50 (1952): 497–502.

44 I. Cresse et al., Dopamine receptor binding predicts clinical and pharmacological potencies of antischizophrenic drugs, *Science* 192 (1976): 481–83.

45 J. D. Griffith, Dextroamphetamine: Evaluation of psychotomimetic properties in man, *Archives of General Psychiatry* 26 (1972): 97–100.

46 It is now known, furthermore, that later antipsychotic drugs (e.g., risperidone) act not only on different dopamine receptors than the earlier drugs but also on other neurotransmitter systems (e.g., serotonin).

47 A. Khan, How do psychotropic medications really work? *Psychiatric Times*, October 1999, 11.

48 See W. H. Morse and R. T. Kelleher, Schedules as fundamental determinants of behavior, in *The theory of reinforcement schedules*, edited by W. N. Schoenfeld (New York: Appleton-Century-Crofts, 1970), 43–61; W. H. Morse and R. T. Kelleher, Determinants of reinforcement and punishment, in *Handbook of operant behavior*, edited by W. K. Honig and J. E. R. Staddon (New York: Prentice Hall, 1977), 174–200; W. H. Morse et al., Control of behavior by noxious stimuli, in *Handbook of psychopharmacology*, edited by L. L. Iverson et al. (New York: Plenum Press, 1977), 7:151–80.

49 Morse and Kelleher, Schedules as fundamental determinants of behavior.

50 Interview with C. R. Schuster by Robert Balster, conducted at the NIDA for the Division 28 (American Psychological Association) Oral History Project, 16 August, 1991. Very early papers coauthored by Seevers include A. L. Tatum and M. H. Seevers, Theories of drug addiction, *Psychological Review* 11 (1929): 447–75; A. L. Tatum et al., Morphine addiction and its physiological interpretation based on experimental evidence, *Journal of Pharmacology and Experimental Therapeutics* 36 (1929): 401–10.

51 M. H. Seevers, Opiate addiction in the monkey: I. Methods of study, *Journal of Pharmacology and Experimental Therapeutics* 56 (1936): 147–56.

52 Interview with C. R. Schuster by Robert Balster, conducted at NIDA for the Division 28 (American Psychological Association) Oral History Project, 16 August 1991.

53 Ibid.

54 G. A. Deneau et al., Self-administration of psychoactive drugs by the monkey: A measure of psychological dependence, *Psychopharmacologia* 16 (1969): 30–48.

55 C. R. Schuster and C. E. Johanson, The use of animal models for the study of drug abuse, in *Research advances in alcohol and drug problems*, edited by R. J. Gibbins et al. (New York: John Wiley and Sons, 1974), 1–31; C. R. Schuster and T. Thompson, Self-administration of and behavioral dependence on drugs, *Annual Review of Pharmacology* 9 (1969): 483–502.

56 S. R. Goldberg, Comparable behavior maintained under fixed ratio and second order schedules of food presentation, cocaine injection or d-amphetamine injection in the squirrel monkey, *Journal of Pharmacology and Experimental Therapeutics* 186 (1973): 18–30. See also, S. R. Goldberg (1976). The behavioral analysis of drug addiction, in *Behavioral pharmacology*, edited by S. D. Glick and J. Goldfarb (St. Louis: C. V. Mosby, 1976), 283–316.

57 C. E. Johanson and W. M. Fischman, The pharmacology of cocaine related to its abuse, *Pharmacological Reviews* 41 (1989): 24.

58 A. Goldstein, Heroin addiction: Sequential treatment employing pharmacological supports, *Archives of General Psychiatry* 33 (1976): 353–58.

59 Also reinforcing this view at the time was the Vietnam experience: while drug use among American soldiers was rampant in Vietnam, in part because of the absence of "countervailing influences in human society," the fact that it did not continue afterward, when soldiers returned home, suggested that drug-seeking behavior was not an abnormal response (see L. N. Robins et al., Narcotic use in Southeast Asia and afterward: An interview study of 898 Vietnam returnees, *Archives of General Psychiatry* 32 [1975]: 955–61).

60 See S. Dworkin et al., The effects of 12-hour limited access to cocaine: Reduction in drug intake and mortality, *Problems of drug dependence*, edited by L. S. Harris (Washington: U.S. Government Printing Office, 1986), 221–25.

61 T. E. Fitch and D. C. S. Roberts, The effects of dose and access on the periodicity of cocaine self-administration in the rat, *Drug and Alcohol Dependence* 33 (1993): 119–28.

62 M. E. Carroll, Concurrent phencyclidine and saccharin access: Presentation of an alternative reinforcer reduces drug intake, *Journal of the Experimental Analysis of Behavior* 43 (1985): 131–44.

63 Quoted in J. P. Morgan and L. Zimmer, Animal studies of self-administration of cocaine: Misinterpretation, misrepresentation and invalid extrapolation to human cocaine use, in *New public health policies and programs for the reduction of drug related harm*, edited by P. Erickson et al. (Toronto: University of Toronto Press, 1997), 265–89.

64 Carroll, Concurrent phencyclidine and saccharin access.

65 M. A. Nader and W. L. Woolverton, Effects of increasing the magnitude of an alternative reinforcer on drug choice in a discrete-trial choice procedure, *Psychopharmacology* 105 (1991): 169–74; M. A. Nader and W. L. Woolverton, Effects of increasing response requirement on choice between cocaine and food in rhesus monkeys, *Psychopharmacology* 108 (1992): 295–300. See also M. A. Nader and W. L. Woolverton, Choice between cocaine and food by rhesus monkeys: Effects of conditions of food availability, *Behavioural Pharmacology* 3 (1992): 635–38; W. L. Woolverton, Determinants of cocaine self-administration by laboratory animals, in *Cocaine: Scientific and social dimensions*, edited by G. R. Bock and J. Whelan (West Sussex: Wiley, 1992), 149–64.

66 D. Morgan et al., Social dominance in monkeys: Dopamine D2 receptors and cocaine self-administration, *Nature Neuroscience* 5 (2002): 169–74.

67 Michael Nader, interviewed in Low rank monkeys more prone to cocaine addiction, *New Scientist*, 20 January 2002.

68 M. E. Carroll et al., A concurrently available nondrug reinforcer prevents the acquisition or decreases the maintenance of cocaine-reinforced behavior, *Psychopharmacology* 97 (1989): 23–29; M. E. Carroll and S. T. Lac, Autoshaping I.V. cocaine self-administration in rats: Effects of nondrug alternative reinforcers on acquisition, *Psychopharmacology* 110 (1993): 5–12. See also M. E. Carroll, The economic context of drug and non-drug reinforcers affects acquisition and

maintenance of drug-reinforced behavior and withdrawal effects, *Drug and Alcohol Dependence* 33 (1993): 201–10.

69 For more on the relationship between the role of conditioning in the making of meaning, see R. J. DeGrandpre, A science of meaning, *American Psychologist* 55 (2001): 721–39.

70 D. G. Levine, "Needle freaks": Compulsive self-injection by drug users, *American Journal of Psychiatry* 131 (1974): 297–300.

71 R. T. Kelleher, Chaining and conditioned reinforcement, in *Operant behavior: Areas of research and application*, edited by W. K. Honig (New York: Appleton-Century-Crofts, 1966), 160–212.

72 See S. R. Goldberg et al., Second-order schedules of drug injection, *Federation Proceedings* 34 (1975): 1771–76; S. R. Goldberg et al., Behavior maintained under a second-order schedule by intramuscular injection of morphine or cocaine in rhesus monkeys, *Journal of Pharmacology and Experimental Therapeutics* 199 (1976): 278–86; J. L. Katz, Second-order schedules of intramuscular cocaine injection in the squirrel monkey: Comparisons with food presentation and effects of d-amphetamine and promazine, *Journal of Pharmacology and Experimental Therapeutics* 212 (19880): 405–11.

73 Barrett, Reflections: The emergence of behavioral pharmacology, http://molinterv.aspetjournals.org/.

74 B. J. Primm and P. E. Bath, Pseudoheroinism, *International Journal of the Addictions* 8 (1973): 231–42. See also S. Peele, Hype overdose, *National Review*, 7 November 1994.

75 J. L. Falk, The discriminative stimulus and its reputation: Role in the instigation of drug abuse, *Experimental and Clinical Psychopharmacology* 2 (1994): 43–52. See also J. L. Falk and C. E. Lau, Establishing preference for oral cocaine without an associative history with a reinforcer, *Drug and Alcohol Dependence* 46 (1997): 159–66.

76 Falk, The discriminative stimulus and its reputation.

77 Ibid., 48.

78 L. Park and L. Covi, Nonblind placebo trial, *Archives of General Psychiatry* 12 (1965): 336–45. The study reported that "all 14 completers [of the 15 who started] were improved, the average initial patient score per item of 1.78, approximately 'quite a bit,' reducing by 0.77 (43%) to an average post-treatment score of 1.01, 'just a little'" (338).

79 S. Siegel, Drug anticipation and drug tolerance, *The psychopharmacology of addiction*, edited by M. Lader (Oxford: Oxford University Press, 1988), 73–96.

80 For example, see H. F. Fraser et al., Methods for evaluating addiction liability: (A) "Attitude" of opiate addicts toward opiate-like drugs, (B) A short-term "direct" addiction test, *Journal of Pharmacology and Experimental Therapeutics* 133 (1961): 371–87.

81 T. R. Kosten, The Lexington narcotic farm, *American Journal of Psychiatry* 159 (2002): 22.

82 Ibid.

83 Joseph Brady and colleagues also created a naturalistic setting for observing drug use by building "programmed residential environments" (see H. H. Emurian, The effects of a cooperation contingency on behavior in a continuous three-person environment, *Journal of the Experimental Analysis of Behavior* 25 [1976]: 293–302).

84 J. H. Mendelson and N. Mello, Experimental analysis of drinking behavior of chronic alcoholics, *Annals of the New York Academy of Sciences* 133 (1966): 828–44. See also G. Bigelow and I. Liebson, Cost factors controlling alcoholic drinking, *Psychological Record* 22 (1972): 305–14; G. Bigelow et al., Effects of response requirement upon human sedative self-administration and drug seeking behavior, *Pharmacology, Biochemistry, and Behavior* 5 (1976): 681–85; I. A. Liebson et al., The token economy as a research method in alcoholism, *Psychiatric Quarterly* 45 (1971): 574.

85 R. R. Griffiths et al., Human drug self-administration: Double-blind comparison of pentobarbital, diazepam, chlorpromazine and placebo, *Journal of Pharmacology and Experimental Therapeutics* 210 (1979): 301–10.

86 Bigelow et al., Effects of response requirement.

87 H. Fingarette, *Heavy drinking* (Berkeley: University of California Press, 1988), 36.

Chapter Eight **Possessed by the Stimulus**

1 William James, *Principles of psychology* (New York: Holt, 1890).

2 H. S. Becker, Becoming a marihuana user, *American Journal of Sociology* 59 (1953): 235–42.

3 H. S. Becker, *The outsiders* (New York: Free Press, 1963), 48–49.

4 M. L. Hirsch et al., The use of marijuana for pleasure: A replication of Howard S. Becker's study of marijuana use, in *Handbook of replication research* (Corte Madera, Calif.: Select Press, 1990).

5 P. Laurie, *Drugs: Medical, psychological and social facts* (Baltimore: Penguin, 1967), 99.

6 See A. Weil, *The natural mind* (Boston: Houghton Mifflin, 1972).

7 I. Chein et al., *Narcotics, delinquency and social policy* (London: Tavistock, 1964) (cited in P. Laurie, *Drugs: Medical, psychological and social facts* [Baltimore: Penguin, 1967], 20).

8 A. Lindesmith, *Addiction and opiates* (Chicago: Aldine Publishing, 1968), 8.

9 T. S. Szasz, *Ceremonial chemistry* (Garden City, N.Y.: Anchor Press, 1974), 52–53.

10 D. Healy, *Let them eat Prozac: The unhealthy relationship between the pharmaceutical industry and depression* (New York: New York University Press, 2004).

11 K. Schulz, Did antidepressants depress Japan? *New York Times Magazine*, 22 August 2004, 39–41.

12 Ibid.

13 Ibid.

14 M. H. Teicher et al., Emergence of intense suicidal preoccupation during fluoxetine treatment, *American Journal of Psychiatry* 147 (1990): 207–10.

15 C. MacAndrew and R. B. Edgerton, *Drunken comportment: A social explanation*
(Chicago: Aldine Publishing, 1969), 4.

16 Szasz, *Ceremonial chemistry*, 11.

17 D. V. Gauvin and F. A. Holloway, Cross-generalization between an ecologically-
relevant stimulus and a pentylenetetrazole-discriminative cue, *Pharmacology,
Biochemistry, and Behavior* 39 (1991): 521–23.

18 C-S. Chen, A study of the alcohol-tolerance effect and an introduction of a new
behavioral technique, *Psychopharmacologia* 12 (1968): 433–40.

19 R. J. Carey, Disruption of timing behavior following amphetamine withdrawal,
Physiological Psychology 1 (1973): 9–12.

20 C. R. Schuster et al., Behavioral variables affecting the development of amphetamine tolerance, *Psychopharmacologia* 9 (1966): 170–82.

21 Ibid. See also C. R. Schuster, Timing behavior during prolonged treatment
with dl-amphetamine, *Journal of the Experimental Analysis of Behavior* 4 (1961):
327–30.

22 Schuster et al., Behavioral variables, 177, 181.

23 S. Siegel, Tolerance to the hyperthermic effect of morphine in the rat is a learned
response, *Journal of Comparative and Physiological Psychology* 92 (1978): 1137–49.
See also H. Kalant, Tolerance and its significance for drug and alcohol dependence, in *Problems of drug dependence*, edited by L. S. Harris (Washington: U.S.
Government Printing Office, 1987), 9–19; D. L. Wolgin, The role of instrumental learning in behavioral tolerance to drugs, in *Psychoactive drugs: Tolerance
and sensitization*, edited by A. J. Goudie and M. Emmett-Oglesby (Clifton, N.J.:
Humana Press, 1989), 12–16.

24 S. Siegel, Heroin "overdose" death: Contribution of drug-associated environmental cues, *Science* 216 (1992): 436–37.

25 N. B. Eddy et al., Drug dependence: Its significance and characteristics, *Bulletin
of the World Health Organization* 32 (1965): 721–33.

26 Laurie, *Drugs*, 9.

27 S. Cohen, Reinforcement and rapid delivery systems: Understanding adverse
consequence of cocaine, in *Cocaine use in America: Epidemiologic clinical perspectives*, edited by N. J. Kozel and E. H. Adams (Washington: U.S. Government
Printing Office, 1984), 151–53.

28 F. H. Gawin, Cocaine addiction: Psychology and neurophysiology, *Science* 251
(1991): 1580.

29 L. D. Harrison, Cocaine using careers in perspective, *Addiction Research* 2
(1994): 1–20.

30 E. M. Adlaf et al., *Drug use among Ontario adults, 1977–1991* (Toronto: Ontario
Addiction Research Foundation, 1991).

31 R. K. Siegel, Changing patterns of cocaine use, in *Cocaine: Pharmacology, effects,
and treatment of abuse*, edited by J. Grabowski (Rockville, Md.: U.S. Government Printing Office, 1984), 92–110.

32 P. G. Erickson, Prospects of harm reduction for psychostimulants, in *Psychoactive drugs and harm reduction*, edited by N. Heather et al. (London: Whurr, 1993), 184–210; P. G. Erickson, *The steel drug: Cocaine in perspective* (Lexington, Mass.: Lexington Books, 1987). See also C. Reinarman, Pharmacology is not destiny: The contingent character of cocaine abuse and addiction, *Addiction Research* 2 (1994): 21–36.

33 C. R. Schuster et al., Measurement of drug craving during naloxone-precipitated withdrawal in "methadone-maintained" volunteers, *Experimental and Clinical Psychopharmacology* 3 (1995): 424–31. See also P. D. Kanof et al., Clinical characteristics of naloxone-precipitated withdrawal in human opioid-dependent subjects, *Journal of Pharmacology and Experimental Therapeutics* 260 (1992): 355–63.

34 S. M. Mirin et al., Psychopathology and mood during heroin use: Acute vs chronic effects, *Archives of General Psychiatry* 33 (1976): 1503–8. See also T. F. Babor, Behavioral and social effects of heroin self-administration and withdrawal, *Archives of General Psychiatry* 33 (1976): 363–77; R. E. Meyer, A behavioral paradigm for the evaluation of narcotic antagonists, *Archives of General Psychiatry* 33 (1976): 371–77.

35 Schuster et al., Measurement of drug craving, 430.

36 R. W. Fischman et al., Effects of desipramine maintenance on cocaine self-administration in humans, *Journal of Pharmacology and Experimental Therapeutics* 253 (1990): 760–70.

37 See R. W. Foltin et al., Effects of methadone or buprenorphine maintenance on the subjective and reinforcing effects of intravenous cocaine in humans, *Journal of Pharmacology and Experimental Therapeutics* 278 (1996): 1153–64.

38 R. Nemeth-Coslett and J. E. Henningfield, Effects of nicotine chewing gum on cigarette smoking and subject and physiological effects, *Clinical Pharmacology and Experimental Therapeutics* 39 (1986): 625–30.

39 Laurie, *Drugs*, 14.

40 S. Schachter and J. E. Singer, Cognitive, social and physiological determinants of emotional state, *Psychological Review* 69 (1962): 379–99.

41 Ibid., 398.

42 Another report, which appeared in *Science* in 1977, illustrated that stimuli can acquire meaning and that this meaning affects the drug experience. Earlier in the century, researchers and clinicians working with drug users, including cigarette smokers and alcoholics, had begun taking note of how environmental stimuli associated with drug use acquired meanings that, when experienced at some later point — perhaps even years later — resulted in increased drug desire and/or drug use. If environmental stimuli mediate drug tolerance, certainly they could also mediate drug desire. Wikler and colleagues noted in 1974, for example, "Obviously any therapeutic approach, whether it be insight, behaviorally or pharmacologically orientated, that does not recognize the powerful, evocative effects of interoceptive and exteroceptive stimuli . . . and that neglects to provide techniques for modifying the strength of these effects will likely be destined for failure." In the 1977 study the idea that a learned association could affect drug

use was formally tested by pairing a compound stimulus (an intense tone and odour) with drug withdrawal in opiate users (withdrawal was induced via the administration of an opiate antagonist). Although the compound stimulus did not by itself produce the same magnitude of withdrawal as did the administration of the antagonist drug, it did produce withdrawal, including increases in respiration, heart rate, and motor responses, as well as a decrease in skin temperature. Subjects were also asked to report symptoms of withdrawal, and at least half reported tearing, sweating, and running noses. Perhaps most important, subjects were generally incapable of distinguishing between drug-induced withdrawal and withdrawal elicited by the compound stimulus presented alone. (See C. P. O'Brien et al., Conditioned narcotic withdrawal in humans, *Science* 195 [1977]: 1000; A. M. Ludwig et al., The first drink: Psychobiological aspects of craving, *Archives of General Psychiatry* 30 [1974]: 539–47; A. M. Ludwig and A. Wikler, Craving and relapse to drinking, *Quarterly Journal of Studies on Alcohol* 35 [1974]: 108–30.)

43 C. Reinarman and H. G. Levine, The crack attack: Politics and media in America's latest drug scare, in *Images of issues: Typifying contemporary social problems*, edited by J. Best (New York: Aldine de Gruyter, 1989), 115–37.

44 Quoted in D. R. Gordon, Crack in the penal system, *Nation*, 5 December 1995, 704. The commission report mirrored a report on cocaine issued to Congress by the Ford White House a quarter-century earlier: "[cocaine] usually does not result in serious social consequences, such as crime, hospital emergency room admissions or death" (Reinarman and Levine, The crack attack).

Chapter Nine **Ideology**

1 Marihuana menaces youth, *Scientific American*, March 1936, 150.
2 E. Said, *Orientalism* (New York: Vintage, 1979).
3 Ibid., 3.
4 Ibid., 333.
5 That Dutch policies failed is a myth promoted by, among other sources, the White House Office of Drug Control. In fact, the Netherlands has a lower number of addicts per capita than France, Britain, Italy, and Switzerland (see Going Dutch, *Economist*, 15 January 2000, 55–56).
6 M. Foucault, *The history of sexuality: An introduction* (New York: Vintage, 1990).
7 Ibid., 72.

Alexander, B. K. *Peaceful measures: Canada's way out of the "war on drugs."* Toronto: University of Toronto Press, 1990.

Becker, H. S. Becoming a marihuana user. *American Journal of Sociology* 59 (1953): 235–42.

Bentall, R. *Madness explained: Psychosis and human nature*. London: Allen Lane, 2003.

Brecher, E. M., et al. *Licit and illicit drugs*. Boston: Little Brown, 1972.

Burroughs, W. *Naked lunch*. New York: Grove, 1992.

Carroll, M. E., et al. A concurrently available nondrug reinforcer prevents the acquisition or decreases the maintenance of cocaine-reinforced behavior. *Psychopharmacology* 97 (1989): 23–29.

Chein, I., et al. *The road to H*. New York: Basic Books, 1964.

Courtwright, D. T. *Dark paradise: Opiate addiction in America before 1940*. Cambridge, Mass.: Harvard University Press, 1982.

Currie, E. *Reckoning: Drugs, the cities, and the American future*. New York: Hill and Wang, 1993.

Davenport-Hines, R. *The pursuit of oblivion*. London: Weidenfeld and Nicolson, 2001.

DeGrandpre, R. J. Constructing the pharmacological: A century in review. *Capitalism, Nature, Socialism* 30 (2000): 75–104.

———. The impact of socially-constructed knowledge on drug policy. In *Drug policy and human nature: Psychological perspectives on the management, prevention and treatment of illicit drug abuse*, edited by W. K. Bickel and R. J. DeGrandpre, 301–22. New York: Plenum, 1996.

———. The Lilly suicides. *Adbusters* 10 (2002): 39–48.

———. *Ritalin nation: Rapid-fire culture and the transformation of human consciousness*. New York: Norton, 1999.

———. A science of meaning. *American Psychologist* 55 (2001): 721–39.

DeGrandpre, R. J., and W. K. Bickel. Stimulus control and drug dependence. *Psychological Record* 43 (1993): 651–66.

DeGrandpre, R. J., and E. White. Drug dialectics. *Arena Journal* 7 (1996): 41–63.

———. Drugs: In the care of the self. *Common Knowledge* 4 (1996): 27–48.

Deneau, G., et al. Self-administration of psychoactive drugs by the monkey: A measure of psychological dependence. *Psychopharmacologia* 16 (1969): 30–48.

Dews, P. B. Studies on behavior. I. Differential sensitivity to pentobarbital of pecking performance in pigeons depending on the schedule of reward. *Journal of Pharmacology and Experimental Therapeutics* 138 (1955): 393–401.

———. Stimulant actions of methamphetamine. *Journal of Pharmacology and Experimental Therapeutics* 122 (1958): 137–47.

Dunhill, A. *The gentle art of smoking*. New York: Putnam, 1954.

Durlacher, J. *Cocaine: Its history and lore*. London: Carlton, 2000.

Dworkin, S. I., et al. The effects of 12-hour limited access to cocaine: Reduction in drug intake and mortality. In *Problems of drug dependence*, edited by L. S. Harris. Washington: U.S. Government Printing Office, 1986.

———. Response-dependent versus response-independent presentation of cocaine: Differences in the lethal effects of the drug. *Psychopharmacology* 117 (1995): 262–66.

Erickson, P. G., et al. *The steel drug: Cocaine in perspective*. Lexington, Mass.: Lexington, 1987.

Fingarette, H. *Heavy drinking*. Berkeley: University of California Press, 1989.

Fisher, S., and R. P. Greenberg. *The limits of biological treatments for psychological distress*. Hillsdale, N.J.: Erlbaum, 1989.

Grinspoon, L., and J. B. Bakalar. *Cocaine: A drug and its social evolution*. New York: Basic Books, 1985.

Healy, D. *The antidepressant era*. Cambridge, Mass.: Harvard University Press, 1997.

———. *The creation of psychopharmacology*. Cambridge: Harvard University Press, 2002.

———. *Let them eat Prozac: The unhealthy relationship between the pharmaceutical industry and depression*. New York: New York University Press, 2004.

Heath, D. B. U.S. drug control policy: A cultural perspective. *Daedalus* 121 (1992): 269–91.

Inciardi, J. A. *The war on drugs II*. Mountain View, Calif.: Mayfield, 1992.

Inglis, B. *The forbidden game: A social history of drugs*. New York: Scribner, 1975.

Jarvik, M. E. Further observations on nicotine as the reinforcing agent in smoking. In *Smoking behavior: Motives and incentives*, edited by W. L. Dunn. Washington: Winston, 1973.

Johanson, C. E., and C. R. Schuster. A choice procedure for drug reinforcers: Cocaine and methylphenidate in the rhesus monkey. *Journal of Pharmacology and Experimental Therapeutics* 193 (1975): 676–88.

Johnston, J. *Chemistry of common life*. Edinburgh: Blackwood, 1855.

Joseph, M. *Speed*. London: Carlton Books, 2000.

Kessler, D. *A question of intent*. New York: Public Affairs, 2001.

Laurie, P. *Drugs: Medical, psychological and social facts*. Baltimore: Penguin, 1967.

Lindesmith, A. R. *Addiction and opiates*. Chicago: Aldine Publishing, 1968.

———. A sociological theory of drug addiction. *American Journal of Sociology* 43 (1938): 593–613.

Ludwig, A. M., and A. Wikler. Craving and relapse to drinking. *Quarterly Journal of Studies on Alcohol* 35 (1974): 108–30.

MacAndrew, C., and R. B. Edgerton. *Drunken comportment: A social explanation*, Chicago: Aldine Publishing Company, 1969.

McKenna, T. K. *Food of the gods: The search for the original tree of knowledge*. New York: Basic Books, 1992.

Musto, D. F. *The American disease: Origins of narcotic control*. New York: Oxford University Press, 1987.

———. America's first cocaine epidemic. *Wilson Quarterly* 13 (1989): 59–64.

Nadelman, E. Position paper on harm reduction. In *The harm reduction approach to drug control: international progress*. New York: The Lindesmith Center, 1994.

Nader, M. A., and W. L. Woolverton. Effects of increasing the magnitude of an alternative reinforcer on drug choice in a discrete-trial choice procedure. *Psychopharmacology* 105 (1991): 169–74.

Olds, J., and P. Milner. Positive reinforcement produced by electrical stimulation of septal area and other regions of rat brain. *Journal of Comparative and Physiological Psychology* 47 (1954): 419–27.

Park, L., and L. Covi. Nonblind placebo trail. *Archives of General Psychiatry* 12 (1965): 336–45.

Peele, S. Addiction as a cultural concept. *Annals of the New York Academy of Sciences* 602 (1990): 205–20.

———. *The meaning of addiction: Compulsive experience and its interpretation*. Lexington, Mass.: Lexington Books, 1985.

Peele, S., and R. J. DeGrandpre. Cocaine and the concept of addiction. *Addiction Research* 6 (1998): 235–63.

Porrino, L. J., et al. The distribution of changes in local cerebral energy metabolism associated with brain stimulation reward to the medial forebrain bundle of the rat. *Brain Research* 511 (1990): 1–6.

Primm, B. J. and Bath, P. E. Pseudoheroinism. *International Journal of the Addictions* 8 (1973): 231–42.

Ray, O. *Drugs, society, and human behavior*. St. Louis: Mosby, 1983.

Reinarman, C., and H. G. Levine. The crack attack: Politics and media in America's latest drug scare. In *Images of issues: Typifying contemporary social problems*, edited by J. Best, 115–37. New York: Aldine de Gruyter, 1989.

Richards, J. F. Opium and the British Indian empire. *Modern Asia Studies* 36 (2002): 375–420.

Robins, L. N., and G. E. Murphy. Drug use in a normal population of young negro men. *American Journal of Public Health* 57 (1967): 1580–96.

Robins, L. N., et al. Drug use by U.S. Army enlisted men in Vietnam: A follow-up on their return home. *American Journal of Epidemiology* 99 (1974): 235–49.

———. Narcotic use in Southeast Asia and afterward. *Archives of General Psychiatry* 32 (1980): 955–61.

Schivelbusch, W. *Tastes of paradise*. New York: Pantheon, 1992.

Schuster, C. R., et al. Behavioral variables affecting the development of amphetamine tolerance. *Psychopharmacologia* 9 (1966): 170–82.

Seevers, M. H. Opiate addiction in the monkey. I. Methods of study. *Journal of Pharmacology and Experimental Therapeutics*, 56 (1936): 147–56.

Shapiro, D. Smoking tobacco: Irrationality, addiction, and paternalism. *Public Affairs Quarterly* 8 (1994): 187–203.

Siegel, S. Tolerance to the hyperthermic effect of morphine in the rat is a learned response. *Journal of Comparative and Physiological Psychology* 92 (1978): 1137–49.

———. Heroin "overdose" death: Contribution of drug-associated environmental cues. *Science* 216 (1992): 436–37.

———. Drug anticipation and drug tolerance. In *The psychopharmacology of addiction*, edited by M. Lader. Oxford: Oxford University Press, 1988.

Sinclair, A. *Era of excess: A social history of the prohibition movement*. New York: Harper-Colophon, 1964.

Singh, L., and T. Brassey. *First report of the Royal Commission on Opium with minutes of evidence and appendices*. London: H. M. Stationery Office, 1894–95.

Sloman, L. *Reefer madness: The history of marijuana*. New York: St. Martin's Griffin, 1979.

Starr, P. *The social transformation of American medicine*. New York: Basic, 1982.

Szasz, T. S. *Ceremonial chemistry*. Garden City, N.Y.: Anchor Press, 1974.

Volkow, N. D., et al. Is methylphenidate like cocaine? Studies on their pharmacokinetics and distribution in the human brain. *Archives of General Psychiatry* 52 (1995): 350–53.

Waldorf, D. Natural remission from opiate addiction: Some social-psychological processes of untreated recovery. *Journal of Drug Issues* 13 (1983): 237–80.

Weil, A. *The natural mind*. Boston: Houghton Mifflin, 1972.

Weil, A., and W. Rosen. *From chocolate to morphine: Everything you need to know about mind-altering drugs*. Boston: Houghton Mifflin, 1983.

Wesson, D. R., and D. E. Smith. *Barbiturates: Their use, misuse, and abuse*. New York: Human Sciences Press, 1977.

Winick, C. The life cycle of the narcotic addict and of addiction. *U.S. Bulletin on Narcotics* 16 (1964): 1–11.

Zinberg, N. E. *Drug, set, and setting*. New Haven: Yale University Press, 1984.

Zinberg, N. E., and Jacobson, R. C. The natural history of "chipping." *American Journal of Psychiatry* 133 (1976): 37–40.

dependence problems, 152–153;
American Psychiatric Association
and, 151; compared to barbiturates,
154; compared to opiates, 152–153;
development of, 150–152; as drug of
misuse, 152–154; as first minor tranquilizer, 150–152; and Wallace Laboratories, 151–152, 165
Miriani Wine Tonic, 21. *See also* Patent
medicines
Morphine: animal research and, 185–
186, 205–206, 229: controlled use of,
106–114; history of, 125–132; initial
subjective experiences with, 214;
withdrawal and, 121, 123
Morphinism, 21, 109, 126–127, 129,
152
Musto, David, 126, 132, 263 n.1, 266
n.86

Nadelman, Ethan, 251 n.60, 252 n.79
National prohibition. *See* Alcohol
Nazism, compared to pharmacologicalism, 238
Nembutal, 52, 155. *See also* Barbiturates
Newsweek, 162; coverage of antidepressants and, 54, 57–58
New York Times, 8, 29, 32, 37, 59, 61,
132, 218; Eli Lilly and, 37; marijuana
hysteria and, 136
Nicotine, 68–99, 122, 189, 203, 222,
232; addictiveness and, 83–86, 89–
100; animal studies of addiction to,
77–78, 90–91; as behavioral habit,
83–94; compared to cocaine and heroin, 83, 96; early use in America,
126–128; manipulation in cigarettes,
82–83, 85–86. *See also* Tobacco
Nicotine transdermal patch, and other
nicotine replacement technologies,
84–85
NIDA (National Institute on Drug
Abuse). *See* U.S. National Institute
on Drug Abuse

Nineteenth century: drug use and abuse
in United States during, 103–106
Nixon, Richard, role in U.S. war on
drugs, 174
Norepinephrine, 9, 55, 57–59, 182–183

Office of National Drug Control Policy,
12
Olds, James, 179–183, 191, 277 n.96.
See also Electrical brain stimulation
Opiate addicts: historical case studies,
108–110. *See also* Halsted, William
Stewart
Opiates: alternatives to prohibition,
149–151; Harrison Act and, 134–135,
139, 141, 143, 243 (app. 1); as most
addictive drug, 105; prohibition and
changing nature of use, 131–135;
Royal Commission on Opium, 124–
125; use in America (nineteenth century and early twentieth), 125–133;
use in India, 111–112
Opioids (synthetic opiates), development of, 149
Opium, 103, 105, 109–114, 149, 153,
155, 189, 235, 243 (app. 1); eating of,
120, 124–126. *See also* Opiates
Orientalism, compared to pharmacologicalism, 239–240
Oxycondone. *See* Oxycontin
Oxycontin, 91, 149, 170, 172, 197

Parke Davis and Company: commerce
with cocaine, 103, 146; commerce
with marijuana, 103; development
and sale of amphetamines, 146
Patent medicines, 21, 52, 52, 103–104,
126, 131–132, 139, 146, 149, 152–
153, 158, 170; AMA control over,
141–142; prescription medicines vs.,
140–143
Paxil, 28, 59, 144, 188, 218; compared
to other SSRIs, 9–10; development
by SmithKline, 54; homicides after

Paxil (*continued*)
taking, 47–49; withdrawal syndrome and, 49. *See also* SSRIS

Peele, Stanton, viii; addiction as concept and, 285; on meaning of addiction, 129

Pentobarbital. *See* Nembutal

Pfizer Pharmaceuticals, SSRIS and, 38, 41. *See also* Zoloft

Pharmacodynamics, 8–9

Pharmacokinetics, 8

Pharmacological determinism. *See* Pharmacologicalism

Pharmacological essence, viii, 27–28, 104, 186, 210–211, 220

Pharmacologicalism, 28, 47, 83, 104–105, 122, 170, 209–210, 221, 242, 271 n.6; cocaine and, 184–187; compared to other ideologies, 238–240; concept of addiction and, 105, 120; definition of, 27; marijuana use and, 213; tobacco wars and, 99

Phencyclidine (PCP), studies of, 200

Physical dependence, 123, 230; Miltown and, 152–153; opiates and, 105; smoking and, 98; SSRIS and, 48–49

Placebo. *See* Placebo effect

Placebo effect, 7, 18, 59–63

Placebo text, 103, 122–137, 188, 201, 205–206, 214–217, 233–234; amphetamines and, 148; definition of, 120–121

Poppy, 105. *See also* Opiates

Prozac, vii, 24, 34, 64, 104, 110, 182; ambiguity of withdrawal experience, 219–220; as cause of suicide and murder, 34–60, 63; compared to pharmacology of other SSRIS, 9–10. *See also* Eli Lilly Pharmaceuticals; SSRIS

Psychiatry, viii, 187, 193, 194, 196, 237

Psychoactive drugs: as angels and demons, 105, 130, 137, 172, 187, 235, 241–242; compared to other sources

of sensory experience, 222; conditioning with, 124, 202–204; construction of meaning of, 211–216; cultural adaptability of, 17–19, 170–173; intensification of use of, 25–28; myth of, 27–28; nature of, ix, 175, 242; social aspects of, vii-viii, 17–25, 27, 28, 32, 83, 88–91, 93, 104, 119, 121, 127, 133, 149, 174, 186–188, 196, 200, 201, 220, 223, 233–234, 237, 238, 240–242; viewed as "medicine," 3; viewed as stimulus, 208–215, 219–226, 231–234

Psychopharmacology, 10, 38, 41, 55, 146, 192, 194, 197, 205, 223, 237. *See also* Behavioral pharmacology

Quaalude. *See* Methaqualone

Rate-dependence, 191–192, 195, 197, 199. *See also* Dews, Peter

"Rat Park," 30

Ray, Oakley, viii, 161

Reagan, Ronald, role in U.S. war on drugs, 174

Ritalin, 3, 13–33; abuse of, 4–12; ADHD and use of, 4; animal studies of, 7; comparisons with cocaine and coca, 7–12; DEA and, 5–6

RJR (R. J. Reynolds Tobacco Company), 72–74, 76, 81

Rolling Stones, 168

Said, Edward, 239

Schell, Donald, 47–48

Schivelbusch, Wolfgang, 21, 87

Schlosser, Eric, viii

Schuster, C. R., 7, 187–188, 190, 196–197, 227–228, 231–232. *See also* U.S. National Institute on Drug Abuse

Science, and myth of pharmacological determinism, 104–105. *See also* Pharmacologicalism

Science, 29, 60, 85, 183, 184, 202, 230

Valium, 13, 28, 39, 52, 76, 95, 104, 110, 197, 218; development of, 167–168. *See also* Benzodiazepines

Volkow, Nora, Ritalin and, 9–11, 247 n.1, 249 n.20, 249 n.31

Volstead Act, 139, 142

Weil, Andrew, viii, ix, 19–20, 122, 214, 222

Wesbecker, Joseph, Prozac and, 35–38, 42

White market drugs. *See* "Ethical drugs"

Wikler, Abraham, 206, 270 n.53, 282, n.42

Withdrawal. *See* Drug withdrawal; Physical dependence

World Health Organization (WHO), Cocaine Project of, 22–27

Xanax, 39, 167, 188, 218. *See also* Benzodiazepines

Yanagita, Tomoji, 197, 251 n.68

Zinberg, Norman, viii, 113–114, 117, 188, 210

Zoloft, 41, 50, 54, 59, 188; compared to pharmacology of other SSRIS, 9–10; link to suicides, 46–47. *See also* SSRIS

Richard DeGrandpre is an independent scholar of drugs and other "technologies of the self." He has a doctorate in psychopharmacology and was a fellow of the National Institute on Drug Abuse. He is the author of *Ritalin Nation: Rapid-Fire Culture and the Transformation of Human Consciousness* and *Digitopia: The Look of the New Digital You*. He has also written numerous scientific, theoretical, and popular articles on drugs and is a former senior editor at *Adbusters* magazine.

Library of Congress Cataloging-in-Publication Data

DeGrandpre, Richard J.
The cult of pharmacology : How America became the world's most
troubled drug culture / Richard DeGrandpre.
    p. cm.
Includes bibliographical references and index.
    ISBN-13: 978-0-8223-3881-9 (cloth : alk. paper)
    ISBN-10: 0-8223-3881-5 (cloth : alk. paper)
1. Drug utilization — United States. 2. Pharmaceutical industry —
United States. 3. Drugs — Social aspects — United States. I. Title.
RM263.D44 2006
615'.1 — dc22

2006014259

CPSIA information can be obtained
at www.ICGtesting.com
Printed in the USA
JSHW010029130723
44440JS00001B/27

9 780822 349075